D1627861

THINKING ABOUT PRESCRIBING

THE PSYCHOLOGY OF PSYCHOPHARMACOLOGY WITH DIVERSE YOUTH AND FAMILIES

THINKING ABOUT PRESCRIBING

THE PSYCHOLOGY OF PSYCHOPHARMACOLOGY WITH DIVERSE YOUTH AND FAMILIES

Edited by

Shashank V. Joshi, M.D.
Andrés Martin, M.D., M.P.H.

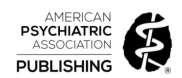

AMERICAN
PSYCHIATRIC
ASSOCIATION
PUBLISHING

If you wish to buy 50 or more copies of the same title, please go to www.appi.org/specialdiscounts for more information.

Copyright © 2022 American Psychiatric Association Publishing

ALL RIGHTS RESERVED

First Edition

Manufactured in the United States of America on acid-free paper
25   24   23   22   21   5   4   3   2   1

American Psychiatric Association Publishing
800 Maine Avenue SW
Suite 900
Washington, DC 20024-2812
www.appi.org

Library of Congress Cataloging-in-Publication Data
Names: Joshi, Shashank V., editor. | Martin, Andrés, editor. | American Psychiatric
    Association Publishing, Publisher.
Title: Thinking about prescribing : the psychology of psychopharmacology with
    diverse youth and families / edited by Shashank V. Joshi, Andrés Martin.
Other titles: Thinking about prescribing (Joshi)
Description: First edition. | Washington, DC : American Psychiatric Association
    Publishing, [2022] | Includes bibliographical references and index.
Identifiers: LCCN 2021040735 (print) | LCCN 2021040736 (ebook) | ISBN
    9781615373888 (paperback : alk. paper) | ISBN 9781615373895 (ebook)
Subjects: MESH: Mental Disorders—drug therapy | Child | Psychopharmacology—
    methods | Cultural Diversity
Classification: LCC RM315 (print) | LCC RM315 (ebook) | NLM WS 350.33 |
    DDC 615.7/8—dc23
LC record available at https://lccn.loc.gov/2021040735
LC ebook record available at https://lccn.loc.gov/2021040736

British Library Cataloguing in Publication Data
A CIP record is available from the British Library.

CONTENTS

Part I: Principles

Part IV: Populations

Part V: Research

Part VI: Becoming

CONTRIBUTORS

John Azer, M.D.
The Austen Riggs Center, Stockbridge, Massachuseutts

Barri Belnap, M.D.
The Austen Riggs Center, Stockbridge, Massachuseutts

Jeff Q. Bostic, M.D., Ed.D.
Department of Psychiatry, MedStar Georgetown University Hospital, Washington, D.C.

Arthur Caye, M.D., Ph.D.
Division of Child & Adolescent Psychiatry, Hospital de Clínicas de Porto Alegre; Department of Psychiatry, School of Medicine, Universidade Federal do Rio Grande do Sul, Brazil

Janice Cho, M.D.
Resident Physician in Psychiatry, University of California, Los Angeles, Los Angeles, California

Andrew Connor, D.O.
Ohana Center for Child and Adolescent Behavioral Health, Community Hospital of Monterey Peninsula, Monterey, California

Takesha Cooper, M.D., M.S.
Program Director, Psychiatry Residency Training Program; Vice-Chair of Education; Equity Advisor; and Chair, Admissions Committee, Department of Psychiatry and Neuroscience, University of California, Riverside School of Medicine, Riverside, California

Jennifer Derenne, M.D.
Clinical Professor of Psychiatry and Behavioral Sciences, Stanford University School of Medicine, Lucile Packard Children's Hospital, Stanford, California

John J. DiLallo, M.D.
Psychiatrist in Private Practice, Dobbs Ferry, New York

Farrah Fang, M.D.
Staff Psychiatrist, Stamps Health Services, Georgia Institute of Technology, Atlanta, Georgia

Carl Feinstein, M.D.
Clinical Professor and Vice Chair, Child and Adolescent Psychiatry, Department of Psychiatry and Neuroscience, University of California, Riverside School of Medicine, Riverside, California; Emeritus Professor of Psychotherapy, Department of Psychiatry and Behavioral Sciences, Stanford University School of Medicine, Stanford, California

Erin Fletcher, M.D., M.P.H.
PGY 3 Psychiatry Resident, Department of Psychiatry and Neuroscience, University of California, Riverside School of Medicine, Riverside, California

Shih Yee-Marie Tan Gipson, M.D.
Instructor, Department of Psychiatry, Massachusetts General Hospital, Harvard Medical School, Boston, Massachusetts

Anne L. Glowinski, M.D., M.P.E.
Weill Institute for Neurosciences, Department of Psychiatry and Behavioral Sciences, Division of Child and Adolescent Psychiatry, University of California, San Francisco, San Fransisco, California

Srinivasa B. Gokarakonda, M.D., M.P.H.
Assistant Professor of Psychiatry, University of Arkansas for Medical Sciences, Little Rock, Arkansas

Simone Hasselmo, A.B.
Yale School of Medicine, New Haven, Connecticut

Amy Heneghan, M.D.
Pediatrician in Private Practice, Palo Alto, California

Donald M. Hilty, M.D., M.B.A.
Professor and Vice Chair of Veteran's Affairs, Department of Psychiatry and Behavioral Sciences, University of California Davis School of Medicine, Sacramento, California

David S. Hong, M.D.
Assistant Professor, Department of Psychiatry and Behavioral Sciences, Stanford University, Stanford, California

Peter S. Jensen, M.D.
Board Chair, The REACH Institute, New York, New York; Adjunct Professor of Psychiatry, University of Arkansas for Medical Sciences, Little Rock, Arkansas

Shashank V. Joshi, M.D.
Professor of Psychiatry, Pediatrics, and Education, Stanford University School of Medicine and Graduate School of Education; Director of Training in Child and Adolescent Psychiatry and Director of School Mental Health at Lucile Packard Children's Hospital Stanford, Palo Alto, California

Mandeep Kaur Kapur, M.D.
Administrative Chief Fellow, Department of Psychiatry and Behavioral Sciences, Division of Child and Adolescent Psychiatry, Stanford University School of Medicine, Palo Alto, California

David Kaye, M.D.
Professor of Psychiatry and Vice Chair of Academic Affairs, Department of Psychiatry, Jacobs School of Medicine & Biomedical Sciences, University of Buffalo, Buffalo, New York

Christian Kieling, M.D., Ph.D.
Division of Child & Adolescent Psychiatry, Hospital de Clínicas de Porto Alegre; Department of Psychiatry, School of Medicine, Universidade Federal do Rio Grande do Sul, Brazil

Jung Won Kim, M.D.
Faculty, Department of Psychiatry, Boston Children's Hospital, Department of Psychiatry and Behavioral Sciences, Harvard Medical School, Boston, Massachusetts

Brandon A. Kohrt, M.D., Ph.D.
Division of Global Mental Health, Department of Psychiatry and Behavioral Sciences, George Washington University, Washington, D.C.

Mari Kurahashi, M.D., M.P.H.
Clinical Associate Professor, Department of Psychiatry and Behavioral Sciences, Stanford University, Stanford, California

Nithya Mani, M.D.
Assistant Professor, Department of Psychiatry and Behavioral Sciences, Stanford University, Stanford, California

Andrés Martin, M.D., M.P.H.
Riva Ariella Ritvo Professor, Child Study Center, Yale School of Medicine; Medical Director, Children's Psychiatric Inpatient Service, Yale New Haven Health, New Haven, Connecticut

Jeffrey A. Mills, Ph.D.
Professor of Economics, Department of Economics, Lindner College of Business, University of Cincinnati, Cincinnati, Ohio

David Mintz, M.D.
The Austen Riggs Center, Stockbridge, Massachuseutts

Katherine M. Ort, M.D.
Clinical Assistant Professor, Departments of Child and Adolescent Psychiatry and Pediatrics, NYU Grossman School of Medicine, NYU Langone Health, New York, New York

Tara S. Paris, Ph.D.
UCLA Semel Institute for Neuroscience and Human Behavior, Los Angeles, California

Kyle Pruett, M.D.
Clinical Professor of Psychiatry, Yale Child Study Center, Northampton, Massachusetts

Sean Pustilnik, M.D.
Department of Psychiatry, MedStar Georgetown University Hospital, Washington, D.C.

Elizabeth Reichert, Ph.D.
Clinical Associate Professor, Department of Psychiatry and Behavioral Sciences, Stanford University, Stanford, California

Magdalena Romanowicz, M.D.
Program Director of Child and Adolescent Fellowship Training, Mayo School of Graduate Medical Education, Division of Child and Adolescent Psychiatry; Assistant Professor of Psychiatry, Mayo Clinic College of Medicine and Science, Rochester, Minnesota

Max S. Rosen, M.D.
Division of Child and Adolescent Psychiatry, Department of Psychiatry, Washington University School of Medicine, St. Louis, Missouri

Sarah Rosenbaum, M.D., M.P.H.
Clinical Instructor, Department of Psychiatry and Behavioral Sciences, Stanford University School of Medicine, Stanford, California

Anthony L. Rostain, M.D., M.A.
Chair, Department of Psychiatry and Behavioral Health, Cooper University Health Care; Professor of Psychiatry and Pediatrics, Cooper Medical School of Rowan University, Camden, New Jersey

Erin Seery, M.D.
Medical University of South Carolina, Charleston, South Carolina

Manpreet K. Singh, M.D., M.S.
Associate Professor, Department of Psychiatry and Behavioral Sciences, and Director of the Stanford Pediatric Mood Disorders Program and the Pediatric Emotion and Resilience Lab, Stanford University School of Medicine, Stanford, California

Jeffrey R. Strawn, M.D.
Professor of Psychiatry, Pediatrics, and Clinical Pharmacology, Department of Psychiatry and Behavioral Neuroscience, University of Cincinnati, College of Medicine, Cincinnati, Ohio

Dorothy Stubbe, M.D.
Associate Professor and Program Director, Child Study Center, Yale University School of Medicine, New Haven, Connecticut

Andrea Tabuenca, Ph.D.
Clinical Assistant Professor, Division of Child and Adolescent Psychiatry, Stanford University School of Medicine, Stanford, California

Ian Tofler, M.B.B.S.
Kaiser West Los Angeles; Visiting Faculty, Department of Psychiatry, Department of Psychiatry, UCLA, Los Angeles, California

Michelle Tom, M.D.
Child and Adolescent Psychiatry Fellow, Department of Psychiatry and Neuroscience, University of California, Riverside School of Medicine, Riverside, California

John T. Walkup, M.D.
Margaret C. Osterman Professor of Psychiatry, Pritzker Department of Psychiatry and Behavioral Health, Ann and Robert H. Lurie Children's Hospital, Chicago, Illinois

Isheeta Zalpuri, M.D.
Clinical Associate Professor and Associate Program Director, Department of Psychiatry and Behavioral Sciences, Division of Child and Adolescent Psychiatry, Stanford University School of Medicine, Palo Alto, California

DISCLOSURE OF COMPETING INTERESTS

The following contributors to this book have indicated a financial interest in or other affiliation with a commercial supporter, a manufacturer of a commercial product, a provider of a commercial service, a nongovernmental organization, and/or a government agency, as listed below:

Peter S. Jensen, M.D.—*Book publishing royalties:* American Psychiatric Association Publishing; Guilford Press, Ballantine Books

Jeffrey A. Mills, Ph.D.—*Support:* Yung Family Foundation.

Tara S. Paris, Ph.D.—*Research support:* National Institute of Mental Health; TLC Foundation for Body-Focused Repetitive Behavior; *Royalties:* Oxford University Press.

Elizabeth Reichert, Ph.D.—*Advisory board:* Little Otter

Manpreet K. Singh, M.D., M.S.—*Research support:* Stanford Maternal Child Health Research Institute and Department of Psychiatry; National Institute of Mental Health; National Institute of Aging; Patient Centered Outcomes Research Institute; Johnson & Johnson;

UNCOVERED

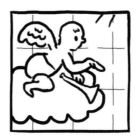

We were elated on first seeing the cover options for *Thinking About Prescribing*. Initially drawn to an all-blue design, we were perhaps giving an unconscious nod to the colors of one of our august institutions. Too august in fact; too serious. We did not want to convey from the get-go a sense of staid *heaviosity* that so often alienates kids from self-important polysyllabic pediatric psychopharmacologists. Instead, we aimed for a cover that transcended "treatise," "tort," or "textbook" trends. We wanted visual messaging that conveyed the playfulness and mystery-solving at the core of our profession. The complementary color scheme and fonts we settled on are child-friendly; the images on the frontispiece a puzzle fit for avid codebreakers. What are angels doing in there? More disturbingly perhaps: what are *grenades*, of all things, doing on the cover of a pediatric book? The nine complementary panels appear to form a sequence of sorts: did the artist aim for a case of Elgar-like *Enigma Variations*? The figures are indeed intended to be enigmatic: to invite questions and head-scratching; to lure the prospective reader in. If we have succeeded as well-intentioned tricksters to draw you in this far, the introduction that follows, *Prescriber, prescribe thyself*, will reveal the underlying mystery—grenades and all. We are deeply grateful to Simone Hasselmo for her artistry, for moving well beyond cartooning the illustrations that grace the cover and enrich the text that follows. We were in awe by what Simone produced: we had merely asked for new perspectives through which to convey complex and abstract concepts. We had asked for different *angles*; Simone instead blessed us with her *angels*.

PRESCRIBER, PRESCRIBE THYSELF
By Way of Introduction

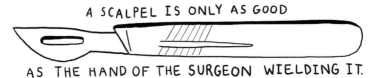

A SCALPEL IS ONLY AS GOOD AS THE HAND OF THE SURGEON WIELDING IT.

It may seem unbecoming to open a book on children's mental health on a surgical note. But there are at least two good reasons to do so. First, there is the answer to that old chestnut "Why did some of us become psychiatrists?" *Because surgery wasn't invasive enough.* Surgery simply did not go sufficiently deep for some of our sensibilities. Second, and to learn from our colleagues in surgery and not just use them as strawmen for a tired quip, let's give them this: Surgeons don't for a second forget that scalpels are instruments, base metals at that. If only we psychiatrists had a similar mindset when prescribing our own pills. Alas, we forget all too often that our potions are partly instruments, base salts at times.

This volume is an invitation—an entreaty—to make good on the fact that our remedies are only as good as the way in which we dispense them, that prescribing psychotropic medications to developing children is as much the cold facts of molecules as it is the warm way in which we envelop them for delivery. It is a reminder that no matter how accurate said delivery may be, it all goes to naught—molecules be damned—if there is no one on the receiving end; a psychotropic not taken is perfectly inert and useless. But our goal should not end at mere "compliance" (an unfortunate term that reeks of power dynamics and hierarchical paternalism); ingesting a pill and letting its molecules fulfill their job description is but the start of a therapeutic process.

Simple conceptualizations of depression as a low serotonin condition or of stimulants as dopamine enhancers are as incomplete today as they are misguided. A chemical's docking, *Apollo*-like, onto a receptor's site to right a neurotransmitter's tenuous balance is as romantic a throwback as a 1960s moon shot. Advances in molecular psychiatry over recent decades have made it clear that psychotropics are more than simple "keys" to neurotransmitter "locks." The contact of molecule and receptor may be a start, but it is the secondary, tertiary, and subsequent messengers where the action truly lies. It is these elusive messengers that get in deep, that get closer to the actual machinery of the cell, that get the job done.

In a similar way, we should be not mere prescribers, the holders of key rings on our proverbial tool belts. We are—or should be, or aspire to be, or reclaim being—pharmacotherapists. Our own job description gets started well before molecules reach their targets; we are cognizant that the moment of chemical bonding is but another start; we remain humble in our commitment, recognizing that to deliver on the full potential of our treatment, we, too, must become and remain secondary, tertiary, and subsequent messenger systems. In his paraphrasing of Donald Winnicott in the book's opening chapter, Kyle Pruett reminds us that "there is no such thing as just a prescription." The prescription, the prescriber, and the prescribed are inherently intertwined; we ignore such bondings (chemical or otherwise) at our own therapeutic detriment.

Entering the Time Frame Continuum

By focusing too narrowly on the dosing of milligrams or the number and class of psychotropic medications, we can easily come to forget that *time* is that other key aspect of our posology. Time is perhaps our most valuable resource, and we would all do well to remember, after Cayer, Kohrt, and Kieling's math (14), that "in psychiatry's measure of time, more is more." For example, in contemplating a patient who does not get better in the way or at the speed that we would hope for, we are comfortable—arguably too comfortable—increasing the milligrams or the number of psychotropics prescribed, and often both at the same time. We can capitulate in a similar fashion when facing some of the many outside influences that can intrude into the confines of our therapeutic relationship: unrealistic expectations for quick fixes or perverse incentives for "biological" treatments, as well as the pervasive influence of the pharmaceutical industry and the tentacular reach of its oversized advertising budget.

This volume is an invitation—an entreaty—to resist being pushed to, yielding to, or (banish the thought) opting for the circumscribed role of "medication prescriber." Our first and best defense against such a misguided interpretation of our role is to remember the centrality of time within and across clinical encounters, to reclaim the dosing of ourselves, of the number and frequency of our visits, of our presence and therapeutic engagement within them. If these words seem too idealistic and removed from the daily realities of a child psychiatrist, contributions in this volume may help move clinicians away from "the myth of the 'med check'" into the reality of the pharmacotherapy visit (6) to bridge the divide between what may be aspirational for some and what is possible for many. Milligrams dispensed are easy; time well spent is hard.

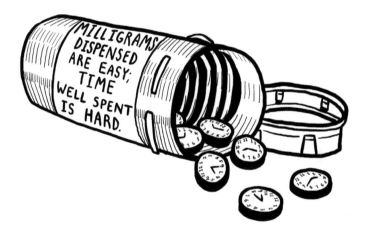

In pediatric psychopharmacology, establishing an appropriate frame is the yang to the yin of its time management. Pruett (1) again provides the pithy prescription for the task: "How you *are* with your patient is as important as what you *do* with your patient." Three very different yet complementary chapters in this edited collection help establish a robust frame through which to be with our patients. Romanowicz, Rosenbaum, and Feinstein (2) have adapted to pharmacotherapy with children and adolescents the "Y-model" first posited by Plakun and colleagues (2009), in which the therapeutic alliance, as the "stem of the Y," provides a common point of entry for any clinical approach. In its original description, that stem bifurcates into psychodynamic and behavioral arms. Belnap, Seery, Azer, and Mintz apply psychodynamic principles to the context of pediatric psychopharmacology in their chapter (3), a task that DiLallo takes on for cognitive-behavioral and motivational interviewing approaches in his (4). As appealing as such a neat tripartite model may sound, it only begins to tell the story when working with children and their families. The "stem" may instead be construed as more akin to a tree trunk and the two arms as but two of the many branches in a complex canopy. Indeed, a multitude of synergistic approaches is what we are routinely called on to muster as pharmacotherapists.

There is an additional and more recent connotation to the "frame" under discussion. And that is the virtual frame through which more of our visits are taking place these days. What started as telepsychiatry in the 1990s, designed to reach remote and particularly underserved locations, has rapidly evolved and made major inroads into routine pediatric psychopharmacology. The COVID-19 pandemic that started in March 2020 did in just a few months for the uptake of "virtual frames" what two decades of telepsychiatry educational efforts could not. Bostic and Kaye (11) have been pioneers and early settlers of these erstwhile barren virtual lands. They are also effective guides, enriching our vocabulary with terms such as *tele-alliance*, *protection of the virtual space*, *telerapport*, *Freudian blips*, *screen empathy*, and *webside manner*. What once was "treatment *not* as usual" has by now become second nature. We should not envision a future devoid of physical visits but rather embrace this new and complementary way of hitting the clinical target as but an additional arrow in our therapeutic quiver. As we embrace e-prescribing over paper scripts (remember those?), and as we swoon over the powers of the pixel, we should not lose sight of the fact that many areas of the world do not have e-prescription capabilities (14), or that families within even high-income nations like ours do not have access to adequate bandwidth or face inequities and barriers to care, including those entrenched through structural racism (13).

At Least Three (Though It Can Still Take Two to Tango)

Pharmacotherapy with adults is largely a dyadic affair between a patient and a prescribing clinician, an approach that at times works in the pediatric realm, particularly with adolescents and transition-age youth (12). However, the vast majority of time, prescribing psychotropic medications to children and adolescents involves other stakeholders—at times several of them—each with competing priorities or agendas to boot. For starters, given the enduring shortage of child psychiatrists, prescriptions often come from partners in a multidisciplinary team, including pediatricians or advanced practice registered nurses (8). In another common approach, treatment may be complemented and synergized among prescribing and nonprescribing clinicians ("split treatment," the commonly used term for this arrangement, is another unfortunate misnomer because it emphasizes the potential divide rather than the intended cohesion) (7). The potential for cooperation and for different vantage points on children, including on their interactions with other children, is multiplied in schools or in congregate care settings such as inpatient units and residential facilities. Two chapters in this collection address the unique challenges and opportunities for pediatric pharmacotherapists working in schools (9) or inpatient environments (10).

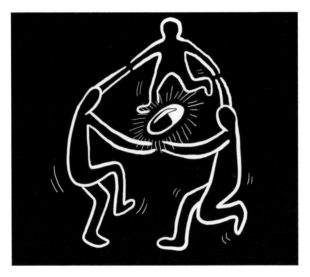

In navigating what can be such tricky shoals, we'd all do well to heed the aphoristic advice by Gokarakonda and Jensen in their chapter (5) that "the messenger may be 'wrong' even if the message is 'right.'" To be the best possible messengers and to maximize the odds of our thoughtfully selected treatments to be consumed, Gokarakonda and Jensen go on to emphasize the role of psychoeducation and cooperation as part of a partnership with common goals. This partnership, when working with children and adolescents, most commonly involves parent(s) or legal guardians. Establishing a caring and trusting relationship with them can be as critical to the success and longevity of our treatment as making the youngster feel at ease with us—and with our psychotropic stand-ins, which we ask them to faithfully ingest.

The richness of our work is in no small measure a reflection of the wide array of ethnoculturally diverse individuals and families we get to work with on a daily basis. And even as we respect their uniquely defining characteristics, we have found it helpful to approach clinical encounters—especially those involving the initial prescription of a psychotropic—through a framework that incorporates the perceived utility of the treatment on the one hand and the stance regarding treatment on the other. We depict the intersection of these two axes in the figure below and go on to provide examples from our clinical practice that exemplify some of the cells in the resulting matrix.

Stance Regarding Treatment

In an optimal situation, if an admittedly idealized one, a child has no preconceived notions about the potential utility of a medication: It is neither helpful nor harmful; it just is. By contrast, when the stance regarding treatment is not entirely neutral but rather ambivalent because ingesting a foreign substance is, if nothing else, a change, at least a modicum of questioning serves a role toward self-preservation. We think of this central cell as *prudent*, one in which a parent (or a child, or the two combined) wants to know more in order to make a well-informed decision. The underlying but often unspoken request may be as simple as this: *Help me gain trust* (in you, in the pill, in whoever you are and whatever this is).

Our hand should tremble (just a bit) before we write a prescription for a young child; a parent should tremble (just a tad more) before first dispensing the medication. The upper-left corner of our proposed matrix is not without its challenges. For starters, there is a fine line between *trusting* and *acquiescing*, and children or parents can be too willing to agree to a treatment without "reading the fine print" first. A lack of tremors on either side suggests the possibility of idealization at best, of recklessness at worst.

Children and parents rarely come to us as blank slates, devoid of memory or expectation, or without fears and desires. We face the *willing* when the prescriber is perceived in a better light than the prescription. When faith in a potion prevails over that in its prescriber, the *questioning* may stick around to accept a trial: not the medication trial so much as our own. The *tentative* may be willing to tolerate psychotropics deemed potentially risky or harmful as long as they can have enough of our trust to go on. We meet the *apprehensive* when it is we who are the ones in question while a psychotropic is given an opportunity to prove its worth.

Moving from any of these contiguous quadrants toward the elusive top-left corner of the matrix—the one in which a predominantly helpful mediation is embraced within an informed and connected treatment relationship—can be as challenging as it is rewarding and conducive to good outcomes. Toward that end, the words we choose in pediatric pharmacotherapy are every bit as critical as the milligrams we dispense. As psychiatrists, we cherish words, though at times we overuse them. Prime examples of such verbal prolixity include the explanation of arcane and outdated mechanisms of action, an emphasis on encyclopedic side effect lists, and a penchant for the legalese of informed consent. To make matters worse, these words have a way of morphing into reams of electronic boilerplate content.

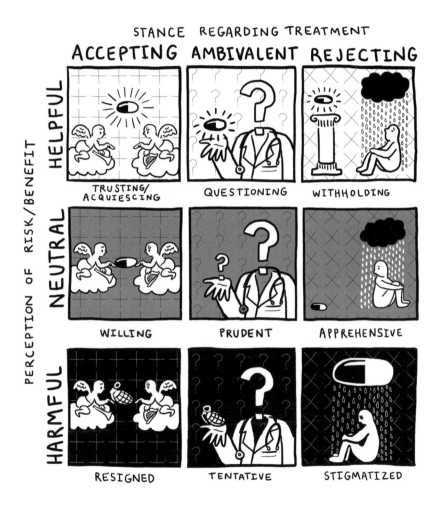

Surely there is a way to reclaim the healing power of pithier word-smithing. And there is. First, go for the object. And the object in this instance is not the medication (it's the child, stupid!). Second, when addressing how treatments work, realize that "chemical imbalance" and the neurotransmitter hi-lo index are more helpful in binding our own anxieties than those of our patients. Accept the fact that we don't really know how our medicines work and step off the podium already. When talking to kids, call the things "medicines" while you're at it, not "medications" or (the horror!) "psychotropics." A "pill" can be "candy," and children do well to take neither one from a stranger. By contrast, a "medicine" is a known entity, and one that generally helps kids feel better.

When addressing side effects, beware of unleashing terms such as "sudden death" and "suicide risk"; these horses are hard to put back in their barns. Not that you should elide them completely; follow instead your own advice to "start low and go slow." Start in fact at the lowest, a truism that often goes unsaid: *the most common side effect is* no *side effect.* And build up from there: there are the relatively common side effects that tend to be minor and well tolerated, and there are the more infrequent and serious ones. Address the ones that are more likely to be pertinent, and remember that some things can't be unheard. After a few minutes, only the most salient words are likely to be heard. You don't have to build Rome in a day—or, by frightening your audience away, demolish it in a day either. Obtain informed consent but stop from making patients and their families feel part of an informed coercion process. And finally, did we mention going for the object? It is right there, staring you in the face. So stop yapping already.

Placebo, Nocebo, No Dice

The placebo effect gets a bad rap, what with all of its muddying of the clinical trials we base so much of our evidence base on (15 and 16). But the placebo effect deserves a closer look as more than methodological noise. The nonpharmacological powers vested in a medication, and the positive meaning and healing expectations attributed to it, can be powerful allies in leading to positive change. By contrast, placebo's younger cousin, the nocebo effect, can be a force to reckon with because it can taint with its negative messaging, dashed hopes, and harmful attributions. When expectations are not only the patient's but those of their parents or guardians, of their schoolteachers or coaches, as well as of their social-media-frenzied feeds, we need to pause to consider the interlocking effects of what Grelotti and Kaptchuk (2011) initially conceptualized for adults, and Czerniak et al. (2020) later refined for children and adolescents, as the *placebo by proxy* or the *nocebo by proxy* effects. We may think of our consulting rooms as a confidential sanctum of privacy, but conversations about treatment rarely end at our doorstep; they are more likely to only get started there, and we risk enlarging our blind spots if we sidestep this chorus of informative or inflammatory influences.

The impact of the placebo (and of the placebo by proxy) is highest in the top row of our proposed matrix. How can we approach its right-most cell, *withholding*, in which a treatment perceived as mostly beneficial is rejected? A self-defeating adolescent in the throes of depression may resist a medication she considers herself unworthy of taking or that may threaten to alter distorted views deemed by then integral to her personality. Gentle yet goal-directed motivational interviewing may permit us to close the gap and "get to yes." A parent or guardian may resist giving a psychotropic out of an understandable abundance of caution, but there are times when untoward hesitation or repeated instances of abandoned treatment may require the involvement of child protective services. No one can force a child to take a medication, and the instance of involuntary administration (as in the case of an intramuscular injection) should remain a (very) last-resort measure within an emergency department or inpatient setting (10). Long-acting depot antipsychotics don't have a safety record in minors to warrant their regular use. In short, protective services, the courts, and injectable medications do have a role in contemporary psychiatry. But they are rarely invoked or useful beyond an acute emergency situation in the case of pediatric pharmacotherapy.

By contrast, the impact of the nocebo (and the nocebo by proxy) is most relevant in the bottom row of the matrix. *Resigned* patients and families may be accepting of treatment that they perceive as potentially hazardous. For many of these all too common scenarios, we provide concrete suggestions we have found helpful in our own practice.

First, it is often our oversharing of details—in the spirit of being transparent and comprehensive—that can corner us into this resigned quadrant. We do not advocate for the outright omission of side effect discussions, but do make a case for being less meticulous and defensive. Take as an example suicide risk in the context of starting an antidepressant. Time and again we hear necessary and well-meaning conversations about the relative risk of emergent suicidal ideation among children taking antidepressants compared with those who are unexposed. So far so good. But what we all too rarely hear is the more relevant comparison—that of higher rates of death by suicide among the untreated. Our cathartic confessionals scare away more often than they meaningfully engage patients and their families: we should resist clinching defeat (in the form of losing a patient to follow up, or tragically, to suicide) out of the jaws of victory (in the form of starting a potentially life-saving medication embedded within a therapeutic relationship).

Second, and relevant to all cells in the matrix, is a reminder that our task is in no small measure one of shared meaning-making. Romanowicz et al. (2) are direct and aphoristic in their advice: "The parent and patient most often seek consultation to receive help with the patient's symptoms, not to receive a DSM diagnosis. Help them co-create meaning and make sense of their symptoms." In an important article, David Mintz (2019, p. 237) expands this notion, alerting us to attend to the meaning of medication, particularly given that "[w]hile all people who take medications may attach pathogenic meanings to them, children and adolescents may be particularly vulnerable, because such effects can be amplified when incorporated into unfolding developmental processes." Moreover, "when harm occurs at the level of meaning, the problem will be most usefully addressed at the level of meaning. Far too often, however, medicated children receive little or no psychological treatment."

A Bitter Pill to Swallow: Stigma

In a sad parallel, the cell relegated to the very end of our conceptual matrix is the *stigmatized* confluence of treatment resisted on the basis of perceived harm. Or so we may be told. In fact, side effects (for example) may be the manifest excuse to turn down treatment, when closer listening may reveal that it is the stigma of mental illness that is the more relevant latent message. To take (or to give) a medication may be seen as tacit endorsement of an unwelcome diagnosis, of "otherness," of frailty or fallibility we would rather ignore. As if the stigma of mental illness was not bad enough, the stigma on psychotropics can increase feelings of exclusion and isolation, of being "broken" and in need of "repair."

There is much that we can do in our daily fight against the stigma of mental illnesses and the medications we often rely on to treat them. Psychoeducation is certainly prominent on the to-do list (5). But there is something else worth considering. It will sound radical, provocative, or boundary-breaking to some, and we respect those views. But for some others, being a bit radical, a tad provocative, a pinch boundary-breaking, and a whole lot legitimate and human, can be game-changing. Specifically, we have used as a tool for good the careful, selective sharing of our own diagnoses, treatments, medicines, family struggles, and recoveries. Whenever we have done this with the patient's wellbeing in mind, when the sharing has been genuine and caring, when we have met with patients and their families in full shared humanity, at those moments, we have been pediatric pharmacotherapists, physicians, and humans at our very best. We are not alone in this endeavor, and we embrace the words of the courageous and pathbreaking Stephen Hinshaw (2017, p. 250) in his sage insight that "fostering humanization may be the single most important weapon in the fight against stigma for…[m]ental disorders don't afflict *them*—a deviant group of flawed, irrational individuals—but *us*: our parents, sons and daughters, colleagues and associates, even ourselves." In short, we have nothing to disclose, but we have much to share.

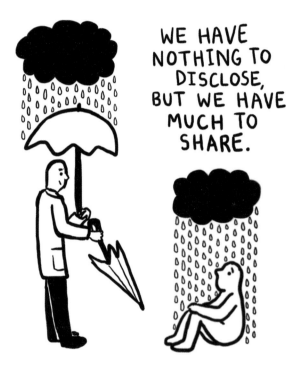

In Closing—and in Dual Dedication

There is much that this volume will demand of its readers. Our intention is to inform and educate so as to elevate our practice rather than to raise expectations that may make us feel inadequate. To the contrary, the penultimate chapter addresses a serious matter in a lighter note; it is, after all is said and done, more than sufficient to be "good enough" pharmacotherapists. By reading these words, you are already proving your good enough–ness. Our aim and our hope is to take you to a place of "good enough +1." That is the goal that as educators of the next generation of practitioners we have dedicated our professional lives to fulfilling (18).

As we look to a future generation—of newer psychotropic agents one day, of children with lessened burdens well before that, and of trainees emerging as inspiring colleagues and friends each and every year—we must thank the generation that preceded and nurtured us. They are conceptually bilingual exemplars, with fluency in both psychotherapy and pharmacotherapy: they embody the principles of psychopharmacotherapy we are hoping to instill in a new generation. Our hope is for this volume to serve as a salve against clinical monolingualism.

This project was first inspired by conversations with two beloved mentors, one in each coast. The chats that Andrés first had in the East Coast in the early aughts led to a chapter in which he was the understudy to Kyle Pruett's visionary thinking and writing (Pruett and Martin 2003). As our thinking evolved, we widened the learning circle, with Shashank joining as a fellow contributor (Pruett et al. 2011). In the West Coast, Shashank learned from, and emulated, another towering figure, Carl Feinstein. Their conversations were not only influential; they were also career-determining and went on to inform an entire new line of thinking and writing (Joshi 2006). The two of us have been blessed by knowing and learning from these two special mentors and friends. They are far from the only mentors we have been fortunate to have, and we cherish the lessons from so many other colleagues, several of whom have contributed to this collective effort.

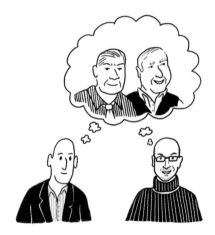

In their chapter in this volume (2), Carl and his coauthors riff off another giant:

As Leston Havens (2004) said, "The first goal is for the clinician to find the patient, and the patient to find the clinician." We have shown…it is not an easy process. Sometimes the clinician gets lost; sometimes the patient is difficult to find.

We concur and can add that finding mentors and inspiring teachers is not easy, either. We are grateful for having found this dynamic duo and learned from the best. We lovingly dedicate this book to them.

This volume is an invitation—an entreaty—to follow in their lead, to be our best professional selves and to do so in order to ease the suffering of the children and families we are privileged to serve. Kyle and Carl have given it their all throughout their careers. We emulate their example each day and invite you to do as well. In short, we invite you, dear fellow prescriber, to prescribe thyself.

Andrés Martin, M.D., M.P.H.
Shashank V. Joshi, M.D.
Illustrations by Simone Hasselmo, A.B.

PRESCRIBING MEDICATIONS IS AS MUCH
THE COLD FACTS OF MOLECULES

AS IT IS
THE WARM WAY IN WHICH WE ENVELOP THEM
FOR DELIVERY.

References

Czerniak E, Oberlander TF, Weimer K, et al: "Placebo by proxy" and "nocebo by proxy" in children: a review of parents' role in treatment outcomes. Front Psychiatry 11(March):169, 2020 32218746

Grelotti DJ, Kaptchuk TJ: Placebo by proxy. BMJ 343:d4345, 2011 21835868

Havens L: The best kept secret: how to form an effective alliance. Harv Rev Psychiatry 12(1):56–62, 2004 14965855

Hinshaw SP: Another Kind of Madness: A Journey Through the Stigma and Hope of Mental Illness. New York, St. Martin's Press, 2017

Joshi SV: Teamwork: the therapeutic alliance in pediatric pharmacotherapy. Child Adolesc Psychiatr Clin N Am 15(1):239–262, 2006 16321733

Mintz D: Recovery from childhood psychiatric treatment: addressing the meaning of medications. Psychodyn Psychiatry 47(3):235–256, 2019 31448987

Plakun EM, Sudak DM, Goldberg D: The Y model: an integrated, evidence-based approach to teaching psychotherapy competencies. J Psychiatr Pract 15(1):5–11, 2009 19182560

Pruett K, Martin A: The psychology of psychopharmacology: thinking about prescribing, in Pediatric Psychopharmacology: Principles and Practice. Edited by Martin A, Scahill LS, Charney D, Leckman JF. New York, Oxford University Press, 2003, pp 417–425

Pruett K, Joshi S, Martin A: The psychology of psychopharmacology: thinking about prescribing, in Pediatric Psychopharmacology: Principles and Practice, 2nd Edition. Edited by Martin A, Scahill LS, Kratochvil C. New York, Oxford University Press, 2011, pp 422–433

PART I

PRINCIPLES

CHAPTER 1

THINK AGAIN ABOUT PRESCRIBING

The Psychology of Psychopharmacology

Kyle D. Pruett, M.D.

> We work in the dark—we do what we can—we give what
> we have. Our doubt is our passion and our passion is
> our task. The rest is the madness of art.
>
> Henry James, *The Middle Years*

The children who come to us, and the families who accompany them, bring ideas, positive and negative feelings, mental images, past experiences, and hopes about who we are, whether we can help, and even the medications we may prescribe. As clinicians, we are no less engaged, often sharing in their doubts and hopes of finding the perfect solution (and potion) for their particular troubles. Yet for all our understanding of pharmacokinetics, drug-environment interaction, and pharmacogenomics, we remain intrigued when an agent happens to work, or not, for this patient, at this time.

Psychopharmacotherapy is the use of a psychoactive medication with psychotherapy. It places emphasis on a therapeutic relationship, on behavior and affects, and on developmental and social determinants. Referred to as "single provider integrated treatment," or "combined treatment," it is increasingly rare in psychiatric practice (Gabbard and Kay 2001; Janicak et al. 2010; Moran 2009) despite its proven efficacy (Gabbard and Kay 2001).

This chapter examines the dynamic implications of medication use within the wider domain of pharmacotherapy. Pharmaco*therapy* includes thorough diagnostic evaluation for children and adolescents referred for consideration of medication treatments. Much more than a "med check," this modality is complex, because prescribing clinicians strive to integrate quality patient care with the ever-changing time, economic, and administrative constraints of practice. As classical psychoanalysis tried to parse the influence of the "gang beneath the couch," we struggle to grasp the significance and influence of the "gang inside the prescription pad." In the sections that follow I discuss the 1) role of the therapeutic alliance, 2) psychological meaning of medication itself, 3) influence of developmental considerations, 4) meaning of the process of medicating, 5) psychological meaning of the context in which prescribing occurs, 6) extramural influences that affect prescribzing, and 7) effects of the shared-case context on prescribing.

Whether one is practicing psychopharmacotherapy or pharmacotherapy, the appropriate framework begins with the therapeutic relationship itself. In my decades of practice, prescribing evolved from a paternalistic and alliance-undermining act to a valued asset in treatment. Those same decades began with a handful of marginally effective (if side effect–ridden) agents for seriously affected children, used primarily in academic settings. Now we have scores of effective therapeutic choices, many marketed directly to parents, prescribed primarily in outpatient settings.

Still, Blackwell's (1973) admonition prevails: "Too often a prescription signals the end of an interview rather than the start of an alliance." This is especially true in the child-parent-therapist triangle, in which the parents' often urgent need for relief adds pressure to "do *something*" before sufficient understanding and therapeutic trust exist. With our increasingly acute clinical populations, a deeper attention to alliance, psychodynamics, diagnoses, and symptoms is crucial.

The Therapeutic Alliance

Joshi and colleagues (Joshi 2006; Joshi et al. 2004) summarized the interpersonal process literature relevant to pediatric pharmacotherapy, highlighting the need to understand both the alliance in the doctor-patient relationship and the dynamics shaping the doctor and parent-caregiver relationships. In preadolescent children, the doctor-caregiver alliance is especially salient (Alexander and Dore 1999). During adolescence, as patients assume more responsibility for their own care, clinicians often need to help parents avoid intrusive or controlling styles and attitudes about taking medication while maintaining a proper monitoring and supervisory relationship. The psychiatrist needs to be seen more as an ally of the teen rather than simply as an agent of caring adults.

The most helpful guidance in forming a good alliance I can recommend is to consider the following: How you *are* with your patient is as important as what you do *with* your patient. Poor alliances lead to premature termination of care (Magnavita 1993), just as good ones, in which patients feel heard and understood, lead to better follow-up and outcome (Zisook et al. 1979). A growing empirical database directly links a strong alliance in pharmacotherapies with positive clinical outcomes (Joshi 2006).

Greenberg and Horvath (1994) suggest that a "good enough alliance" (with both patient and parent or caregiver) is paramount for the therapy to proceed. Whereas the alliance in adult psychotherapy is established relatively early (by the third to fifth session) (Alexander and Dore 1999), a meta-analysis of outcomes in child and adolescent psychotherapy linked later-session relationship measures more strongly with outcomes than earlier-session measures (Shirk and Karver 2003). An early alliance is important for successful collaboration between parents and caregivers (Joshi 2006):

> Alliance development is a series of windows of opportunity, decreasing in size with each session.…[T]he foundation for collaborative work entails adjustments in both the client's and therapist's procedural expectations and goals. The longer the participants find themselves apart on these issues, the more difficult it becomes to develop a collaborative framework. (p. 240)

Havens (1978, 1988, 2000) reminds us that to many patients, the doctor's trustworthiness and decency are not givens, and that "behavior problems" in general and mental illness in particular are tricky subjects to discuss. He suggests that the investigative language and tone we use deliver vitality to the relationship: "[The language we use to inquire] is as important as the matter being investigated or treated.…[I]n fact, the two bear a symbiotic relationship to each other" (Havens 1978, p. 336). He reminds us that patients enter wondering whether the "mind doctor" will be concerned, engaging, suspicious, judgmental, or, worse, indifferent. He advises listening carefully to receive the patient's ideas without being intrusive and avoiding the "look of mock concern" so abhorrent to teenagers (Havens 1978).

Havens offers three "psychological analgesics" that can facilitate the approach to, and the management of, painful topics. These "analgesics" might be "prescribed" for difficult matters, including the need to take psychotropic medication:

1. *Protect self-esteem.* Self-esteem is vulnerable because patients are affected by having to come to a psychiatrist. Patients may also be affected if their parents feel guilty for being the "cause" of the problem through bad parenting, contributing genetic vulnerability, or both.
2. *Emote a measure of understanding and acceptance.* When successful, the patient's problem is grasped intellectually, and the patient's and family's predicament is understood from their point of view.
3. *Provide a sense of future.* Many families have experienced frustration and failure in finding solutions, resulting in diminished hope. Discussion about expectations for treatment that still acknowledges fears or even hopelessness may preserve opportunities for change: "It may seem hopeless to you for *now*" (Havens 1978, p. 340).

The Psychological Meaning of Medication Itself

A 14-year-old girl who had initially responded well to a brief course of pharmacotherapy began to complain that she felt like a "poser" because of taking a selective serotonin reuptake inhibitor (SSRI):

> I know I'm less depressed and irritable. My boyfriend says I'm easier to be around, but I'm not sure this is really *me*. I feel like this poser [posing as another]. Like, every time I take my pills it reminds me that I'm this screw-up who can't manage her feelings on her own. I hated feeling suicidal, but hey—maybe that's more me.

Besides pointing the way to the psychological work that she needed to do on her depression, she articulated a concern many of our patients and their parents have about medicine as change agents: "Will it change *me*, my or others' ideas of me, and not just my symptoms or behavior?"

> A 10-year-old had a behavior-changing response to stimulant medication that allowed him to transfer to a better school, sustain new friendships, and return to his beloved violin lessons. His father, who'd suffered similarly but gone untreated, was concerned that all we'd done

was a "naughty-ectomy, not real therapy." His son, somehow aware of his father's concerns, would occasionally taunt him: "Just call me Speedo [aware he was on a stimulant]—I am what I take!"

Medications and their representations shape-shift in our patients' imaginations as they search for the meaning of "taking pills." They have been depicted in my patients'—and their parents'—dreams and daydreams variously as poisons, magic potions, "mind restraints," aphrodisiacs, handcuffs, binoculars, microscopes, brain "implants," and contraceptives, to mention a few. There is no shortage of grist for the metaphor mill; each one is important to pursue (Mintz and Belnap 2006; Pescosolido 2007; Rappaport and Chubinsky 2000).

For psychiatry residents and fellows, Joshi (2006) reminds us that effective medication regimens may often collapse during the transitions in care common on 6-month "psychopharm rotations." In a study examining patient outcomes during transfer to a new pharmacotherapist (Mischoulon et al. 2000), nearly one-third of psychiatric residents' patients were negatively affected by treatment transfer or termination, regressing clinically or requiring medication changes. The relationship with the prescribing physician was obviously important to patients, such that forced termination had negative effects similar to those of transfers to a new psychotherapist. The authors recommend that sufficient notice be given to help patients deal with the forthcoming loss or change and describe specific suggestions to aid in processing this transition (Mischoulon et al. 2000). In my teaching experience, we encourage trainees to inform families and patients midway into a clinical rotation to allow sufficient processing by all parties. We also strongly discourage use of the term "psychopharm rotation," just as we eschew the term "med check" with youth. These terms fall far short of what actually happens in the room, whether working in pharmacotherapy or psychopharmacotherapy.

The timing of the prescription in ongoing psychotherapeutic work is rich with meaning—why now and not before or later? Should we attempt to relieve symptoms pharmacologically before they are understood by both patient and clinician? When symptoms are severe and acute, the need to medicate often precedes full understanding. In less acute circumstances, premature prescribing may undermine patients' sense that they can cope with these symptoms:

> "Don't you think I can do this by myself?" asked a 13-year-old girl, after we began to discuss an anxiolytic to help her manage her recurring panic attacks away from home. We examined her idea that I was giving up on her ability to understand herself and her behavior by even suggesting medication. In case I'd missed the point, she acted out sufficiently

to scare her parents. Subsequently, she re-engaged in psychotherapy and observed that the more aware she was of her "triggers," the less medication she required.

Beyond connections between timing and meaning, however, another question hectors the act of prescribing: Will medication mean *treat* or *treatment* to this particular patient? Gratification and frustration are balanced and rebalanced in successful psychopharmacotherapy, but awareness of this paradox helps therapist and patient avoid therapeutic diversions (Boris 1994).

Developmental Considerations

Remaining alert to changes in the meaning of the medication to patients as they move into new developmental terrain is especially relevant for clinicians working with children and adolescents. The significant changes in bodily preoccupation, impulsive discharge, and mood lability that occur in pubescence cast any past agent that may have affected weight (gain or loss), endocrine function (galactorrhea), skin appearance (acne), genital arousal or dysfunction, or mood itself in a new light. What may have been acceptable side effects before become intolerable as they emerge during, or simply complicate, already exquisitely sensitive developmental tasks. This is made more complex by the fact that nearly all "side" effects, from extrapyramidal symptoms to nausea, are less well tolerated in younger populations.

Salient for the child and adolescent population—and their caregivers— are the physical properties and dosing requirements of the medications themselves (Table 1–1). For many patients, especially younger ones, function follows form. The prevalence of normative magical thinking makes the color, shape, design, and form (liquid vs. solid) part of the child's attitude toward the medication.

> K. swallowed her clonazepam, but no other solid tablets, because her initial was "cut into it for me."

> The pink color of a schoolboy's guanfacine "always makes [him] think of peppermint candy." This cocktail of wish and suspicion, sweetened with the candy association, was sufficiently positive to help him adhere to taking it regularly. The "candy connection," however, deeply worried his mother, a recovering casualty of the drug culture.

Methylphenidate has generated the most imagery because of its widespread use:

Table 1–1. Children's thinking about medication

Physical properties of the medicine itself

Form	Liquid, tablet, capsule, or injectable forms may each carry different meanings (e.g., liquid is for "babies," injections are "punishments")
Size	The bigger the pill (or its milligram value), the bigger the problem, or conversely
Labeling and printing	Personalized associations to imprinted numbers or letters
Color	Associations to candy or poison

Timing of the dosage

Frequency	More frequent, more trouble, or conversely, more help
AM or PM	AM for school, PM for sleeping or dreaming troubles
During school	Concern about stigma
Self or parent administered	Self is good and mature, whereas parent is now doctor's agent

Source. Adapted from Pruett et al. 2010.

> Charlie, 8, devised a morning ritual involving an empty prescription bottle that he kept in his shoe. It reminded him when dressing to remind his mother, who "forgets half the time." Why a shoe? He heard his father tell his grandmother how Charlie's meds helped him "keep his feet on the ground." Charlie thought, "Just like shoes." How does he feel about taking meds? "They're little mines with codes stamped on them for each little monster inside me that they're going to blow up that day. Then I'm not such a problem!"

Asking about remembering rituals—or lack thereof—gives some understanding of deeper attitudes and ambivalence about specific drugs and their roles. What Charlie did *not* like about taking medication, however, was the way he got his midday dose at school:

> The nurse puts all our pills on her metal cart in these little cups with our names on them. She wheels it down the hall to our classroom door. Six boys and two girls go to the door and wait in line, and she watches us swallow the pills—right there. The whole class watches. It's stupid—I feel so weird.

Medication needn't mean shaming. Longer-acting stimulant preparations are rendering midday doses at school far less common, lessening the social toll associated with daily visits to, or from, the school nurse.

Potential meanings of dosing frequency also are not wasted on children. If children find their medicines helpful, and the medicines are given in the context of a supportive alliance, more frequent dosing can actually be reassuring. In less positive circumstances, when the effects are more ambiguous, more frequent dosing can be intrusive, resented, or read as a sign of "being sicker."

Closely tied to frequency is dosage size. Older children and younger adolescents can become preoccupied with the mathematical value of the dose, assuming that the smaller the number, the less "sick" they are. The converse is also true.

> A young adolescent girl was on her third attempt to find the right medicine for her elusive mixture of panic and depression. She was working hard in her psychotherapy but was getting discouraged. When she read the label, she realized that she was getting "*hundreds* of milligrams!" of a new drug, and since it was "only helping *a little bit!*," she concluded that she must be much sicker than she or the therapist thought.

The cost of medication as experienced by the family has meaning for the child or adolescent patient because of their dependent status. When children overhear or directly encounter their family's discussion about prescription costs, especially in the face of spotty coverage by disparate insurance plans, the child can feel like a further burden on their family. To avoid this further complication of adherence, it is best discussed privately and preemptively with the parents.

The Psychological Meaning of the Process of Medicating

If *primum non nocere* is our maxim primum, second is giving care with confidence and hope: "State of mind in which expectation is colored by hope and faith is an effective [therapeutic] force with which we have to reckon" (Freud 1905, p. 289). The power of this shared state of mind between therapist and patient influences medication choice for the patient's symptom relief. It is this confident, hopeful mindset that we have attempted to factor in, or out, using placebo controls in regulated drug trials.

The problem—and intrigue—with placebos is that they work *through* their meaning. Although they are pharmacodynamic blanks, they have been shown to be 55%–60% as effective as codeine and aspirin for analgesia (Kirsch 1997). Cognitive neuroscience suggests a mode of action more complex than the previously favored endorphin release theory. Ex-

pectancy theory suggests that what the mind believes about the immediate future is based on conditioning from past experience, mediated
through immune-endocrine system interaction (Kinsbourne 1999).

So why the placebo's seedy reputation? Placebos muddy the waters
of efficacy studies because their high "rate of relief" casts doubt over more
chemically active agents that performed acceptably (Puig-Antich et al.
1987). They also carry with them the folklore of the persuasive, patent
medicine–hawking "doc" who sold "proven effective" placebos *and* alco-
hol- and morphine-laced compounds (all for about the same price) to
loyal, witness-bearing clientele.

The classic prospective study by Park and Covi (1965) highlighted
placebo effects of medicating anxious patients. Though a "small *n*" study
with no child participants, its findings remain theoretically compelling:

> Fifteen newly admitted [outpatient] neurotics…, mean age 35, were
> seen in an hour-long interview for evaluation of anxiety. In a follow-up
> 15–30 minute interview, they were placed on a waiting list for interven-
> tion, and introduced in a standardized way to a nonblind placebo trial.
> They were told the placebo was 'a sugar pill with no medicine in it' that
> had helped people with similar conditions. Pink capsules in a t.i.d. dos-
> age were prescribed for a week, with a subsequent interview and symp-
> tom checklist. (p. 335)

All but one patient completed the treatment course, and all but one of
the completers experienced "some to a lot" of improvement. One-third
wished to continue the placebo, refusing to transfer to an active agent, two
felt "cured," and almost half of the completers believed it was a "real"
drug. Half of the believers experienced side effects.

The authors concluded that "1) patients can be willing to take placebo
and improve despite disclosure, and that belief in the pill as drug was not
a requirement for improvement; and 2) improvement was not related to
belief in the nature of the pills, but did appear related to certainty of belief" (p. 344). Placebos apparently need not be "lies that heal" (Harrington 1997) because the treating doctors were "optimistic about the
study, yet anxious about telling the patients that they would receive placebo. The [resulting] combination of enthusiasm and alertness must have
had a strong positive impact on the patients" (p. 343). N.B: *Placebo* is Latin
for "I shall please." Ethical considerations would probably preclude a
similar trial in children, though the forces at work in the therapeutic alliance could be similarly influential in pharmacotherapy with children
and adolescents.

Confident hope is a powerful and useful element in the process of
medicating: "placebos can elicit (both) solace and side-effects" (Schow-

alter 1997, p. 682). Parents respond powerfully to confident hope regarding medication. When parents are supportive and respectful of the child-clinician alliance, adherence and outcome improve. But when their response is fueled more by their own wishes, denial, or projections, outcomes can be undermined. Toffler et al.'s (1999) "achievement by proxy" formulation describes the negative influence on children when their growth and development become a means to a parental end, focusing on the circumstance of high-achieving children and adolescents. Clinicians need to be aware that analogous "treatment by proxy" dynamics can also shape clinical relationships with parents.

The Psychological Meaning of the Context in Which Medication Is Prescribed

There is, to paraphrase D.W. Winnicott, no such thing as just a prescription. Prescriptions are never written in a vacuum, devoid of relational or diagnostic context or marketing influence. The dominant context in which we prescribe is the parental one. The parent must consent, facilitate payment and access, usually dispense, monitor, renew, ensure adherence, deal with resistance, and often explain to a balky child yet again why they "have to" take pills.

Thoughtful appreciation of *all* parental attitudes is a prerequisite for successful medication usage and clinician efficacy. Mothers and fathers have overlapping but distinct concerns about their children's health and well-being (Pruett and Pruett 2010). Each parent's concerns are best understood in the context of the parents' relationship with each other, not simply with the child. Typically, one parent is more forgiving, the other more judgmental—one more optimistic, the other less hopeful—and the clinician will likely hear at least one "I told you it wasn't just in our son's head!"

Clinicians can safely assume that parents are well down their own road of frustrated and spent solutions when they meet for the first appointment. Parents may feel relief when medication is suggested because of the affirmation of the seriousness and accuracy of their concern for their child's difficulties. They may also feel less judgmental and self-deprecatory about failures to date, seeing medication—and its prescriber—as potential new allies. Such alliances are subject to the usual projections and fantasies that parents have about the people to whom they turn for help with their children—positive idealization when the medicines "work," doubt and conflict when they do not. The latter may only show itself in "forgotten renewals" or missed "med checks."

A newer player in the parental-clinician domain is the influence of direct-to-patient marketing of genetically guided prescribing recommendations. Some parents are arriving with personal pharmacogenomic profiles of their child's drug-metabolizing enzymes, which they have been assured "will help the prescriber choose the best medication with the fewest side effects." We know that genetic variations can determine impaired response to drugs, and this approach holds promise, as seen in "poor metabolizer" variations in atomoxetine breakdown. The American Society of Pediatric Hematology/Oncology, however, cautions against routine clinical application of these data because of the lack of high-quality pediatric research (Schuft 2019).

Given the rate at which primary care physicians and advanced practice registered nurses are currently prescribing psychoactive medication to adults, it is likely that parents have had their own experiences with mood- and behavior-altering medicines. A child's positive experience with medication can motivate the parent to investigate their own needs, especially if there are symptom similarities (e.g., fathers of sons with successfully treated ADD and ADHD are especially common).

Less supportive medication attitudes can foul, prevent, or prematurely terminate an alliance. Unexamined loss and grief over having a child "so sick" as to warrant a diagnosis or medication are common. Parents may see this as the start of a lifelong journey with chronic illness.

We know from antibiotic and insulin adherence studies that the more serious a parent feels their child's illness to be and the better understanding they have of the illness itself, the stronger the treatment adherence. Research illuminates several useful techniques to enhance adherence. Hack and Chow (2001) suggest the following:

1. It is important to attend first to the alliance through actively engaging patients and families in ways to communicate adherence success. Daily medication journals or charts are useful tools.
2. The alliance can be strengthened and adherence improved by scheduling sufficient time for office visits, planning for the next appointment as soon as feasible.
3. Written instructions and clinician availability by phone, e-mail, or health information portals decrease miscommunication about dosing and side effects.
4. Because duration of treatment and frequency of dosing contribute to adherence, less frequent dosing can improve adherence substantially (Liptak 1996).

5. Timing and simplicity of the dosing regimen can be tailored to enhance adherence; pairing doses with everyday activities such as meals, homework, or regular screen time can create reminders (Weinstein 1995).
6. Palatability (apparently more important to adults than to children; El-Chaar et al. 1996) may matter more to a particular child; liquid availability and flavoring options exist (provided by most pharmacies) if pill size, consistency, or taste is an issue.
7. Although cost is generally not correlated with adherence (Matsui 1997), it remains a burden for many families. If there is a good alliance, the resultant atmosphere of trust and safety allows families to more comfortably discuss financial stressors (Hack and Chow 2001).

What parents *do* understand about their child's diagnosis and needs warrants discussion in its own right, not simply in terms of the therapist's wish for adherence. As information floods families, we hear questions about "chemical imbalance." Although informed patients typically promote positive outcomes (Healy 1997), this particular concept should be used cautiously. It may mask meanings anywhere from a legitimate request for thoughtful diagnostic clarification to avoiding personal or emotional issues or signal a more superficial "boutique approach" to well-being and personal enhancement (Parens 1998). Valenstein's (2002) sobering discussion in *Blaming the Brain* of the scientific understanding of the role of "biochemical imbalance" in mental illness keeps us wary of prematurely attributing any shared meaning to this phrase.

Schools are important contexts for medicating therapists to consider. Because children's and adolescents' distress are often externalized, attentional and disruptive behavior disorders are frequently more obvious at school than at home. School officials may share in the "delusion of precision" (Gutheil 1982), perceiving drugs as uniformly effective agents, if the pharmacotherapist would just prescribe them. Schools feel mounting pressures to control the child's behavior or disruptiveness for reasons beyond concern for the well-being of a particular child: overcrowding, understaffing, the meritocracies of mandatory testing, and pressure from other parents, to name a few. Parents may or may not cooperate or agree with the school's concerns, facilitating or frustrating appropriate use of medications in an individual case. Parents may also feel that a different classroom or teacher, approach, or curriculum would be more effective than medication as a sole intervention.

Appreciation of these larger system interactions when considering medication will likely improve the efficacy of intervention. The reverse is also true: to *not* prescribe under such systemic pressures can be seen, or experienced, as withholding, not caring about, or being insensitive to the degree of child or parental distress.

Social media and internet information platforms increasingly influence older school-age and adolescent populations. Patients now arrive for consultation with narratives from their peers and browser-generated "information" about "meds that work and meds that suck." Clinicians who inquire "What have you heard about the medicines we're thinking of trying?" are usually rewarded with helpful context and "attitude" about potential medications.

Extramural Influences That Affect Prescribing

The combined corporate influences of the pharmaceutical and managed care industries can shape and even preclude the therapeutic alliance. They are strange bedfellows to the clinician and the prescribing process because their missions are typically disparate. Making a living while doing good would seem the common goal, yet the corporate structures and ethics that vaunt profitability over access flirt with incompatibility in the practitioner's realm of *primum non nocere*.

In 2019, the pharmaceutical industry spent $30 billion a year on promotion and advertising in the United States; 68% of that total was spent on advertising campaigns in our journals, at our meetings, and through direct contact between physicians and their tenacious, highly incentivized sales forces (Mole 2019). The sales force is well trained, chosen for its tenacity, and supported by strong incentives. In 2020, there were about 81,000 "reps," 1 for every 8 practicing physicians in the United States (Sufrin and Ross 2008). Some academics have had sufficient concern about the easy traffic between residents, "drug reps," teaching hospital administrations and their research-funding base, and the pharmaceutical industry that they suggested regular and ongoing vigilance of the "pharmaceutical-academic complex" (Angell 2000).

In 2008 and 2009, a few high-profile exposés of egregious profiteering on the part of some nationally recognized academic experts encouraged the FDA to tighten up things, and the Pharmaceutical Research and Manufacturers of America endorsed 1) science-based, rather than ad-libbed, promotion of products; 2) articulation of "negative effects" when present; 3) only "'modest" (by local standards) comped dinners; and 4) reps speaking with clinicians only if spoken to by clinicians first.

When the Affordable Care Act was signed into law in 2010, it created the Open Payments database in the hope that documenting conflicts of interest in research funding and kickbacks to prescribers would loosen Big Pharma's grip on prescription promotion, but little changed. Each year from 2014 to 2018, drug and medical device companies spent between $2.1 billion and $2.2 billion paying doctors for speaking and consulting, as well as on meals, travel, and gifts for them. These figures do not include research spending, but they do include royalties (Ornstein et al. 2019).

The reason for this caution grows: Marketing works. A pharmacotherapist is more likely to prescribe a drug over the next few days after its pharmaceutical representative takes them to lunch or supplies them with literature (Orlowski and Wateska 1992). Even though prescribers see themselves as intellectually independent of corporate influence, the language they use to describe a drug's properties to themselves and their patients is derived more from advertising than from the more objective scientific literature (Lexchin 1997). Regardless of how physicians see themselves, their patients and families may see them as being unduly influenced. Furthermore, patients express concern about their physicians' susceptibility to such pressure (Mainous et al. 1995).

Direct-to-patient (DTP) marketing—primarily to parents—has been so effective that it gives new meaning to the word "compliance." The National Institute for Health Care Management cited $2 billion as the direct-to-consumer marketing tab back in 2000 and saw it as closely tied to increases in prescription drug sales, including psychoactive ones (Findlay 2000). That number is now closer to $30 billion (Schwartz and Woloshin 2019). Some of the information in DTP marketing frequently raises a parent's level of concern about a child's behavior, prompting him or her to seek consultation sooner rather than later. But it has also led to inappropriate direct-to-physician voice mail and e-mail requests that a specific agent be prescribed over the phone or by return email for a child never seen by the clinician.

Managed care is another prominent member of the "gang inside the prescription pad." The limits on approval, duration, or nature of therapeutic contact or arbitrarily covered medications and services themselves have turned prescription writing into one of the only reliably reimbursable acts therapists can perform on behalf of their patients and their livelihood. The current 15-minute "med-check" session standard diminishes the therapeutic alliance to an encounter between a "med checker" and a "customer" with a target symptom. Policy statements from the American Academy of Child and Adolescent Psychiatry and the American Psychiatric Association oppose "the use of brief medication visits" because of the failure to include the "role of psychosocial intervention, including psychotherapy…in the treatment plan" (American Academy of Child and Adolescent Psychiatry 2001; see also Torrey et al. 2017).

Some have pointed to the concept of the "med check" as inherently inaccurate (Moran 2009). Others have challenged the concept altogether when working with youth (see Rosen and Glowinski in Chapter 6, "#KeepItReal," of this book).

Gabbard and Kay (2001) observed that it is "not really possible to know" what is transpiring between a therapist and patient during a session coded as a "medication visit," suggesting important psychotherapy may also be going on during these encounters.

> It's not as if the patient says "I'm only in for a med check, so I'll only talk to you about benefits and side effects of my meds."…[This highlights the importance that] basic psychodynamic principles—transference, countertransference, resistance, and therapeutic alliance—play in *all* of our interactions with patients. Regardless of modality, as psychiatrists, we need to be integrators *par excellence*.

Pressure from the managed care domain to do something "effective and do it fast" may be at work in the ongoing increase of prescriptions of psychoactive medication to preschoolers (Zito et al. 2000) and possibly the increasing trend toward polypharmacy.

The American Psychiatric Association work group behind "Beyond 'Med Management'" (Torrey et al. 2017) has suggested that 1) the "med-check" label be replaced with the term "psychiatric care visit," 2) the moniker "prescriber" give way to "psychiatric care provider," and 3) symptom rating scales, previous use of medications, aims for the visit, and family history data be collected by a trained psychiatric medical assistant or even user-friendly software (Torrey et al. 2017). These suggestions would increase the amount of focused, comprehensive thinking clinicians could do about prescribing.

The Shared Case: From Split Treatment to Shared Treatment

As reimbursement systems change and evolve, it has become common practice for the child and adolescent psychiatrist to take on the role of medication prescriber, while psychotherapy is offered by a separate (usually nonmedical) clinician. Larger team practices can ameliorate some boundary troubles, but liability, clinical, boundary, transference and countertransference, and systems issues still swirl about the axis connecting these symbiotic components of treatment. The only way to prevent split treaters from splitting the treatment is through effective and frequent communication.

A 13-year-old girl was referred for a pharmacotherapy consultation because of her therapist's concerns about increasing inability to concentrate at
school, inattention to her homework, and increasing social isolation. A diagnosis of ADHD seemed likely from teacher questionnaires. On interview,
her thought rituals, obsessive anxiety-containing behavior patterns, and
need to have "everything just right" (which she reported took hours) before
she could even start her homework suggested a prominent anxiety component (in which SSRIs might be more appropriate than stimulants). When I
e-mailed the therapist to share my initial impressions and suggest that we
discuss this further, she replied with additional information about a strong
family history for ADD and was reluctant to accept my recommendation
but agreed to talk on the phone. Discussion led to resolution, avoiding a potentially ensnaring boundary complication for this young girl who was already sufficiently anxious and confused, a miniscule time expenditure
compared with the costs of ineffective treatment.

The upfront commitment to clear treatment planning and diagnosis
is a universally effective vaccine against interdisciplinary collaboration
dysfunction. Sharing information about each other's practices, training,
practice patterns, and settings can create mutual respect that protects
against future conflict or splitting by some patients or families. Discussion
of medication changes before they are instituted results in less confusion
and resistance. Fax or secure e-mail communications are sufficient for
most shared data. Clarifying at the outset what is salient for collaboration
about this particular child and family is key, including level of vigilance,
adherence, or potential for misuse, among others. These issues argue
for changing the name from *split* treatment to *shared* treatment. See Chapter 6 of this book for further discussion on this topic by Mari Kurahashi
and colleagues.

Clinicians wisely prescribe in the context of medications already being prescribed, sharing recommendations with the primary care physician to avoid potential drug interactions and side effects that evolve over
the course of treatment, preventing misattributions by the psychotherapist to changes in sleep, sexual behavior, irritability, and other symptoms.
A thorough, culturally informed biopsychosocial psychiatric evaluation,
not simply a symptom search, lays the foundation for a holistic understanding of what medications mean psychologically to a patient and to
their family during the course of treatment.

Future Research

Unanswered questions remain regarding how digital technologies, including e-prescribing, paid advertising on such platforms, and social
media are affecting patient adherence and clinician prescribing prac-

tices. Drug pricing—especially when it seems erratic or arbitrary—is another domain that influences and confuses clinicians and patients' families and as such is in need of careful study. Advances in personalized medicine and the influence of pharmacogenomics need clarifying for child and adolescent populations.

Conclusion and Recommendations

- When thinking about medicating, remember that it is the patient, not the drug, that deserves our major attention. Decisions about prescribing medication need to be made in the context of the therapeutic alliance, with less emphasis on the probability of reimbursement.
- Keep in mind that the formulation always precedes the prescription, not vice versa (with the possible exception of emergencies). Thorough clinical conceptualization is not gilding the drug-treatment lily. It is necessary for making good treatment choices, evaluation, and ongoing reevaluation of drug choice and combined treatment effectiveness.
- Resist intimidating time constraints, especially in appointments at the beginning of the consultation. If you have done your diagnostic work and built your alliances accordingly, the relationship will matter more than the time spent sustaining it (Tasman and Riba 2000; Tasman et al. 2000).
- Create and sustain all the relationships necessary to address the child's needs, including parents and other caregivers, teachers and other school staff, collaborative therapists, primary care providers, and others important to the patient.
- Do not prescribe for a patient you cannot remember between appointments. You are forgetting them because neither of you is sufficiently invested in a relationship worth remembering—an infrastructure of insufficient substance to support pharmacotherapy or *any* therapy, for that matter.
- Be perpetually aware of the seductions of marketing. They *are* getting to you and affecting your judgment about drug choice.
- Use "chemical imbalance" discussions with caution, because it may be difficult to predict what they mean to any given patient or their parents.
- Neither over- nor undersell any one drug as part of the treatment regimen. Medications carry sufficient "magic" on their own. Telling parents and patients there are other choices invites them to be collaborators in psychoeducation, not just pill consumers.

- Treat your patients as though the therapeutic relationship matters more than the pills. It usually does.
- Remember the words of Jeree Pawl, president emerita of Zero to Three: National Center for Infants, Toddlers and Their Families: "How you are matters as much as what you do."

References

Alexander L, Dore M: Making the Parents as Partners principle a reality: the role of the alliance. J Child Fam Stud 8:255–270, 1999

American Academy of Child and Adolescent Psychiatry: Prescribing psychoactive medication for children and adolescents. Revised and approved by the Council on September 20, 2001. Available at: www.aacap.org/AACAP/Policy_Statements/2001/Prescribing_Psychoactive_Medication_for_Children_and_ Adolescents.aspx. Accessed April 10, 2020.

Angell M: Is academic medicine for sale? N Engl J Med 342(20):1516–1518, 2000 10816191

Blackwell B: Drug therapy: patient compliance. N Engl J Med 289(5):249–252, 1973 4713764

Boris H: Sleights of Mind: One and Multiples of One. Northvale, NJ, Jason Aronson, 1994

El-Chaar GM, Mardy G, Wehlou K, Rubin LG: Randomized, double blind comparison of brand and generic antibiotic suspensions, II: a study of taste and compliance in children. Pediatr Infect Dis J 15(1):18–22, 1996 8684871

Findlay S: Prescription drugs and mass media advertising. Washington, DC, National Institute for Health Care Management Research and Educational Foundation, 2000

Freud S: Psychical (or mental) treatment (1905), in The Standard Edition of the Complete Psychological Works of Sigmund Freud, Vol 7. Translated and edited by Strachey J. London, Hogarth Press, 1953

Gabbard GO, Kay J: The fate of integrated treatment: whatever happened to the biopsychosocial psychiatrist? Am J Psychiatry 158(12):1956–1963, 2001 11729008

Greenberg L, Horvath AO (eds): The Working Alliance: Theory, Research, and Practice. New York, Wiley, 1994

Gutheil TG: The psychology of psychopharmacology. Bull Menninger Clin 46(4):321–330, 1982 7139146

Hack S, Chow B: Pediatric psychotropic medication compliance: a literature review and research-based suggestions for improving treatment compliance. J Child Adolesc Psychopharmacol 11(1):59–67, 2001 11322747

Harrington A (ed): The placebo Effect: An Interdisciplinary Exploration. Cambridge, MA, Harvard University Press, 1997

Havens L: Explorations in the uses of language in psychotherapy: simple empathic statements. Psychiatry 41(4):336–345, 1978 715094

Havens L: Coming to life interview, National Public Radio, 1988. Available at: https://www.youtube.com/watch?v=SBSVyL6avyc. Accessed April 12, 2020.

Havens L: Forming effective relationships, in The Real World Guide to Psychotherapy Practice. Edited by Sabo AN, Havens L. Cambridge, MA, Harvard University Press, 2000, pp 17–33

Healy D: The Antidepressant Era. Cambridge, MA, Harvard University Press, 1997

Janicak P, Marder S, Pavuluri M: Principles and Practice of Psychopharmacotherapy. Philadelphia, PA, Lippincott Williams & Wilkins, 2010

Joshi SV: Teamwork: the therapeutic alliance in pediatric pharmacotherapy. Child Adolesc Psychiatr Clin N Am 15(1):239–262, 2006 16321733

Joshi S, Khanzode L, Steiner H: Psychological aspects of pediatric medication management, in Handbook of Mental Health Interventions in Children and Adolescents: An Integrated Developmental Approach. Edited by Steiner H. San Francisco, CA, Jossey-Bass, 2004, pp 465–481

Kinsbourne M: Mind and nature: essays on inner subjectivity. J Nerv Ment Dis 189:140–147, 1999

Kirsch I: Specifying nonspecifics: psychological mechanisms of placebo effects, in The Placebo Effect: An Interdisciplinary Exploration. Edited by Harrington A. Cambridge, MA, Harvard University Press, 1997, pp 166–186

Lexchin J: What information do physicians receive from pharmaceutical representatives? Can Fam Physician 43:941–945, 1997 9154366

Liptak GS: Enhancing patient compliance in pediatrics. Pediatr Rev 17(4):128–134, 1996 8637819

Magnavita JJ: The evolution of short-term dynamic psychotherapy: treatment of the future? Prof Psychol Res Pr 24:360–365, 1993

Mainous AG III, Hueston WJ, Rich EC: Patient perceptions of physician acceptance of gifts from the pharmaceutical industry. Arch Fam Med 4(4):335–339, 1995 7711920

Matsui DM: Drug compliance in pediatrics: clinical and research issues. Pediatr Clin North Am 44(1):1–14, 1997 9057780

Mintz D, Belnap B: A view from Riggs: treatment resistance and patient authority, III: what is psychodynamic psychopharmacology? An approach to pharmacologic treatment resistance. J Am Acad Psychoanal Dyn Psychiatry 34(4):581–601, 2006 17274730

Mischoulon D, Rosenbaum J, Messner E: Transfer to a new psychopharmacologist: its effect on patients. Acad Psychiatry 24:156–163, 2000

Mole B: Big Pharma shells out $20B each year to shmooze docs, $6B on drug ads. ARSTechnica, 2019. Available at: https://arstechnica.com/science/2019/01/healthcare-industry-spends-30b-on-marketing-most-of-it-goes-to-doctors. Accessed September 2, 2020.

Moran M: Psychiatrists lament decline of key treatment modality. Psychiatr News 44(13):8–25, 2009

Orlowski JP, Wateska L: The effects of pharmaceutical firm enticements on physician prescribing patterns: there's no such thing as a free lunch. Chest 102(1):270–273, 1992 1623766

Ornstein C, Weber T, Grochowski Jones R: We found over 700 doctors who were paid more than a million dollars by drug and medical device companies. Pro Publica, October 17, 2019. Available at: www.propublica.org/article/we-found-over-700-doctors-who-were-paid-more-than-a-million-dollars-by-drug-and-medical-device-companies. Accessed March 29, 2020.

Parens E: Is better always good? The Enhancement Project. Hastings Cent Rep 28(1):S1–S17, 1998 9539044

Park LC, Covi L: Nonblind placebo trial: an exploration of neurotic patients' responses to placebo when its inert content is disclosed. Arch Gen Psychiatry 12:336–344, 1965

Pescosolido BA: Culture, children, and mental health treatment: special section on the National Stigma Study—Children. Psychiatr Serv 58(5):611–612, 2007 17463339

Pruett K, Pruett M: Partnership Parenting: How Men and Women Parent Differently—Why It Helps Your Kids and Can Strengthen Your Marriage. New York, Da Capo/Perseus, 2010

Pruett K, Joshi SV, Martin A: Thinking about prescribing: the psychology of psychopharmacology, in Pediatric Psychopharmacology: Principles and Practice, 2nd Edition. Edited by Martin A, et al. New York, Oxford University Press, 2010, pp 422–433

Puig-Antich J, Perel JM, Lupatkin W, et al: Imipramine in prepubertal major depressive disorders. Arch Gen Psychiatry 44(1):81–89, 1987 3541830

Rappaport N, Chubinsky P: The meaning of psychotropic medications for children, adolescents, and their families. J Am Acad Child Adolesc Psychiatry 39(9):1198–1200, 2000 10986818

Schowalter JE: Psychopharmacology: the mind-brain frontier. Paper presented at the annual meeting of the American Association of Child and Adolescent Psychiatry, Toronto, Ontario, Canada, 1997

Schuft K: Young blood: challenges and benefits of pharmacogenomics in pediatric practice. Expert Insights. Wolters Kluwer, April 8, 2019. Available at: www.wolterskluwer.com/en/expert-insights/young-blood-challenges-and-benefits-pharmacogenomics-in-pediatric-patients. Accessed March 15, 2020.

Schwartz LM, Woloshin S: Medical marketing in the United States, 1997–2016. JAMA 321(1):80–96, 2019 30620375

Shirk SR, Karver M: Prediction of treatment outcome from relationship variables in child and adolescent therapy: a meta-analytic review. J Consult Clin Psychol 71(3):452–464, 2003 12795570

Sufrin CB, Ross JS: Pharmaceutical industry marketing: understanding its impact on women's health. Obstet Gynecol Surv 63(9):585–596, 2008 18713478

Tasman A, Riba MB: Psychological management in psychopharmacologic treatment, and combination pharmacologic and psychotherapeutic treatment, in Psychiatric Drugs. Edited by Lieberman J, Tasman A. Philadelphia, PA, WB Saunders, 2000, pp 242–249

Tasman A, Riba MB, Silk KR: Using the interview to establish collaboration, in The Doctor-Patient Relationship in Pharmacotherapy: Improving Treatment Effectiveness. Edited by Tasman A, Riba MB, Silk KR. New York, Guilford, 2000, pp 182–192

Toffler I, Knapp P, Drell M: The "achievement by proxy" spectrum: recognition and clinical response to pressured and high-achieving children and adolescents. J Am Acad Child Adolesc Psychiatry 38(2):213–216, 1999

Torrey C, Griesemer I, Carpenter-Song E: Beyond "med management." Psychiatr Serv 68(6):618–620, 2017

Valenstein E: Blaming the Brain. New York, Free Press, 2002

Weinstein AG: Clinical management strategies to maintain drug compliance in asthmatic children. Ann Allergy Asthma Immunol 74(4):304–310, 1995 7719889

Zisook S, Hammond R, Jaffe K, Gammon E: Outpatient requests, initial sessions and attrition. Int J Psychiatry Med 9(3–4):339–350, 1979 757223

Zito JM, Safer DJ, dosReis S, et al: Trends in the prescribing of psychotropic medications to preschoolers. JAMA 283(8):1025–1030, 2000 10697062

CHAPTER | 2

THE MANY FACETS OF ALLIANCE

The Y-Model Applied to Child, Adolescent, and Young Adult Pharmacotherapy

Magdalena Romanowicz, M.D.
Sarah Rosenbaum, M.D., M.P.H.
Carl Feinstein, M.D.

Overview of the Psychology of Psychopharmacology and Developmental Considerations

Effective psychotherapists and pharmacotherapists share two important attributes: technical knowledge and skills. Whereas technical and scientific knowledge can be taught and examined during medical education, the therapeutic skills, also known as "nonspecific" treatment factors or "common factors," are more elusive and harder to describe. Yet based on a recent literature review (De Nadai et al. 2017), these common factors benefit children receiving psychotropic medications as well as their families and their clinicians.

Even very young children are not passive recipients of medications and create meaning around them, unique to their developmental level. They might refuse to take the medicine or develop negative associations about the medication if their physicians fail to help them make sense of their symptoms and develop a meaningful narrative.

> A 3-year-old boy with a significant peanut allergy is undergoing peanut desensitization therapy. His parents report that he is very defiant around taking his daily dose of peanuts and that they are also worried about op- positional and hyperactive behaviors that are present throughout the day. They add that he had a significant anaphylactic reaction when he was 2.5 years old. During a psychiatric evaluation, the physician explores the topic with the child: she carefully explains how the process of desensiti- zation works in a developmentally appropriate way, and they draw a picture of the process together. On follow-up, his parents share that with this new understanding, he is less resistant to his therapy, which he no longer perceives as a threat.

This vignette illustrates a number of important concepts that we will discuss in this chapter. Interview and treatment strategies that foster a ther- apeutic alliance differ for various developmental stages in pediatric pa- tients and must simultaneously acknowledge both the chief complaint and the narrative of the parents. There are a number of patient- and parent- generated variables that precede any actual intervention but contribute to outcomes. These variables include motivation for treatment, attitudes to- ward medications (the child thought the peanuts were going to hurt him), framing of the chief complaint (the parents wondered if their child was op- positional), concerns about stigma, and external pressures from family, the internet, or culture. When so much meaning is generated by simple pea- nuts, one can only imagine what happens when a child is asked to take a psychotropic medication with a name that is difficult to pronounce in or- der to help with feelings and behaviors that are difficult to understand.

Clinicians, children, and their parents all uniquely interact with the en- vironment and are influenced by a variety of internal and external psy- chosocial factors that impact both the treatment alliance and treatment outcomes. The complexity of these interactions makes the task of assessing the efficacy of psychotropic medications difficult (De Nadai et al. 2017). Even well-designed, evidence-based clinical trials struggle to account for factors associated with nonadherence, suboptimal adherence, and drop- outs (Matsui 2009). In child and adolescent psychiatry, adherence is a sig- nificant issue because only 50% of patients report taking commonly used psychotropic medications such as selective serotonin reuptake inhibitors and stimulant medications as prescribed. Most children do not continue their antidepressants for more than 6 months despite a recommendation by their doctors to do so. Overall, children have lower adherence than adults, and adolescents are even less likely to take their medications as prescribed compared with younger children (Costello et al. 2004; Matsui 2007). Despite the widespread challenges with adherence in child and adolescent populations, the motivations for stopping medications are understudied.

"Nonspecific" treatment factors, also referred to as "common factors," including a number of psychosocial variables such as motivation for change, expectation for positive outcome, and therapeutic alliance, have been shown to have a major impact on treatment outcomes in psychotherapy with adults. However, the impact of these common factors on treatment outcomes for children and adolescents has been largely unexplored, and most of the writing to date on this topic has been extrapolated from studies with adults. The application of this literature to the pediatric context is further complicated by the need to account for the alliance with the parent or caregiver and for developmental factors that impact motivation, levels of understanding of illness, and treatment planning. The specific mechanisms by which a therapeutic alliance is formed between clinician and patient remain an underdescribed topic in the literature. Furthermore, how the therapeutic alliance and other common factors influence treatment outcomes is difficult to study, especially when it comes to child and adolescent patient populations.

Most psychopharmacological trials to date either have neglected to account for common factors or have conceptualized them as confounds (Miller et al. 2009). Nevertheless, some empirical data from adult trials suggest that in the psychopharmacological treatment of patients with depression, therapeutic alliance accounts for 19%–56% of the treatment outcome (Krupnick et al. 1996; Weiss et al. 1997). Many experienced therapists appreciate how fragile and yet crucial early alliance is in psychotherapy. Likewise, when it comes to pharmacological treatment of patients with depression, an early treatment alliance with the prescriber is predictive of positive antidepressant treatment outcomes in adults (Blatt and Zuroff 2005).

De Nadai et al. (2014) suggest that a strong therapeutic alliance creates a stable platform from which the child or adolescent patient and their clinician can communicate. The existence and stability of this shared and mutually created starting point foster a sense of trust that ultimately allows for better engagement of a patient in therapeutic interventions and techniques and in turn more positive treatment outcomes. In psychopharmacological treatments, a strong therapeutic alliance helps foster both medication adherence and positive treatment expectations (Thompson and McCabe 2012). For children and adolescents, clinicians must be sensitive and responsive to the nuances in patients' perceptions of them that are colored by developmental stage and youth subculture particulars. These are difficult to anticipate but must be taken into account. For example, in the treatment of adolescents, potential factors influencing the initial attitude toward an alliance with a new doctor might include the doctor's appearance, demeanor, manner of speech, knowledge of youth subcultures, and office furnishings.

Another complicating factor in child and adolescent psychopharmacology is that the alliance that must be built and sustained is almost never only between the clinician and the child but, crucially, must also be between the clinician and the child's parents (Joshi 2006). Patients trust their clinicians for a host of reasons—both conscious and unconscious—that are difficult to quantify with parent-completed patient satisfaction rating scales. These scales often gather material that patients are comfortable sharing with anyone but may not identify more personal responses that result in a favorable or unfavorable response to their clinician. There is significant room for improvement in how we study common factors in child and adolescent psychopharmacology, but progress in understanding them will be important in improving treatment outcomes.

The "Stem of the Y" Model: Implications for Treatment

Let's start with posing a question: How do patients and parents "know" that they have a good doctor in front of them? This subjective assessment begins immediately, even before entering an office or sharing their presenting concerns. Based on research with adults, a person determines whether they trust a new clinician within the first 100 milliseconds (ms) of meeting the clinician (Wampold 2015); 100 ms is enough time for the parent to take a glance at the approaching doctor and see how they are dressed, whether they smiled, and perhaps whether they addressed the child in the waiting room. For a child, it might be as simple as whether the clinician has interesting toys in their office; a teenager may value whether their doctor looks cool or fashionably dressed. A study by Chung and colleagues (2012) showed that a doctor's clothing is an important nonverbal communication that has an impact on the patient-clinician relationship, especially in the initial stages.

As the treatment progresses, the therapeutic relationship evolves with all its different layers and expectations. Wampold (2015) describes it as an unusual relationship based on an agreement of confidentiality (with some statutory limits; i.e., safety, child abuse) and the fact that the main premise of treatment is that the patient is encouraged to say anything in the sessions, even if it is embarrassing or offensive, without being judged by the clinician. The clinician, rather than responding judgmentally, chooses to explore with the patient the motivations and reasons to bring personal, family, or peer information into the treatment conversation. Frank and Frank (1991) discuss the importance of a patient's expectations for treatment. They describe the process of remoralization for patients who arrive at their sessions demoralized, but also underscore how important it is for patient and clinician to co-create meaning and make sense of the patient's symptoms. This supportive and interested response nurtures rapport, and treatment begins.

In discussing the therapeutic alliance in this chapter, we can only touch on the numerous important topics that address how the clinician brings this about: What exactly does the clinician do to help the patient feel they are caring, trustworthy, and credible? What does the clinician do so that the patient and their parents believe that their problems are understood? How exactly does the clinician explain their approach to treating the patient's symptoms? For psychopharmacological treatments, how does the clinician make sure that their patient adheres to the treatment with fidelity? We underscore that the answers to these questions are complex and often unique to each set of patients, parents, and clinicians. Although therapeutic encounters are governed in part by a collection of well-defined rules (the treatment frame), each successful clinician-patient relationship has a unique combination of common factors, specific to a particular dyad or triad.

The method in this chapter will be to first list and then define the common factors that should be addressed, based on the stem-of-the-Y model proposed by Plakun et al. (2009). We will formulate in general terms the principles and methods that treating clinicians (psychopharmacotherapists) can put into practice to optimize treatment outcomes, moving beyond the fatalistic idea that the doctor's capacity for the therapeutic alliance is some sort of fixed innate "talent" such as being "empathic." However, as Kubie (1971) describes in his timeless paper "The Retreat From Patients," there is a difference between learning psychiatry and the process of becoming a psychiatrist. The latter is not something that a learner can gain only from books, lectures, or abstract conversations but rather from "experiencing repeatedly within themselves the turmoil of personal growth and change, as these are induced by repeated experiences of interacting with and adjusting to patients as they change." Considering the many forms of psychiatric disorder and the many vicissitudes in treatment progress and setbacks, it is not a small task to learn from repeated encounters with our patients as they fall ill, respond to treatment, relapse, and retreat from and return to care. This process of "interacting with and adjusting to patients as they change" can be especially challenging when caring for children, who not only change with the ebb and flow of their symptoms but are also constantly evolving and growing over the course of normal development.

Learners need a place to start on their way to becoming child psychiatrists and finding the golden grail of balance between being empathic and objective in their patient encounters. In 2009, Plakun, Sudak, and Goldberg published an important paper, "The Y Model: An Integrated, Evidence-Based Approach to Teaching Psychotherapy Competencies." With a number of psychotherapy schools competing with each other for primacy in residency training, the intent of Plakun et al.'s paper was to provide an integrated model for core competencies across the main schools of psychotherapy: the stem of the Y represents the alliance and other foundational elements shared across the schools, while the branches of the Y represent the divergent theories underpinning cognitive-behavioral therapy and psychodynamic therapy.

Here we focus on specific elements of the stem of the Y in the context of pharmacotherapeutic encounters. These elements include establishing rapport, fostering an atmosphere of safety and trust, forming consistent boundaries and a treatment frame, relating with accurate empathy and genuineness, engaging in reflective listening, and providing education about diagnosis and treatment (Plakun et al. 2009). Additional elements were added by Peterson (2019) in his editorial "Common Factors in the Art of Healing." Peterson emphasized that for patients to adhere to prescribed treatment, a genuine relationship needs to be established. Empathy, warmth, genuineness, having a positive regard for the patient, and unconditional acceptance all foster this relationship. This atmosphere allows for clinician and patient to engage in the co-creation of a coherent narrative or conceptual framework. Together, doctor and patient look for context and create a therapeutic framework that includes a process for communicating about goals of treatment and adherence (i.e., what to look for in treatment changes, side effects, and target symptoms). This positive treatment alliance contributes to the necessary platform from which clinicians can engage with their patients in health-promoting activities such as validation, advice giving, instruction, learning, and practice. These practices, in turn, help patients confront their fears and stigma as well as process negative or hostile information or misinformation they may have encountered on the internet or from members of their families or communities.

Treatment Frame

The establishment of the treatment frame is one of the foundational elements of any therapy or psychopharmacological encounter. When working with children and adolescents, the message must be developmentally appropriate depending on the age of the patients. For children and adolescents of all ages, it is critical that the clinician introduce themselves and explain what they do. The clinician should also always lay out what will happen in the office visits, including fixed structural elements such as time and length of appointment, steps in the diagnostic process (who meets with whom when), what types of information will be collected, and what tests will be done and why. The clinician should make it clear how to contact him or her. Issues of confidentiality should be explicitly and clearly explained. Parents often demand certain types of information later in the treatment or are surprised that the clinician did not, for example, disclose to them that their teenager has been using marijuana. It is much easier if limits to confidentiality are clearly outlined at the beginning of the treatment. Providing context and a rationale for why certain information is being collected may also help prevent negative feelings about questions that patients or parents might experience as intrusive.

Last, it is important to keep in mind that the information that the clinician is asking for is often difficult for patients and parents to share. They might feel ashamed, guilty, and responsible for their symptoms or those of their child. The clinician should explicitly invite the child and parent to explore their many and varied questions, opinions, preferences, preformed notions, expectations, motivations, and fears, be it during consultation or during follow-up appointments. Sometimes it is as simple as a reminder that to help patients with their symptoms, pain, and inhibition, the clinician needs to gather as much information as they can. Often it is more complex and requires that clinicians create and maintain an atmosphere devoid of judgment, that they monitor for their own countertransference reactions, and that they engage in regular peer consultation and supervision.

Alliance

Therapeutic alliance issues are particularly important and evident with adolescent patients; however, they must not be overlooked when treating younger children as well. How children and adolescents view their clinicians very much depends on their stage of development and their level of understanding about the purpose of the appointment and what it entails. Parents of preschool and latency-age children pay close attention to how the clinician attends to their child (e.g., whether the doctor sat at their child's level when they said hello and spent dedicated time with them). Younger and older children, each from their own perspective, can sense when the doctor puts their parent(s) at ease, and this can facilitate their own degree of cooperation and openness with their doctor. Conversely, adolescents and school-age children often get locked into a struggle with their parents when it comes to acknowledging or accepting the way their parents describe their symptoms and problems. This can cause them to view the clinician as an agent of the parents rather than a help to them. In this type of situation, appointments can become a punishment or stigmatizing humiliation imposed by the parents, and patients may refuse to participate in treatment.

Ideally, the patient should be involved in formulating a shared treatment goal. However, there are, for example, adolescent patients who have no motivation to change because of the severity of their depression, shame or denial about their symptoms, secret problems that their parents are not aware of, or difficulty communicating with their parents. In particular, adolescents often disagree with the presenting complaint as described by their parents. Given this impasse, there is no motivation for treatment, and developing a treatment alliance is a challenging clinical problem that positions a clinician in an uneasy triangle between the perceived problem identified by the parent and either the absence of concern or the presence of a completely different problem as perceived by the patient. Reaching for a prescription plan to bulldoze through this predicament is often not the best solution. There must be some degree of alliance around a shared treatment goal, or no matter what the doctor prescribes, treatment will be undermined by nonadherence, patient dropout, or, at best, a prolonged and painful stalemate.

Instead, a good starting point for building a therapeutic alliance is taking an empathic stance toward all parties involved and communicating genuine interest in the presenting symptoms as described from the child's and the parents' perspectives. Sometimes adolescents agree to start taking medications just to take their parents off their proverbial backs during the appointment but later refuse to take medications or pretend to be diligently taking them when, in fact, they are not. Clinicians should be wary of initiating pharmacological treatment with an adolescent who does not accept the need to take medication or experiences seeing a psychiatrist as stigmatizing or shameful. Rather, there should first be a concerted effort by the clinician to therapeutically engage the adolescent in seeking relief for something that bothers him or her and ultimately to form a treatment alliance around that.

Often, patients and parents are much more interested in the symptoms being experienced than the formal psychiatric diagnosis provided by the clinician. During appointments, patients and parents should be asked about what bothers them most and which behaviors, states of mood, and impairments in functioning have been of greatest concern. It is important that the clinician clarify the relationship between symptoms experienced or expressed by the patient and parent and the formal psychiatric diagnosis. Without a basic level of agreement and acceptance between the doctor's diagnosis and the way the patient and parent understand the target problems and treatment goals, the family may see the clinician as simply "treating the diagnosis." This may be experienced as stigmatizing, off-putting, incomprehensible, or simply "psychiatric jargon" by the patient or parent, and, not uncommonly, by some collaborating medical specialists or primary care providers. It is crucial to explain to the patient and parent why providing a diagnosis helps with the treatment. This disconnect between patient, parent, and clinician, in which the well-intentioned clinician seeks to adhere to evidence-based practice by prescribing medications indicated for specific DSM diagnoses without finding some bridge to the narrative of the patient or parent, can make the doctor seem aloof and not patient-centered.

Motivational Interviewing

Making use of motivational interviewing prior to beginning any medication can help improve a patient's motivation and sense of agency to participate in treatment. These techniques help to better understand, validate, and express empathy for both the patient's goals and resistances (Dean et al. 2010; Haynes et al. 2008). Motivational interviewing has been shown to improve alliance and adherence in psychopharmacotherapy with adults (Byrne and Deane 2011). This is likely due at least in part to the opportunity this orientation offers patients to describe their symptoms and goals in their own words and their reasons for and against making an effort to change their current state.

Motivational interviewing also helps link the patient narrative with the formal diagnosis. Reliance on the use of standardized symptom rating scales without also considering the patient's narrative and motivations for change can be off-putting and alienating unless the reason for administering them is explained. For some patients and parents, these standardized questions reinforce culturally influenced negative biases about psychiatrists, diagnoses, and mental illness, in addition to an intense fear of risking exposure and stigma by answering them honestly. And yet at the same time, there are patients who appreciate using scales and surveys as a way to organize their thoughts or start a difficult conversation, which can, in turn, in the dialogue in the office, be a means to engage them in a deeper understanding of their motivations to change. Please see Chapter 4 of this book by John Dilallo for more on motivational interviewing with youth.

Genuineness

It is particularly important that psychiatrists not mystify the process of examining and diagnosing patients by acting aloof or unengaged, especially when dealing with children and adolescents. The beliefs that the doctor must be a cipher, never use the pronoun *I*, never express an opinion or conjecture about the patient, and never show an emotion are archaic. *Genuineness* implies steering away from the use of formulaic questioning techniques (referred to by many patients as "psychiatrese" or "psychobabble") to maintain the natural flow of conversation and to follow the needs of the patient from moment to moment. It is also very important for the clinician to ask questions that help elicit a better understanding of the patient and their situation better (being explicit about the process), as opposed to rhetorical questions or vague, general, or standardized questions that are of little meaning to the patient. Finally, genuineness also refers to the doctor being genuine in their own personhood, relating to patients in a manner that is authentic to their character and nature, while simultaneously remaining careful not to violate boundaries or to impose unwanted, unrequested, or unnecessary personal information.

Reflective Listening

Although Plakun et al. (2009) did not explicitly describe reflective listening as a component of the stem of the Y, it deserves mention here as we discuss how to establish and foster the therapeutic alliance. Reflective listening is closely connected to the concept of reflective functioning formulated by Peter Fonagy (Fonagy et al. 1991). Fonagy hypothesized that secure attachment between parent and child depends on the parents' ability to see their child as a separate entity from themselves with separate mental states and in turn to sufficiently attune their responses to their child's mental states. Similarly, in therapeutic encounters with patients, clinicians should demonstrate their intent to attune their care to the needs of the patient and parent. The doctor can attempt to accomplish this by, for example, summarizing what they heard and then checking with patients and their parents to confirm whether this is, in fact, what they are thinking, feeling, or trying to convey. The parent and patient must feel listened to, respected, and treated courteously as they articulate the chief complaint that led them to seek treatment. They also must feel that their clinician has a good understanding of their narrative of symptoms and causes. There will inevitably be some misunderstandings and misattunements. It is not a small task to try to understand someone who has a mind of their own in connection to our own mind and emotions. It is therefore essential that the clinician repeatedly and iteratively reflect back and clarify what they heard with both the child and their parents.

Mentalization

In child and adolescent psychiatry, another complicating factor is that although our patient is the child or teen in front of us, we are also expected to effectively communicate with their family. To accomplish this, the clinician uses three main overlapping skills: reflective listening, empathy, and cognitive perspective taking. All three skills are conceptually related to an important psychological construct known as *mentalization*, around which a dedicated therapy known as mentalization-based therapy has been developed (Fonagy et al. 2002). Mentalization, a concept that has many links to the account of reflective functioning described earlier by Fonagy et al. (1991), is the ability to recognize internal mental states in oneself as well as within another person with whom one has an interaction. The capacity to mentalize is very important when dealing with parents and patients, all of whom come to us with separate minds of their own. Acknowledging and respecting the distinct perspectives the patient and parents might have allows the clinician to acknowledge the autonomy of the patient while respecting the wishes of the parents. The capacity to mentalize also enables the clinician to take a compassionate and caring stance toward the patient's and parents' plights and dilemmas. It does not imply that a clinician must always agree with their patients or their states of mind but instead that the clinician is better equipped to understand these states of mind and express empathy explicitly and with genuineness and care.

Common Factors

In his paper on common factors, Peterson (2019) describes "interpersonal attunement and alliance between clinicians and their patients" as the "true science and art of healing." Notice that the author describes the common factors not only as the art of patient-clinician interactions but also as "true science." In pharmacotherapeutic encounters, an effective therapeutic alliance starts with the process of making and delivering a diagnosis but, equally important, also requires the establishment of consensual treatment targets and goals. A formal psychiatric diagnosis disconnected from the patient's narrative may not only feel alienating but also stigmatizing and have the effect of "pathologizing the patient," who may, for example, feel "normal" except for occasional social difficulties. It is critical to explain to the patient and parents why the clinician considers the diagnosis important and relevant to helping the patient recover from the problems in their narrative that brought them to treatment. Parents might, for example, be seeking treatment to keep their child from having behavior or disciplinary problems at school. In this context, simply providing a diagnostic label for the child's psychiatric condition that can be shared with the school may be perceived as receiving a stigmatizing label that only further risks their child's future reputation. Following a thorough evaluation, clinicians should not hold back from sharing their impressions or conveying accurate diagnostic findings with the family. However, to sustain the therapeutic alliance through this stage of the treatment, clinicians must also address and convey an understanding of the patient and family's priorities and the symptoms they care most about or that concern them the most. The formal diagnosis may be the least palatable element in the formulation of the treatment plan.

Patients also often come to consultation appointments with preconceived notions and preferences for or against medications. Some might have heard about specific side effects or even rumors of danger in relation to particular medications from relatives, friends, the internet, or hostile publications promulgated by pseudoscientific organizations. Listening to and working through these opinions, beliefs, and values is critical. Similarly, it is important for the clinician to "get on the same page" with the patient and parents regarding the schedule and frequency of follow-up clinic visits and what to expect from each visit. Busy, tightly scheduled psychiatrists often struggle with hearing the patient's interval history narratives about symptoms, adaptation, possible side effects, new problems, new stressors, and conjectures of causality. It can be challenging for the doctor to acknowledge all of these variables and reflectively listen to patients month after month, especially if there are rigid time limitations placed on follow up visits. However, an exclusive reliance on standardized diagnostic behavioral checklists risks alienating some parents, who feel that their specific concerns are not being addressed. This can lead to poor medication adherence, treatment dropouts, or less-than-satisfactory treatment outcomes. These hurdles may be forestalled when patients and parents feel heard and understood. Therefore, alongside choosing the right medication, genuine thoughtfulness, reflective listening, cognitive perspective taking, and mentalization remain integral to successful psychiatric treatment.

Putting It All Together: Stem of the Y With Clinical Examples

As Leston Havens said, "The first goal is for the clinician to find the patient, and the patient to find the clinician" (Havens 2004, p. 56). We have shown in this chapter it is not an easy process. Sometimes the clinician gets lost; sometimes the patient is difficult to find. Stem-of-the-Y principles help to guide and provide a framework for the treatment process, but its authors did not intend for them to replace years of mentoring and supervision. These principles are best conceived as a "scaffolding" that helps to keep the therapeutic process moving forward successfully. Here we present two clinical cases to show what the process of building therapeutic alliance looks like in practice with a young child (age 0–5 years) and teenager (age 13–18 years).

> Dr. T was a first-year child and adolescent psychiatry fellow. She was about to meet her first 4-year-old patient, K, and was carefully placing magnetic blocks in her office while making a quick list of differential diagnoses in her head. When K entered the office, she immediately went toward the dollhouse. "It's pink!" she squeaked. Her exhausted-appearing mother fell on the couch. She remarked to Dr. T that she looked too young to be a doctor and asked if she had kids of her own. Dr. T reflected back her concerns that a youthful appearance might suggest inexperience and that not having kids of her own might mean that she did not know what it meant to take care of a young child. She shared with the mother that although she did not have this personal experience, she

was an expert in child psychiatry and was there to help both the mother and K.

K's mother started by listing a number of behavioral struggles. Dr. T listened intently and then looked at the child and asked, "K, do you know why you are seeing a doctor today?" K shook her shoulders. Again looking directly at K, Dr. T explained to her that she was a doctor who played with children. She clarified that her office was a place where K could talk about all kinds of things. She added that her mommy was worried about K's body getting very angry and hurting other people and she brought K to the doctor to help her with that. K looked at Dr. T as she was talking and smiled. Toward the end of the appointment, Dr. T wondered if she could obtain collateral information from K's preschool before making the final diagnosis. K's mother agreed but stressed that she was hoping to get some kind of medication soon because she was barely managing with three children in the house. Dr. T reflected back that it was very difficult to manage three young children and went on to explain what the process of making a diagnosis entailed, reassuring her that it did not have to take a long time and clearly conveying that it required that Dr. T gather necessary information. She also clarified with K's mother what symptoms she was hoping the medication would target. K's mother listed a number of symptoms, including inattention, hyperactivity, and restlessness as well as oppositional and defiant behaviors. She added that she herself had ADHD and took medication that she found helpful.

In this case, we present a number of important elements of alliance building discussed in this chapter. Verbal and nonverbal communications that have the potential to influence both alliance and eventual adherence start with the first 100 ms of the initial meeting, when the patient and parent experience their first impressions of the clinician in front of them. We would like to highlight how critical it is for the clinician to address any concerns that families might have at this juncture. The mother in our vignette might not have shared any of her initial reservations had the clinician not created an atmosphere of acceptance and nonjudgment. Through reflective listening, Dr. T was able to establish a sense of trust that allowed the mother to shift away from her concerns about Dr. T's competency to her concerns about her daughter. This case also demonstrates that a positive alliance does not equate with giving in to whatever requests the patient or parents make of the clinician. When the mother in the vignette expressed that she was expecting to receive a prescription for medication during the appointment, the clinician empathized with her and then explained the rationale for not writing a prescription right away. The mother and Dr. T were then able to begin a conversation about the symptoms of greatest concern to the mother as well as the mother's own personal beliefs and experiences.

J, 18 years old, has been in and out of various forms of psychiatric treatment for as long as he can remember. At 13 years old, he was diagnosed with major depressive disorder. He did not think that therapy was for him and often forgot to take his medications or stopped them altogether because he thought they were not working or gave him side effects. He tried to self-medicate with marijuana and occasional beer with his friends. J thought that the combination of the two would actually take the edge off his anxiety and allow him to sleep at night. His parents were not aware of this. They were worried about J's lack of motivation and his constant irritability. They were hoping he could go to college but were not sure if he would be able to keep up with his classes without their support and supervision. These concerns led them to Dr. Z, who asked J to tell him a little bit about himself as a person. He wondered what he liked to do with his friends, what music he listened to, and whether he was into any sports. As it turned out, they both loved the rapper-producer Post Malone. Dr. Z made it clear to J that because he was 18 years old, he was in charge of all decisions related to his treatment. He did wonder if perhaps J wanted his parents to be involved in some capacity, especially because they lived together. J agreed to his parents being told his diagnosis and their helping with treatment planning but made it clear that he did not want them to learn about his drug and alcohol use.

J spoke with Dr. Z about his difficulty with adherence in the past, his hopelessness regarding treatment effectiveness, and his lack of motivation to engage in any treatment. Dr. Z empathized with J. He commented on how difficult his experience had been. He wondered what kept him going, what got in the way of healing, and what supports J had around him. He also asked questions about target symptoms. What benefits did J experience from marijuana and beer that in his opinion kept him using? Was he interested in quitting, and if so, why? With J's permission, his parents were invited to the office to share their perspectives as well. Everyone participated in the process of crafting a treatment plan. J realized that this interaction was different from those in the past. This treatment plan was his. He knew how to contact Dr. Z if he needed to change it. Follow-up appointments were scheduled to discuss how J was doing.

This is a case of an older teenager, entering adulthood, that highlights the important subject of patient autonomy. As an 18-year-old, J was legally in charge of his medical decisions. However, because he was still living with his parents, who were also paying for all of his medical expenses, they wanted to be involved as much as they could. Dr. Z was able to "get on the same page" with the patient and the parents by first listening to the teenager's expectations and then being clear regarding what the parental involvement was going to entail. From the very beginning, with the assist of motivational interviewing, the doctor was able to create a collaborative atmosphere. He made sure that the patient understood that treatment planning was a process involving a number of follow-up appointments rather than one with a quick fix. He asked questions about J as a person that allowed him to feel that he was appreciated as more than a list of symptoms on a checklist, and this process also helped with alliance building. Importantly, for a teenager who had spent years in ineffective treatment, partially because of nonadherence, the techniques used by Dr. Z did not take a long time to implement.

Discussion and Areas for Future Research

The twenty-first century has been filled with new discoveries about the neurobiology and genetic underpinnings of psychiatric disorders, new psychotropic medications, and new interventional techniques such as brain stimulation treatments. Eric Kandel once said, "A brain scan may reveal the neural signs of anxiety, but a Kokoschka painting, or a Schiele self-portrait, reveals what an anxiety state really feels like. Both perspectives are necessary if we are to fully grasp the nature of the mind, yet they are rarely brought together" (Kandel 2012, p. 16). We are hopeful that the impressive progress of modern biological psychiatry will continue to improve our understanding of the brain and psychiatric illness. However, in parallel to this march forward, we hope that beginning and expert pharmacotherapists alike continue to strive to understand and cultivate the therapeutic relationship that allows us, in the words of Kandel, "to fully grasp" with empathy and in collaboration what matters most to patients and their families.

Arthur Kleinman (Gardner and Kleinman 2019) has argued that the field of psychiatry is currently in crisis and that we have gone too far in creating a division between the biological and the psychological elements of treatment. Factors related to clinical care, research, and education have all contributed to this growing division. The ubiquitous use of electronic health records that rely on checklists, the need to chart during patient encounters, administrative pressures for significantly shorter visits, and managed care have reshaped clinic encounters. Scientific journals and research grants largely favor studies focused on biologically based research. As emphasized by Plakun et al. (2009), the teaching of psychotherapy and stem-of-the-Y practices have also been marginalized in psychiatric training programs. Because the missions of clinical care, research, and education are all closely interconnected, the best way forward in addressing knowledge gaps is to make sure that none of these domains are neglected.

Zulman et al. (2020) recently presented five actionable practices that have the potential to enhance physician presence and meaningful connection in all specialties of medical practice with adults. Interestingly, although this research does not explicitly reference stem-of-the-Y practices such as empathy or reflective listening, there is a significant overlap between the five suggested practices and the skills we have discussed in this chapter. Based on a rigorous mixed methods study, the authors identified that clinicians should listen to patients without interruptions, develop treatment plans collaboratively with patients, notice patients' emotions, and reinforce patients' stories. The brilliant study by Zulman et al. (2020) should be replicated with child and adolescent patient populations. Unfortunately, to date, only a handful of studies have addressed the subject of alliance formation with school-age children and adolescents (Feinstein et al. 2009; Joshi 2006), and no studies have explored this topic in the care of young children. This creates a gap in our training and evidence-based practice because the therapeutic alliance plays a crucial role in treatment outcomes. It remains unclear whether common factors are an adjuvant treatment to pharmacotherapy or whether they have unique effects independent of medication use (De Nadai et al. 2017). However, their importance for improving treatment outcomes is well established.

We would be remiss if we left the impression that the stem-of-the-Y approach to teaching psychotherapy in residency and fellowship programs is sufficient in itself for teaching clinicians how to improve the treatment alliance with patients. For teaching purposes, single clinical case studies are still vital material, especially if written by a master clinician. Unfortunately, these are far too rarely published by academic journals. It is valuable, even inspiring, for learners to read in depth about the ways master clinicians approach patients. Quantitative studies that are preferentially published by most academic journals rarely capture the important nuances of the individual clinician-patient relationship.

It is also vital that training programs foster a culture in which educators interested in teaching based on stem-of-the-Y techniques are valued and supported by their departments. Teaching should be provided via many different means: supervision on individual cases, mentoring, lectures, and grand rounds, among others. Trainees should be encouraged to observe experienced clinicians interview patients on inpatient units and be provided the opportunity to shadow attendings in their outpatient practices. In-depth case discussions can be facilitated by having attendings present cases to trainees and share with them the evolution of their thought processes, occasional struggles, and ongoing care for their patients and families.

The process of becoming a psychiatrist who is skillfully able to use stem-of-the-Y techniques in patient encounters happens slowly, "one patient at a time" (Kubie 1971). Continuous practice is key.

Conclusion and Recommendations

Elements of the stem of the Y, such as establishing rapport, fostering an atmosphere of safety and trust, forming consistent boundaries and a treatment frame, relating with accurate empathy and genuineness, engaging in reflective listening, and providing education about diagnosis and treatment, are facets of every pharmacotherapeutic encounter.

- A strong therapeutic alliance creates a stable platform from which you can better communicate with your patient. It allows for positive engagement with your patient in treatment interventions and improves treatment outcomes (De Nadai et al. 2014).
- Children and adolescents are known to adhere poorly to prescribed medications. A therapeutic alliance with each pediatric patient greatly facilitates adherence as well as positive participation in the treatment. Explain what a pharmacological treatment or test entails and why you are recommending it using language that is appropriate to the developmental level of your patient. Make sure to obtain assent from the child or adolescent in addition to consent from the parents.
- The therapeutic alliance is almost never between you and the child alone. Forming and maintaining an alliance with parents and guardians is also essential to treatment. The patient is their child. They have primary responsibility for the welfare of their child and almost always are the ones who will make the decision about whether treatment is started, changed, or continued. It is critical to explain to parents what treatment entails and why you are prescribing it and to set aside time to make sure you address their questions and concerns.
- The blend of professionalism and genuineness in your personal demeanor and your office setting are important nonverbal factors that influence the formation and maintenance of a therapeutic alliance.
- Remember that treatment often begins before the patient comes to your appointment. It starts with the family's and patient's expectations, preconceived notions, stigma, internet searches, and conversations with other family members and friends. It is important that you explore all this during consultation appointments in an atmo-

sphere of safety and trust. Use reflective listening to demonstrate that you are really hearing their narratives.

- The parent and patient most often seek consultation to receive help with the patient's symptoms, not solely to receive a DSM diagnosis. Help them co-create meaning and make sense of symptoms.
- In cases of family conflict and parent-child relationship issues, empathic and reflective communication with all the parties involved and genuine interest in both patient and parent narratives of illness are a good starting point in alliance building.
- Be genuine in your communications. Take responsibility for what you say. This might include using the pronoun *I* when asking questions or conveying your opinions, observations, expressions of empathy, or interpretations. This includes using reflective listening to confirm "being on the same page" and sharing emotion, if deemed therapeutic for the patient and family.

References

Blatt SJ, Zuroff DC: Empirical evaluation of the assumptions in identifying evidence based treatments in mental health. Clin Psychol Rev 25(4):459–486, 2005 15893862

Byrne MK, Deane FP: Enhancing patient adherence: outcomes of medication alliance training on therapeutic alliance, insight, adherence, and psychopathology with mental health patients. Int J Ment Health Nurs 20(4):284–295, 2011 21729254

Chung H, Lee H, Chang DS, et al: Doctor's attire influences perceived empathy in the patient-doctor relationship. Patient Educ Couns 89(3):387–391, 2012 22445730

Costello I, Wong IC, Nunn AJ: A literature review to identify interventions to improve the use of medicines in children. Child Care Health Dev 30(6):647–665, 2004 15527475

Dean AJ, Walters J, Hall A: A systematic review of interventions to enhance medication adherence in children and adolescents with chronic illness. Arch Dis Child 95:717–723, 2010 20522463

De Nadai AS, King MA, Karver MS, Storch EA: Addressing patient motivation, therapeutic alliance, and treatment expectancies in interventions for anxiety disorders (Chapter 56), in The Wiley Handbook of Anxiety Disorders. Edited by Emmelkamp P, Ehring T. New York, Wiley, 2014

De Nadai AS, Karver MS, Murphy TK, et al: Common factors in pediatric psychiatry: a review of essential and adjunctive mechanisms of treatment outcome. J Child Adolesc Psychopharmacol 27(1):10–18, 2017 27128785

Feinstein NR, Fielding K, Udvari-Solner A, Joshi SV: The supporting alliance in child and adolescent treatment: enhancing collaboration among therapists, parents, and teachers. Am J Psychother 63(4):319–344, 2009 20131741

Fonagy P, Steele M, Steele H, et al: The capacity for understanding mental states: the reflective self in parent and child and its significance for security of attachment. Infant Ment Health J 12(3):201–218, 1991

Fonagy P, Gergely G, Jurist EL, Target M: Affect Regulation, Mentalization, and the Development of the Self. New York, Other Press, 2002

Frank JD, Frank JB: Persuasion and Healing: A Comparative Study of Psychotherapy, 3rd Edition. Baltimore, MD, Johns Hopkins University Press, 1991

Gardner C, Kleinman A: Medicine and the mind—the consequences of psychiatry's identity crisis. N Engl J Med 381(18):1697–1699, 2019 31665576

Havens L: The best kept secret: how to form an effective alliance. Harv Rev Psychiatry 12(1):56–62, 2004 14965855

Haynes RB, Ackloo E, Sahota N, et al: Interventions for enhancing medication adherence. Cochrane Database Syst Rev Apr 16;(2):CD000011, 2008 18425859

Joshi SV: Teamwork: the therapeutic alliance in pediatric pharmacotherapy. Child Adolesc Psychiatr Clin N Am 15(1):239–262, 2006 16321733

Kandel E: The Age of Insight: The Quest to Understand the Unconscious in Art, Mind, and Brain, from Vienna 1900 to the Present. New York, Random House, 2012

Krupnick JL, Sotsky SM, Simmens S, et al: The role of the therapeutic alliance in psychotherapy and pharmacotherapy outcome: findings in the National Institute of Mental Health Treatment of Depression Collaborative Research Program. J Consult Clin Psychol 64(3):532–539, 1996 8698947

Kubie LS: The retreat from patients: an unanticipated penalty of the full-time system. Arch Gen Psychiatry 24(2):98–106, 1971 5539862

Matsui D: Current issues in pediatric medication adherence. Paediatr Drugs 9(5):283–288, 2007 17927300

Matsui D: Strategies to measure and improve patient adherence in clinical trials. Pharmaceut Med 23:289–297, 2009

Miller FG, Colloca L, Kaptchuk TJ: The placebo effect: illness and interpersonal healing. Perspect Biol Med 52(4):518–539, 2009 19855122

Peterson BS: Common factors in the art of healing (editorial). J Child Psychol Psychiatry 60(9):927–929, 2019 31407818

Plakun EM, Sudak DM, Goldberg D: The Y model: an integrated, evidence-based approach to teaching psychotherapy competencies. J Psychiatr Pract 15(1):5–11, 2009 19182560

Thompson L, McCabe R: The effect of clinician-patient alliance and communication on treatment adherence in mental health care: a systematic review. BMC Psychiatry 12:87, 2012 22828119

Wampold BE: How important are the common factors in psychotherapy? An update. World Psychiatry 14(3):270–277, 2015 26407772

Weiss M, Gaston L, Propst A, et al: The role of the alliance in the pharmacologic treatment of depression. J Clin Psychiatry 58(5):196–204, 1997 9184613

Zulman DM, Haverfield MC, Shaw JG, et al: Practices to foster physician presence and connection with patients in the clinical encounter. JAMA 323(1):70–81, 2020 31910284

CHAPTER 3

PSYCHODYNAMICS OF MEDICATION USE IN YOUTH WITH SERIOUS MENTAL ILLNESS

Barri Belnap, M.D.
Erin Seery, M.D.
John Azer, M.D.
David Mintz, M.D.

In this chapter we consider the psychodynamics of medication use in children with serious mental illness. We must first begin with defining the term *serious mental illness*. The phrase itself evokes many connotations. One might envision that serious mental illness equates with conditions such as schizophrenia, bipolar disorder, anorexia, severe depression, or autism spectrum disorders. However, the National Institute of Mental Health (2020) only defines serious mental illness within the lens of functional impairment. What makes a condition functionally impairing? From what we know of adult psychiatric illness, symptoms tend to be more impairing and more difficult to treat in the context of diagnostic comorbidity or early adversity or trauma and are especially challenging for those with few current psychosocial supports (Weinberg et al. 2019). Many children whose primary struggle lies in their ability to manage and use negative feelings have a poor long-term prognosis. Often it is not just the index problem but also the psychosocial and developmental context that is primary. It can then be especially challenging as a psychiatrist or mental health clinician to attend to the complexity of the presenting problem if one is viewed only as a "prescriber."

Psychodynamic psychopharmacology (Mintz and Belnap 2006, 2011) is a discipline that places the role of meaning and interpersonal factors at the center of psychopharmacological treatment. Traditional approaches to the prescribing relationship can be problematic because they tend toward generalizing the unique suffering of each individual in an attempt to standardize care and outcomes among patients. A psychodynamic understanding attempts to offer a complementary element to treatment that elevates the encounter between an individual and psychopharmacological treatment. This approach has been particularly important in understanding treatment-resistant conditions, which do not respond to the usual interventions as expected and in which a differentiating perspective may become critical for full access of treatment possibilities. Psychodynamic psychopharmacology can also have an important role in the understanding of children with mental health challenges deemed to be "serious illnesses." For these children and adolescents, the focus can be placed on ameliorating the distressing symptom, at times for the benefit of the family or school system, without as much attention to the function the symptom serves, the developmental context of the symptom, or how the symptom impacts the identified patient.

Conceptions of childhood have varied surprisingly over the span of humanity. They have coalesced into a primary understanding of childhood in the light of adulthood. That is to say, the structure, form, and function of adulthood contextualize our notions about childhood. We have used the ideal adult behavior as a standard against which to measure our children as healthy or deficient. For children designated as having serious mental illnesses, there is a complicated path to adulthood. The recent evolution of dynamic systems theory, in its attempts to incorporate chaos theory, has challenged our thinking by emphasizing how each child's developmental path is unique (Demos 2019). This has relevance as we attempt to appreciate the impact of medications on children, because the theory suggests that the introduction of such a factor has extensive permutational capacity in one's life and consequently challenges our preconceived notions of development and childhood.

Developmental Considerations

There has been an explosion of research about how we grow from infancy to adulthood. Attachment theory, mentalization, and the work of Tronick (Beeghly and Tronick 2016), Damasio, and many others have introduced us to a brain that is an amazing problem-solving tool. The new theories focus on the brain's problem-solving capacity and the relationships that support its development. A child is not alone on this developmental path; instead, their capacities are dependent on the parent-child dyad. The parent is an engaged companion to that growth and provides opportunities for the skillful development of the child's brain. The focus of the new theories about children's health and illness is on what factors contribute to the movements between mutual regulation to mutual dysregulation. The ordinary failures and misattunements that can make up 70% of the interactions between a healthy parent and child are the resources that develop the brain as a tool for solving problems (Gold 2017, p. 94). To label dysregulation as pathology or "serious mental illness" interferes with the necessary growth of the child because these moments, though emotionally intense and behaviorally symptomatic, are essential to learning how to solve problems that are appropriate for the child's developmental age.

Based on her research, Virginia Demos has helped us focus on two organizing principles of human development and health that when interfered with can be assumed to contribute to mental illness: 1) the need for psychic coherence and 2) the preference of each person to be an active agent in the course of both internal and external events of their life (Demos 2019, p. 33).

Attachment and mentalization have moved the relationship between parent and child to the forefront of development. Neurology has increased our awareness of the intricacies of lower brain and higher brain functioning and has broadened our appreciation of how self-regulation is learned in relationship with another person and is state dependent.

The new research suggests that infant development lays down the fundamentals of affect sequences that will determine the child's or adult's expectations of others and the child's capacity for trust in their own agency. Agency is learned through the iterative experience that requires one to develop three skills: "awareness of distress" (A), the "intention to want to lessen it" (I), and "the effort of mobilizing a response" (M), or AIM (Demos 2019, p. 60). Each step is essential, and the process needs to proceed in that order.

The evolutionary functions of feelings are to motivate the child and others to care about something of importance to an individual in his or her immediate context. The child or adult may not know what the feeling signals until 1) it is shared with others and 2) the possible sources are investigated and mapped out jointly. This is especially important when shame, blame, or failure is the primary issue. Sometimes a child is bringing feelings of sadness to a parent to investigate what the parent knows about how one uses sadness in one's own life, according to his or her chosen ideals and values. In this moment, the child not only is looking for mentoring but also is seeking to understand her parent's internal world and decision-making process.

A parent who believes her role is to intervene before the child has a capacity to notice and signal his distress, though well intentioned, undermines the capacity for the child to lay down important brain circuits necessary to experience himself as an agent who can regulate his own emotions. Self-regulation is learned because stress is identified and then engaged with effectively. Intentions are not as effective in affecting the course of child development as parents or adults might imagine. In the best of situations, parents are "guilty" of not reading their infants or children accurately most of the time. Parents need to be able to feel guilty without being blamed so they can see guilt as a vital resource in learning with children how to read things wrongly, readjust perceptions, and reestablish a better attunement (Gold 2017). This is how resilience is achieved. This is the process that is necessary to learn to gauge reality well—the reality about both oneself and others. Getting it wrong and creating a space for the parent to be curious about the infant or child's feelings is the path to reestablishing mutual regulation and is also good enough to enable the infant to develop the skills and capacities that will create confidence that he can restore a positive experience that has gone badly.

By learning to recognize the parent's unique patterns and needs, the child gains competence at attuning herself to her parent and at holding the parent in mind more skillfully. This can make the child more effective in being an agent in the return to mutual regulation. The conversations between parents and children about the many possible ways to respond to feelings and the different effects such responses can have on getting things done in the world are the process through which children achieve emotional maturity and sophistication. They are also the process by which they learn who they are, and that who they are may well be different from who their parents are and from whom their parents want them to be. This process of differentiation is a vital phase of growing up. However, in this process, a child may encounter a parent's own difficulty with affective expression. The child may learn that certain emotional expressions are not tolerated. This will shape how the child understands and responds to these emotions.

This process can become confusing when affective learning is intertwined and equated with illness. For example, anger can be both an aspect of a psychiatric disorder and an expectable consequence of feeling let down or betrayed. A child may learn that certain feelings are pathological and can lose access to the important information they provide (Mintz 2019). Children do not understand causal relationships in the manner that adults do (Whiteman 1967). Children's concepts of illness are thought to proceed through a developmental sequence that is connected to Piaget's (1948, 1960, 1969) understanding of how children conceptualize causal relationships (Bibace and Walsh 1980). To better understand how children understand causality related to personal illness and illnesses of friends or relatives, Robert Bibace and Mary Walsh studied 72 medically and emotionally healthy children ages 3–13 years (Bibace and Walsh 1980). They identified six types of explanations expressed by children that proceeded from primitive to complex and followed a chronological course, with older children tending to have a more advanced understanding than younger children. Young children ages 2 and 6 years tended to explain illness through phenomenological or magical causes. For example, a child in this age range may explain illness as being caused by God. Children ages 7–10 years tended to conceptualize illness as manifesting from contamination or internalization. It can be developmentally "normal" for children in this age range to believe that illness is the result of having done something wrong, to perceive illness as a source of shame and guilt, and to view hospitalization and medical treatments as parental rejection or punishment (Beverly 1936; Bibace and Walsh 1980; Koopman et al. 2004; Perrin and Gerrity 1981; Shapiro 1996). This was replicated in a survey of medically hospitalized children who were asked, "Why do children get sick?"; 90% of respondents stated it was "because they are bad" (Beverly 1936). Around age 11 years, developmentally normal children are just beginning to arrive at psychophysiological explanations for illness. This is considered the most mature developmental level, in which the person has the ability to understand several causes for illness, including that one's thoughts and feelings can impact a person's functioning (Bibace and Walsh 1980).

There is little if any research regarding how children with serious psychiatric illness perceive their illness and treatments. For children who manifest disruptive behaviors as a feature of their symptomatology, it can be easy to see how the child's environment can unintentionally reinforce and ingrain a sense of "badness" into their developing identities. One might expect these children to hold significant shame and guilt, which might contribute to continued serious impairment in functioning and dysfunctional ideas about the need and use of medications.

An Approach to Psychopharmacological Interventions

Focusing on the arousal state allows us to target psychopharmacological interventions in ways that can support the growth of children with serious mental illness. The "low brain" regulates arousal and identifies feeling states as being "calm," a state of "alarm," or a state that researchers call "terror." Cognitive function declines in parallel. Minds think best in a calm state and much less so in a state of terror. This has led Perry (2006, 2009) to develop a "bottoms up" strategy to interventions. The first objective is to return the child and parent to the calm state, then move to strengthening the relationship between child and parent, and finally to reason. Perry classifies this framework as "Regulate–Relate–Reason."

When parents offer ideas and words to a child who is terrified, these words cannot be heard as they are intended. Instead, when terrified, children experience parental appeals to reason as punishment, leading to confusion and a deepening of the sense of being out of control. This might be akin to spending time explaining to a child why he must not set fires while standing in the middle of a burning room. Recognizing this, parents are encouraged to reframe the seemingly "defiant child" in this state as "helpless" and dysregulated. Parents faced with a terrified helpless child often find themselves regressing to the same or similar state and default to authoritarian efforts to establish control, which only deepen the vicious cycle. This presents a challenge to the clinician working with this dyad. At stake is what kind of affect sequence the mind will come to expect. Will a child learn to expect that positive experiences that turn bad only lead to further negative feelings? The experience with caregivers of restoring mutual regulation after a period of mutual dysregulation stimulates the lower brain to create neural connections that predict the possibility that positive experiences that become negative can be expected to return to positive feelings. When the child experiences himself as an active agent in that transformation, he develops a sense of agency, optimism about the world, and the belief that he can survive the intensity of his internal world. He learns that he can put intense feelings to good use, which will reward him and improve the relationships with those he loves and depends on. Depression, boredom or lack of motivation and desire, and a fear of his internal states, come from not being able to be an active agent in the restoration of mutual regulation. Clinicians can play a vital role in this process. Instead of stopping a behavior, the reframing of containment means that caregivers use the capacity to recognize the child's feelings accurately. This recognition needs to manifest itself as a spontaneous gesture that indicates to a child that it is safe to show his feelings because parents are able to take in what the child is feeling. This is Fonagy's concept of "marked mirroring" (Fonagy et al. 1991). Prescribers are engaged with a seriously ill child at points of crisis. Psychodynamically oriented prescribers can prescribe in a manner that allows problematic symptoms and developmental concerns to both be addressed. Prescribers can define for the family how to set limits in a way that balances safety with the need to engage developmental priorities. A practical application of this understanding is recognizing what the child does when he feels helpless and what the parent does when she is trying to use his agency, instead of labeling him as "defiant." Good limit setting is the product of a good fit between our expectations of a child and what the child can do at that moment (Gold 2017, p. 115).

With help, parents and other caregivers can be encouraged to identify their own "hot spots"—times when they cannot easily tolerate their own feelings or when they regress to the same arousal state as the child who is in distress. Hot spots interfere with the ability to remain curious about a child's feelings. Parents need support to deal with their hot spots, and as clinicians, we might become caught up as well. As a practitioner working with these patients, it is common to receive reports from parents and schools with pejorative descriptions of the child's underlying character. The child assimilates these messages and is at risk of developing an identity as a "bad child" rather than progressing to a more complex view of the cause of her condition. Although we can use developmental norms to estimate an adolescent's expected level of understanding for his or her condition, a particular child may be more or less advanced than age-matched peers. In practice, it is important to avoid potentially reinforcing shame- and guilt-based understandings of illness because the patient may internalize these beliefs into her own self-perception, and this may further contribute to psychiatric distress and an adversarial relationship with psychiatric treatment. The more complex relational view also protects parents from an identity as "bad" or "inadequate." To provide effective care, we must be able to tolerate and listen to parents' experiences so they have a place separate from the interactions with the child to get support and rediscover what they need to hold their child in mind so as to see the child as the child sees herself. Parents can feel empowered by understanding how they played a part in a pattern of trouble with their child and can appreciate the intimacy and feeling of engaged collaboration from achieving a return to mutual regulation. In supporting conversations, the clinician can both strengthen the parent-child relationship and establish themselves as an ally in this process.

In a calm state, in which parent and child have established mutual regulation after a period of mutual dysregulation, the pair can regrow the pathways in the brain interrupted by early environmental trauma and maltreatment that occur as a part of daily life even in the best of family situations. The effect of betrayal of trust is toxic helplessness. The process of re-establishing trust in the process of trying to hold each other in mind "grows the brain" because it creates expectations and capacities that will become new and healthier neural pathways.

It can be helpful to take a humble stance with both patient and parent in regard to the efficacy of most psychiatric medications. Medications alone do *not* "fix it" but support the capacity of the patient and his caregivers to engage in the exploration of "why my child is—or why I am—expressing this feeling in this particular way and at this time," requiring recognition of both the arousal state and the hot spots that move either parent or child out of the calm state and into fear or alarm states.

Implementation

The core concepts summarized in Figure 3–1 and discussed below help define the role of the clinician in applying the basic principles of development to the setting of a prescriber's office.

CASE EXAMPLE

Tommy is a 13-year-old adolescent with a history of oppositional defiant disorder, ADHD, and unspecified psychotic disorder referred to care for aggressive outbursts and mood lability at home and school. He has had several psychiatric admissions for aggressive and paranoid behavior and tried several medications, though his symptoms have not been well controlled. He is currently prescribed valproate 500 mg bid and aripiprazole 15 mg qam. A recent valproate level was low, indicating poor adherence. Tommy has been suspended from school several times and is now at the point of possible expulsion.

Tommy is brought to the evaluation by his mother, Alice, who reports feeling at a loss for how to manage her son's behavior and feeling the pressure of the school system and the state's child welfare agency to improve her son's behaviors. She remarks how "none of these medications are helping; he acts just like his father did, and nothing helped him." Tommy's father, Bruce, was previously diagnosed with schizoaffective disorder, ADHD, and alcohol abuse. Tommy witnessed domestic violence between his parents and now has limited contact with his fa-

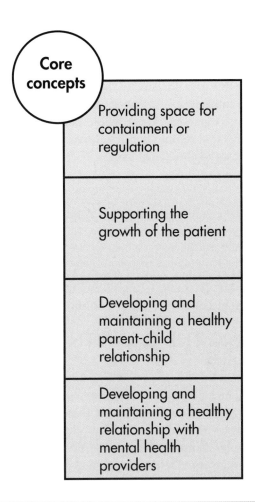

Figure 3–1. Core concepts in defining the role of the clinician in applying the basic principles of development to the setting of a prescriber's office.

ther. Tommy has a marked nonverbal response to the mention of his father; he sits with his fists clenched and pounds his foot on the floor. He frequently looks to the clock on the wall but for the majority of the evaluation keeps his eyes downcast. Tommy's responses are limited initially; he says mostly, "I don't know," and rolls his eyes to questions directed toward him. After his reaction to his mother's mention of his father, Tommy states, "I keep thinking about my dad, but I know my mom doesn't like me talking about him. If I wasn't so messed up, he might've stuck around."

PROVIDING SPACE FOR CONTAINMENT AND REGULATION

As clinicians, we must first ask ourselves the following questions: Why is Tommy acting this way now and in this context? What specific behavior is leading to mutual upset between him and his mom? What does *aggression* mean to his mom? What would help his mom hear Tommy talk about feelings that remind her of her husband (or her prior experiences) and stay trusting and curious?

> Tommy seems to be expressing something he does not think his mom wants to hear. [Already in this brief vignette, we understand that aggression relates in some way to Tommy's father; it stirs a reaction from both Tommy and his mother.] When the doctor asks if he thinks anyone else in the family has things to say that no one wants to hear about, he says, "Yes." His mom agrees with him. They both talk about having things to say that they think others do not want to hear. Tommy says this happens at school, too. He thinks his teacher is frustrated with him but does not want to tell him.

SUPPORTING THE GROWTH OF THE PATIENT

Elicit the patient and parent in discovering something about the problem by asking, "What is bothering you that we can learn about together?" Consider with Tommy and his mother what behaviors reflect a problem in the environment for growth that have developmental value and that will change after the developmental need is met, and what behaviors are representative of "illness." Consider how Tommy's identification with his father has a positive developmental aim, although it is manifesting through problematic behaviors. How else might Tommy understand what it means to be a man? For Tommy, his aggression has many meanings, one of which may be related to disruptive mood dysregulation disorder, psychosis, or bipolar disorder, but other meanings are connected to his identity and place within his family. Tommy may be responding to the perceived efforts at dismissing his positive developmental aims by being less adherent to prescribed medications and increasing defiant behaviors.

One might intervene in the following way:

> CLINICIAN: Tommy, I see those fists that you had the first day we met. It looks like your fists want to say something. What would your fists want to say if they could speak?

TOMMY: My fists want a lot of different things. I think today they want him to come back, for my mom to not be so sad, and for everything to be okay.

DEVELOPING AND MAINTAINING A HEALTHY PARENT-CHILD RELATIONSHIP

It is important to consider what success looks like to each of the stakeholders. On initial discussion, success for one might signal defeat to the other. For example, Alice might want Tommy to be less argumentative so that she feels respected, and Tommy may want to feel heard without having to destroy things. This important conversation will happen over and over as mutual goals are explored. This discussion with child and parent on equal footing when it comes to saying what they feel and care about has the potential to revitalize parents' ideas about who they are, what they value, and why. Discussion is the vehicle by which a child learns "how to decide" what he values and how to differ from others in a way that has dignity and produces mutual respect. But these discussions evoke fear, which can create arousal states incompatible with a reasoning discussion. A clinical intervention is working when the child's problem pushes the family to close the gap between developmental age and chronological age of the patient; this may mean facing a painful engagement but promises the rewards that result from the intimacy of working on something very hard together.

DEVELOPING AND MAINTAINING A HEALTHY RELATIONSHIP WITH MENTAL HEALTH PROVIDERS

It can be intimidating to work with children with serious mental illnesses if we approach them from a position of having to know all the answers at once. The method of working with patients and families discussed in this chapter empowers the family system to begin to examine the sources of the problem and collaborate with the clinician as an ally in that journey. This opening up of the family's experience is not something that can be done in a 15-minute "med check" but it can have an effect over several brief, focused psychopharmacotherapy sessions if the clinician is open to discovering and learning with patients and families along the way. We as clinicians can get caught in our own hot spots of attempting to fix a symptom before we have fully understood the problem that created it. There are many systems pressures that create this feeling within us. We might feel, as Tommy's mother initially did, that we must prescribe a medication to keep Tommy in school. With an imprecise understanding of the problem, we hinder our ability to diagnose and prescribe effectively. Every time the doctor returns the family to a place of trusting the ways Tommy's feelings have meaning, he or she promotes the family's resilience and their own capacity to find a way to work together on the painful but developmentally important problems that face them. If Tommy can trust himself and the clinician, he can accept a medication to help manage what is difficult to bear, without blaming his feelings or believing that his feelings mean he is "bad" or "damaged goods."

Treatment of symptoms can end when the patient and family can ask for support without predicating it on illness. Health care providers can support the family's resilience, thereby lessening the tendency in a family to equate "need" with illness.

Discussion

When a child is very ill, the circle of people who hold the child in mind is wider; it includes the parents and many others—school psychologist, therapist, teacher, department of child services, siblings, friends, and significant others. Group stressors and supports also reach beyond the family of origin. The sources of stress or maltreatment and support are wider than the family.

The goal of a successful treatment is to ensure a healthy environment that nourishes and provides opportunities for growth that are appropriate to developmental age. This requires making the relationship between child and caregivers a priority to avoid developmentally needed behaviors being mistaken for symptoms of disease. Children and families need help even in cases when there is no disease state. As clinicians, we need to attend to our own hot spots to avoid being caught up in a dysregulated dynamic with the parent, school system, and child.

For children, a successful treatment is marked by the capacity to say of an emotion, "I am worried, afraid, happy, or sad, but I recognize this feeling, I can name it, and I can consider its origins and what I want to do in response to it. I am not overwhelmed by it." With help, a child can turn *processing difficulties* into *strategies* by focusing on the special way the child understands information coming in and planning the responses that go out (Gold 2017, p. 84). For parents, it is important to have the ability to do the same and to stay curious when possible or recover curiosity when lost. Parents who can model the capacity to have guilt and use it to take responsibility by forming new strategies to solve a problem in the future give their children a valuable learning opportunity that promotes the re-silience of their children. Resilience is the goal of treatment.

As physicians, parents, and teachers, we need to develop our ability to recognize disruption and arousal states in children so that we can appropriately switch our focus to getting the child and parents into a calm state, correctly identify the need for control, and address that need in a way that targets the child's developmental level. Sophisticated use of an "overall" diagnosis creates a safe, blame-free environment where both the feelings of the child and the difficult feelings of the parents in reaction to their child will be accepted. At stake is the possibility for the way the child sees himself or herself internally to match how others see him or her. This promotes the two key human needs of "coherence" and the ability to be an active agent in framing what happens in one's life—both externally and internally.

The clinician can empower the parent to repair disruptions. The goal is for a dance of mutual regulation to replace the dance of mutual dysregulation (Gold 2017, p. 104).

References

Beeghly M, Tronick E: Self-regulatory processes in early development, in The Oxford Handbook of Treatment Processes and Outcomes in Psychology. Edited by Maltzman S. New York, Oxford University Press, 2016

Beverly B: The effect of illness upon emotional development. J Pediatr 8:533–543, 1936

Bibace R, Walsh ME: Development of children's concepts of illness. Pediatrics 66(6):912–917, 1980 7454481

Demos E: The Affect Theory of Silvan Tomkins for Psychoanalysis and Psychotherapy. New York, Routledge, 2019

Fonagy P, Steele M, Moran G, Higgitt A: The capacity for understanding mental states: the reflective self in parent and child and its significance for security of attachment. Infant Ment Health J 12:201–218, 1991

Gold C: The Developmental Science of Early Childhood: Clinical Applications of Infant Mental Health Concepts From Infancy Through Adolescence. New York, WW Norton, 2017

Koopman HM, Baars RM, Chaplin J, Zwinderman KH: Illness through the eyes of the child: the development of children's understandings of the causes of illness. Patient Educ Couns 55(3):363–370, 2004

Mintz D: Recovery from childhood psychiatric treatment: addressing the meaning of medications. Psychodyn Psychiatry 47(3):235–256, 2019 31448987

Mintz D, Belnap B: A view from Riggs: treatment resistance and patient authority, III: what is psychodynamic psychopharmacology? An approach to pharmacologic treatment resistance. J Am Acad Psychoanal Dyn Psychiatry 34(4):581–601, 2006 17274730

Mintz D, Belnap B: What is psychodynamic psychopharmacology? An approach to pharmacologic treatment resistance, in Treatment Resistance and Patient Authority: The Austen Riggs Reader. Edited by Plakun EM. New York, WW Norton, 2011, pp 42–65

National Institute of Mental Health: Serious mental illness. Bethesda, MD, National Institute of Mental Health, 2020. Available at: www.nimh.nih.gov/health/statistics/mental-illness.shtml. Accessed February 17, 2020. Accessed February 17, 2020.

Perrin EC, Gerrity PS: There's a demon in your belly: children's understanding of illness. Pediatrics 67(6):841–849, 1981 7232049

Perry B: Applying principles of neurodevelopment to clinical work with maltreated and traumatized children: the neurosequential model of therapeutics, in Working With Traumatized Youth in Child Welfare. Edited by Webb NB. New York, Guilford, 2006, pp 27–52

Perry B: Examining child maltreatment through a neurodevelopmental lens: clinical applications of the neurosequential model of therapeutics. J Loss Trauma 14:240–255, 2009

Piaget J: The Origins of Intelligence in Children. New York, International Universities Press, 1948

Piaget J: The Child's Conception of the World. Patterson, NJ, Littlefield Adams, 1960

Piaget J: The Psychology of the Child. New York, Basic Books, 1969

Shapiro T: Developmental considerations in psychopharmacology: the interaction of drugs and development, in Diagnosis and Psychopharmacology of Childhood and Adolescent Disorders, 2nd Edition. Edited by Werner J. New York, Wiley, 1996, pp 80–95

Weinberg E, Seery E, Plakun EM: A psychodynamic approach to treatment resistance, in Treatment Resistance in Psychiatry. Edited by Kim Y-K. Singapore, Springer, 2019, pp 295–310

Whiteman M: Children's conceptions of psychological causality. Child Dev 38:143–155, 1967

CHAPTER 4

"WHAT'S IN IT FOR ME?"

Adapting Evidence-Based Motivational Interviewing and Therapy Techniques to Adolescent Psychiatry

John J. DiLallo, M.D.

Importance of Therapeutic Communication in Adolescent Psychopharmacology

It stands to reason that anyone who freely decides to take psychotropic medication (or to participate in any form of mental health treatment) and who subsequently adheres to a treatment regimen must have some internalized, autonomous rationale for doing so. However, upon first evaluating adolescents who are already taking psychotropic medication, psychopharmacologists commonly encounter youth whose understanding of the rationale for their medication seems incomplete. Initial questions such as "Can you tell me about why you take this medication?" or "Can you tell me why you were brought here to see me?" sometimes produce less substantive responses than would be expected from a young person who is actively engaged in their treatment plan. Delving deeper into self-judging responses such as "Because I do bad things" or "Because I have a chemical problem" could reveal cognitive distortions affecting self-esteem or the experience of medication as a form of punishment. Alternatively, a simple "I don't know" response, though seemingly bland and detached, could represent anything from a telling moment of distraction, to shame-driven avoidance of self-disclosure, to limited insight or a low expectation that psychiatric care will be helpful. Arguably, leaving any such underlying issues unaddressed would appear to decrease the likelihood of both adherence to treatment and positive functional outcome.

Conceptually, the process of engaging individual youth in psychiatric treatment falls somewhere within the doctor-patient relationship. As part of the "art" or "process" of clinical practice, engagement generally is not assigned importance either in clinical trials of medication efficacy or in the various quality improvement metrics to which prescribers may be subjected. At the regulatory level, a psychotropic medication achieves an FDA-sanctioned indication (or "label") based on its rate of reported symptom reduction among people identified with a matching complaint or condition. But even a clearly indicated medication will not help at all if a patient does not take it as prescribed. In the real world of psychiatric practice, a medication is prescribed to an individual person with a particular set of values, co-existing problems, and personality traits whose life is embedded in particular cultural and socioeconomic environments. What it truly means to be "doing better" may differ significantly from person to person, and a large part of being helpful is clarifying what a meaningful improvement, from the perspective of a specific individual, would look like.

DiLallo and Weiss (2009) described the promise of motivational interviewing (MI)—as a patient-centered, collaborative communication style—to improve medication adherence and overall treatment engagement among adolescent psychopharmacology patients. MI already had been applied with success to treatment adherence in adolescent medical conditions such as type 1 diabetes (Channon et al. 2007). More recently, two empirical trials of motivational interventions have reported positive results targeting adherence to psychotropic medication among teen cohorts: one consisting of teens taking any type of mood medication (antidepressant, mood stabilizer, or both; Hamrin and Iennaco 2017) and another made up of teens diagnosed with bipolar disorder (Goldstein et al. 2020). Meanwhile, the search for non-process-oriented explanatory factors correlating to adolescent medication adherence has appeared less definitive. A recent literature review identified 15 empirical studies of psychotropic medication adherence among adolescents, with nonadherence rates ranging from 6% to 62% (median, 33%). However, no firm conclusions regarding the impact of factors such as diagnosis, medication type, side effects, perceived treatment effectiveness, or family-related factors could be reached (Häge et al. 2018).

In tandem with MI, contemporaneous process-oriented developments pertaining to psychiatric practice include 1) the growth of "transdiagnostic" therapy models that have emerged from cognitive-behavioral therapy (CBT) and 2) an ongoing literature concerning effective communication in clinical medicine. A 2009 meta-analysis of medical communication (Zolnierek and DiMatteo 2009) reported a 19% higher risk of treatment nonadherence among patients whose physicians communicated poorly than among patients whose physicians communicated well, as well as significant improvements in patient adherence resulting from physician training in communication. Specific to psychiatry, a 2011 conceptual review of "good" communication identified five guiding principles for use across treatment settings (Priebe et al. 2011). The first four principles—a focus on patient's concerns, positive regard and personal respect, appropriate involvement of patients in decision making, and genuineness and personal touch—appear to recapitulate core aspects of motivational methods. The fifth guiding principle—applying elements of evidence-based psychological treatment models to induce therapeutic change—however, pertains more to the process-oriented descendants of CBT that are examined in this chapter.

This chapter explores motivational and therapeutic strategies for engaging psychiatrically impaired youth in treatment, with an emphasis on adherence to treatment with psychotropic medication. Current knowledge about adolescent development is reviewed in support of these strategies, which ultimately help young people discover their particular answer to the question "What's in it for me?" Three evidence-based treatment models are explored for tools to help pharmacotherapists engage their adolescent patients. Selected tools include collaborative motivational strategies for behavioral change as prescribed by MI, treatment orientation and commitment strategies used in dialectical behavior therapy (DBT), and the eliciting of values and value-determined actions as practiced in acceptance and commitment therapy (ACT).

Developmental Considerations: Engaging the Adolescent Brain

Cultivating motivation, engagement, and treatment adherence in adolescent psychiatry is enhanced by knowledge of adolescent development. In recent years, the physical and psychological processes long described in adolescents have been complemented by findings in brain development research (summarized in Casey et al. 2008). The following brief synopsis may provide a useful orientation to this vast area, if we bear in mind that the vast majority of adolescents prove to be resilient and proceed through developmental struggles successfully.

The adolescent body normally undergoes significant physical growth together with increasing motor coordination, pubertal changes, and the emergence of enhanced sexual sensations. For the first time, plans that might previously have been fantasized about—independent movement, sex, aggression—are now within an individual's capacity for action. Urges and emotions may run high, and in comparison with the thought process of adults, adolescent cognition is relatively "limbic": impulsive, emotional, concrete, egocentric, self-conscious, and reactive to peer influence. Likewise, in clinical psychiatry, we may see distress generated by these developmental changes and a spike in the incidence of anxiety and depressive disorders.

Behaviorally, the Eriksonian process of identity formation (vs. role confusion) can be witnessed as an adolescent "trying out" various peer relationships, romantic interests, and new roles within their social milieu. Adolescents may be observed impulsively taking risks, testing limits, and protesting or breaking rules as they seek to define "who I am." As the capacity for abstract thought increases, so may the penchant for verbally justifying impulsive or disruptive behavior. Clinically, we see a rise in the incidence of addictions and conduct disorders as these processes sometimes veer into areas of trouble.

Underlying these observations is an adolescent brain that contains the highest amount of gray matter in its lifetime: peak levels occur by about age 11 years in anatomical girls and age 12.5 years in anatomical boys. At this point, synaptic pruning and neural myelination ramp up and continue at a faster pace until roughly age 25 years, when the majority of "adult" neural networks have been constructed. Adolescent brain development begins in the rear (motor and sensory areas), then proceeds through the center (including limbic areas), and finally moves to the front, where the last brain areas to mature are the temporal lobes and the prefrontal cortex. These final areas are considered essential to such important functions as memory consolidation (to begin the cortical processing of "raw" sensory memories into narrative memory), perspective taking (for theory of mind, empathy), and development of executive functions used by well-functioning adults (planning, prioritizing, working memory, motivation, attention, persistence, and emotion regulation).

Thus, adolescence appears to be a lengthy developmental stage during which advanced capacities for feeling and taking action come online well before capacities for impulse control and self-regulation. Related research on adolescents has also found that

- Adolescent cognition shows greater reliance on limbic emotional regions than on prefrontal control regions.
- The adolescent limbic system appears hypersensitive to both rewards and threats, with implications for addictions and social behavior.
- The presence of peers increases risk taking by adolescents.
- Adolescent onset of substance use confers a greater risk of addiction than substance use beginning in adulthood (Substance Abuse and Mental Health Services Administration 2014).

To effectively engage an adolescent facing emotional and behavioral challenges, a prescriber must be mindful of this dynamic developmental stage. Helping a patient to discover "what's in this [medication or treatment plan] for me" depends first on an attitude of nonjudgmental acceptance: respecting the adolescent patient's needs for autonomy in their choices and flexibility regarding their impulses. To reduce the chances of harm, however, this attitude must be balanced with more deliberate guidance and limit setting, steering the patient safely toward discovering which life changes will bring the most positive meaning to their emerging identity.

Three Process-Oriented Clinical Models for Promoting Engagement and Treatment Adherence Among Diverse Youth

Following the emergence of CBT from behavior therapy in the 1970s, evidence-based therapy models gradually shifted focus to target the mental processes involved in specific psychiatric disorders. More recently, "transdiagnostic" therapy models have evolved to target specific mental processes across disorders, with the chief aim of improving client functioning and only a secondary focus on symptom reduction (Hayes and Hofmann 2017). Examples include DBT (Linehan 1993) and

ACT (Hayes et al. 2012), both of which have been adapted for use with adolescents from diverse cultural backgrounds (Hayes and Ciarrochi 2015; McCauley et al. 2018; Miller et al. 2007). Both models aim to shift focus beyond the patient's mental contents (thoughts, feelings, and behaviors) and toward the patient's relationship to these experiences after they have been brought into reflective awareness (e.g., through the practice of mindfulness). Significant overlap between general CBT and MI has been noted, and efforts have been made to integrate the two models, with CBT providing more of the content or "what" of treatment and MI more of the "how" (Naar and Safren 2017).

For many psychiatric clinicians, the time and energy required to master MI, DBT, and ACT, together with the limits often imposed on the prescriber's clinical role by systemic factors, makes rigorous training impractical. However, the potential for these clinical modalities to enhance pharmacological practice is great, so time studying them is well spent. Each provides a clear model of psychological functioning that is readily applied to diverse adolescents across diagnostic categories and varied clinical settings (clinic, inpatient ward, school or other community context). Each also provides useful strategies that are adaptable to increasing patient engagement in treatment and adherence to medication. Before we move on to specific motivation and engagement strategies, let's begin with a brief overview of each of the three treatment models, not only to orient clinicians to their theoretical contexts but also to enable the self-identification from psychopharmacologist to embrace a framework of "pharmacotherapist."

1. MI developed as a nonconfrontational approach to decreasing the harmful behaviors found in substance use disorders, and it is based on the stages of change (SoC) model of Prochaska and DiClemente (1983) (Table 4–1). *Motivational interviewing* is defined by its authors as a client-centered, directive method for enhancing intrinsic motivation to change by exploring and resolving ambivalence (Miller and Rollnick 2002, 2013). It seeks to elicit the pro-change components that exist already within a patient's thinking and to promote their growth. In general, this process begins by guiding the patient in determining their personal goals and then exploring the discrepancies between where the patient is and where they would like to be with respect to these. MI can boost the effectiveness of the therapeutic alliance by enhancing three major elements: empathy that is accurate to the patient's experience, patient confidence in their ability to improve, and positive expectations regarding the recommended treatment. The nonconfrontational stance of MI can be particularly

Table 4–1. Stages of readiness for change

Patient's stage of change	Clinician intervention
Precontemplation	Engagement
Contemplation	Persuasion
Preparation	Planning "menu"
Action	Active treatment
Maintenance	Relapse prevention

Source. Adapted from Prochaska et al. 1992.

effective in counseling adolescents, whose developmental needs may predispose them to ambivalence toward authoritative advice.

2. DBT was developed initially to treat women with borderline personality disorder (Linehan 1993) and later adapted to work with adolescents who struggle with recurrent thoughts of suicide, engage in nonsuicidal self-injury (NSSI), or make suicide attempts. Emotional dysregulation is formulated to be the core element of the behavioral disturbances of these groups. It is explained in some theoretical models as the developmental result of a temperamentally sensitive individual exposed to an invalidating emotional environment. In other words, an emotionally sensitive child growing up in a family that conveys powerful messages that the child should not have the feelings he or she does (e.g., a family that maintains denial in regard to trauma like sexual abuse) may suffer identity confusion and great distress. Clinicians recognize the pattern of recurring crises that such patients often bring to their treatment. Some patients may miss appointments whenever they are not in a crisis and then focus only on relieving their immediate distress when they do attend. The orientation and commitment strategies used in DBT help to reframe the problem as one of managing negative emotions and the solution as requiring a more behaviorally structured and longitudinal approach toward change. The main content of DBT consists of skills in four areas: distress tolerance, emotion regulation, mindfulness, and interpersonal effectiveness. DBT skills are taught under the a priori view that patients are doing the best they can, and yet they must learn skills to do even better.

3. ACT is rooted in a behavioral paradigm that its authors call *functional contextualism*, which emphasizes behavior as having a particular purpose within a specific environment. Various cognitive habits and other behaviors that are intended to avoid difficult emotions can

lead an individual to an entrenched psychological rigidity, which may be directly harmful itself or may greatly limit the individual's ability to adapt to changing demands. By contrast, the primary goal of ACT is to promote psychological flexibility, which allows an individual to choose behavior according to his or her personal values in a manner that holds the most positive meaning for that person even when this entails discomfort. Learning to accept and "sit with" negative emotions, rather than avoid them, is paramount. ACT helps individuals formulate personal values according to what they most want their lives to be about and then make values-based action plans to reach goals. A particular therapy session focuses on one or more cognitive-behavioral skill areas, chosen according to where a person seems to be stuck. The six skill areas for adults are flexible attention to the present moment, cognitive defusion, self-as-context, acceptance, values, and committed action. For adolescents, these skill areas have been developmentally adjusted to include values plus three modes of reflective thinking, which are referred to as the discoverer, the noticer, and the adviser (the DNA-V Model; see Hayes and Ciarrochi 2015).

Each of these three process-based models contains unique elements valuable to pharmacotherapy practice. In the next two sections, selected strategies from among them are divided roughly into those pertaining more to "what" to do versus "how" to do it. As in all things, practice makes perfect or, at least, more effective.

Motivation and Cognitive-Behavioral Strategies in Adolescent Psychopharmacology, Part I: The "What"

Despite having many distinct features, MI, DBT, and ACT all share a fundamental emphasis on facilitating behavioral change. To adapt these models for pharmacotherapy practice, therefore, the clinician must orient the treatment plan in terms of the *functional outcomes* that are most desired by the patient. Nonbehavioral goals such as "feeling less depressed" or "worrying less" are insufficient for this purpose, so redefining the objectives of treatment in terms of behavioral change is a primary task. Behavioral impairments related to psychiatric disorders—such as avoidance, rumination, distractibility, impulsivity, aggression, and self-harm—may be reframed as impediments to reaching desired behavioral goals and therefore as targets for change. In many cases, clear behavioral goals cannot be readily elicited at the outset of treatment, so full engagement requires a gradual operationalizing of the patient's thinking about his or her reasons for seeking help.

Although desired behavioral changes provide the orientation for treatment, helping these changes to happen depends on the recruitment of inner motivation. Specific strategies help patients to discover what matters most to them and to find ways to live according to these values in spite of their symptoms. As noted earlier, MI was developed initially to help reduce substance abuse and DBT to decrease NSSI and lifestyle-interfering behaviors. These behavioral targets apply in relevant prescribing situations, yet even patients for whom harm reduction is a primary goal must connect with their particular underlying reasons for making these changes.

An individual's success in doing what matters most to him or her—known in ACT as "values-based action"—results in a life of "vitality," which ACT proposes as the missing ingredient in the often-lamented clinical definition of health as merely the "absence of disease." Increasing vitality may sound like a lofty goal for psychopharmacological treatment, but boosting hope and self-efficacy are basic elements of effective therapeutic relationships across cultures (Frank 1973; Frank and Frank 1991). The following strategies aim to guide pharmacotherapists in this process.

FRAMING A MOTIVATIONAL TREATMENT PROCESS

An initial psychiatric evaluation entails screening for all types of mental disorders followed by the detailed exploration of symptoms, their duration, and exacerbating and ameliorating factors. MI and ACT both encourage us to supplement these inquiries with data about the patients' personal aspirations along with their perceptions related to the possibility of behavioral change. As with diagnostic assessment, this process is ongoing, and modifications are made over time as new data present themselves. Initial inquiries might be as follows:

- "For this evaluation, I will need to ask you a lot more questions about problems that people sometimes have. But first I'd like to understand if there is anything you've been working on lately for yourself or maybe any changes you'd like to make for the future."

- "So, if you were to look ahead a few months from now, say, next [spring, summer, or fall], are there any specific things you would want to be different in your life, like maybe in school or in your personal relationships?"
- "If treatment with medication could be helpful to you, what would that allow you to do?"

MEETING PATIENTS "WHERE THEY ARE"

As noted, MI is based on the SoC model of Prochaska and DiClemente. Likewise, engagement efforts must begin by responding to patients "where they are" with respect to stage of readiness for change and adjusting communication accordingly (Prochaska and DiClemente 1983) (Table 4–2). Initial SoC assessment requires reflection on the whole of the patient's communications facilitated by questions such as

- "Your parents seem to be worried about you. Do you think they should be?"
- "You mentioned wanting to get better at [personal goal]. On a scale of 1 to 10, with 10 being the highest, how important to you is accomplishing this goal?"
- "What kind of obstacles might get in your way?"
- "Can you think of anyone or anything that might help you reach this goal?

IDENTIFYING AREAS OF EMOTIONAL AVOIDANCE

Thinking behaviorally requires the pharmacotherapist to create a new benchmark for treatment response, distinct from symptom reduction as often measured by conventional rating scales. In fact, overemphasizing the nonbehavioral goals mentioned earlier—feeling less depressed or less worried—would run contrary to the therapeutic process advocated by both DBT and ACT, which contend that patients must learn to *accept* unpleasant emotions whenever avoidance gets in the way of doing what matters most in their lives. Clinicians should call attention to the habitual behaviors a patient may be using to avoid unpleasant emotions and determine what important social or occupational aspirations are likely being undermined. Related questions might include the following:

Table 4–2. Motivational interventions according to stage of change

Patient's stage of change	Clinician intervention	As developed for treatment of substance abuse	Adaptations to adolescent psychopharmacology
Precontemplation	Engagement	Increase awareness of consequences of substance use. Develop discrepancies and elicit ambivalence toward change. Harm reduction model entails acceptance and nonconfrontation.	Develop discrepancy by eliciting patient's personal goals and comparing with current functioning as affected by psychiatric symptoms.
Contemplation	Persuasion Risk-reward analysis	Amplify ambivalence. Roll with resistance. Increase confidence in ability to decrease substance use. Provide menu of treatment options.	Early introduction of treatment options, including medication. Instill realistic, positive expectations for medication and other therapies.
Preparation	Planning "menu"	Negotiate a treatment plan, including biological, psychological, and social components. Obtain informed consent. Negotiate patient's commitment to a full trial of selected treatment options.	Elicit patient's rationale for taking a medication and the meanings it has for concept of self. Emphasize autonomy, safety, and benefit of adherence to full trials of medication and other therapies.
Action	Active treatment	Reaffirm commitment. Track level of substance use and related behavior. Reinforce any harm reduction achieved.	Review medication response and adverse effects. Identify any factors affecting nonadherence. Develop "reminder rituals" as needed.
Maintenance	Relapse prevention	Encourage active problem solving using cognitive techniques. Revisit ambivalence as it arises. Revert to previous-stage interventions if relapse occurs.	Review adherence, response, pros and cons of maintenance dosing, and meaning of long-term therapy for patient's identity.

Source. Reprinted from DiLallo JJ, Weiss G: "Motivational Interviewing and Adolescent Psychopharmacology." *Journal of American Academy of Child and Adolescent Psychiatry* 48(2):108–113, 2009. Copyright 2009, American Academy of Child and Adolescent Psychiatry/Elsevier. Used with permission.

- "No one likes to feel [negative emotion]. Is there anything you do to avoid feeling that way that could be causing problems in other parts of your life?"
- "What do you think would be different about your life if that [reported feeling] were not there?"
- "If a medication were to help with that [reported feeling], would that help you to do anything differently?"

ASKING PERMISSION AND FOSTERING AUTONOMY

Eliciting a patient's explanation of their presenting problem fosters a sense of autonomy, as does asking permission before giving the patient medical information. Establishing that the patient is in control helps to avoid power struggles, *particularly for adolescents in the precontemplation or contemplation stages*. Except in urgent situations, medication options are best mentioned only as part of a menu of possibilities for outpatient treatment in the event that a patient decides to make a change. Adolescents also may be reminded that no one can force them to take a pill for psychiatric reasons and that agreeing (or not) is an important decision they will need to make.

- "The note I read from your previous psychiatrist said that you were diagnosed with [diagnosis]. Do you think that is accurate for you?"
- "Would you like to discuss how that diagnosis is made?"
- "Most people find it helpful to have all the facts before they make a decision. Please let me know if at some point you want more information about medications and other treatments that could help you change this situation."

PROVIDING TREATMENT ORIENTATION AND USING COMMITMENT STRATEGIES

DBT shows how structured expectations for participation in treatment can help dysregulated individuals (i.e., those prone to emotional cognition, such as adolescents) to engage. Prototypical DBT includes firm expectations for attendance, safety and communication agreements, and homework. Likewise, in adolescent psychopharmacology, a treatment agreement should be negotiated, with emphasis on regular attendance of appointments, communication with parents and the doctor regarding side effects and any safety issues, prohibition of sharing medication (diversion), and consultation with the doctor before any decision to discontinue the medication. Establishing realistic expectations for treatment may help prevent nonadherence due to erroneous notions of a "quick fix." Patients should understand that medication treatment is a process that may take weeks or months to work. (See the chapters in this book by Romanowicz et. al., Pruett, and Strawn et al. for ways to promote the placebo effect and enable a possible earlier response.) Gradual dose adjustments may be required before a response is seen, and possible side effects may necessitate starting over with a new medication. Patience, frustration tolerance, and careful self-observation may be required in order to find the best medication and dose. Defining clear targets for medication effectiveness and homework in the form of self-monitoring for these targets can help prevent ambiguous expectations and outcomes.

- "You seem to have mixed feelings about taking medication. Before you decide about that, I think you should also understand that we will use the best science available to select the right medication. However, it may require some trial and error. Because everyone responds differently to a particular medicine, you and I may need to meet a number of times to get it right."
- "We have discussed how SSRIs [selective serotonin reuptake inhibitors] can sometimes (rarely) cause suicidal ideas in young people. I respect your concerns about privacy regarding your parents. However, I can't prescribe an SSRI for you safely unless you are willing to tell your parents about any strange or dangerous thoughts that might occur. Is that something you are willing to do?"
- "That last time you tried a psychostimulant, you really weren't sure if it was helping. Can we identify two or three problems on this list of ADHD symptoms where you would expect to see a change if the medication were helping you?"

DBT also advocates salesperson-like strategies for eliciting commitment to treatment, including "foot in the door" (asking for a minimal duration of participation and then increasing the expectation over time) and "door in the face" (starting with a very large participation demand and settling for something less). With the possible exception of psychostimulant trials, young patients can be advised to commit to a period of up to 3 months before they conclude whether or not medication will be helpful to them. Three months could be considered a "door in the face" amount, in that the commitment for half that time is probably enough. In early SoC situations, arguing matter-of-factly that the patient may not really need treatment may be attempted to intensify their ambivalence. This "devil's advocate" DBT technique is an amplified version of an MI strategy called "rolling with resistance," in which validating the patient's arguments against change, while keeping the door open for future conversation, may lead the patient to generate "pro-change" arguments on his or her own. Some suggestions to apply these techniques are listed below.

- "Taking medication is a serious decision, and finding the best medication can require a lot of patience. I recommend that you commit yourself to the process for at least 2 or 3 months or otherwise hold off until you feel more ready."
- "Well, you certainly express some valid concerns about not wanting to take medicine. Maybe it's better for you to keep doing psychotherapy (as the only treatment) for a while before you consider taking it."
- "Would you like to find out more about medication options now, in case you want to consider these in the future?"

HIGHLIGHTING DISCREPANCIES TO HELP RESOLVE AMBIVALENCE

MI emphasizes that the seeds of motivation already exist within a patient's thinking and that they must be found and then cultivated to help the patient move forward. Clinicians can begin by eliciting the pros and cons of a problem behavior while watching for any patient-expressed language that argues for change (i.e., "change talk"). After any type of personal goal is identified, the clinician can explore the discrepancy between where the patient is and where he or she would like to be in regard to it. Highlighting such discrepancies often amplifies the patient's ambivalent attitudes, pro and con, leading toward resolution and change. To foster the patient's autonomous thought process, clinicians should maintain a nonjudgmental stance, acknowledge the negative consequences of the patient's current behavior in a matter-of-fact manner, and "roll with resistance" (as described earlier).

- "You seem to really want that diploma, but that won't happen unless you start going to class and doing your homework. Can you tell me what you like about not doing these things?"
- "So, it sounds like you really want to find more kids you are comfortable with and expand your circle of friends. But you also said you don't like talking to unfamiliar people at school because it causes anxiety. Have there been times when you were able to meet new people even though you felt uncomfortable?"

- "I think that medication could probably help if you want to increase [pro-change behavior]. But it sounds like you have firmly decided that medication is not for you."

DEFINING PERSONAL VALUES

As treatment progresses, ACT takes personal goals to a deeper level, instructing us to elicit patients' underlying personal values and to help them live according to what matters the most to them regardless of specific mental health symptoms. Values can be identified in a number of life domains, such as family, friendships, career, interests, and health. As described earlier, aiming to enhance patient vitality through values-based action can orient us toward meaningful interventions at any stage of psychopharmacology treatment, including the maintenance phase, when symptoms are more under control and appointments less frequent.

Values are abstract concepts, so they can be trickier to grasp for younger patients. For all age groups, values may be explained as "things that we want our life to be about," life priorities that an individual can invest effort in. And unlike the fixed traits that we cannot choose about ourselves—such as our height, eye color, or particular aptitudes—values are things we do get to choose, to determine what kind of person we most want to be. Values are ideals that can guide us like points on a compass as we navigate the various trials of our lives. Also, we do not get to choose our values just once but any time that reorienting ourselves needs to occur.

Goals are the behavioral building blocks for living out our values, but goals should not be mistaken for values because they may not be as genuine. "Getting straight A's in school" is a potentially problematic goal. It could derive from an autonomous value such as "learning as much as I can" or from a more imposed value such as "satisfying my parents." Guiding the patient toward healthy values is another aspect of the process. When time permits, printed values exercises such as the "Bull's Eye," "Life Compass," and "Problems and Values Worksheet" are well worth exploring (see Harris 2009). Otherwise, conversations aiming toward value definition go something like these:

- "You mentioned sometimes feeling bad about yelling at your teacher. Can you tell me what kind of person you would like to be when you are in a conflict with a grown-up?" (assertiveness, respect, kindness)
- "You seem to really care about getting a good job some day. Can you tell me why that is important to you?" (independence, achievement)

- "You said that when your friends at school stir up too much drama it can make you feel depressed. Can you tell me about what kind of things you think friends should do for each other?" (caring, trustworthiness)
- "The situation you are describing sounds very stressful. Can you tell me what type of person you would like to be in situations like this? Or perhaps what words you might like your friends to use to describe you when you are not there with them?" (many possible values)

Motivation and Cognitive-Behavioral Strategies in Adolescent Psychopharmacology, Part 2: The "How"

An established literature addresses "common factors" of effective alliances across therapy models, including such qualities as genuineness, trust, compassion, and particularly the ability to instill hope (De Nadai et al. 2017; Frank and Frank 1991; Reisner 2005). Among these elements, MI, DBT, and ACT prioritize particular qualities of relationship and focus.

MAINTAINING OPENNESS

A nonjudgmental, open, and collegial stance is paramount to forming the "collaboration of experts" advocated by motivational models. Measured doses of irreverence and self-disclosure ("being real") may also promote therapeutic alliances with young people. Importantly, the psychiatrist must regard the patient as the essential source of solutions to the problem behavior and as the only true expert in regard to what making change will entail. In practice, this perspective engenders a *genuine curiosity* on the part of the clinician that guides each step of the clinical process. Meanwhile, the psychiatrist's specific expertise is limited to more general clinical information, given preferably at those times when the patient chooses to receive it. Except in situations of imminent harm, the adolescent patient is regarded always as autonomous and ultimately responsible for any choices made in regard to treatment or behavioral change.

KEEPING THE FOCUS ON CHANGE

In tandem with an open attitude of curiosity and acceptance, the clinician uses a highly directive conversational technique, delving further into any change-related content that may emerge. MI refers to "change talk" as any self-expressed language that could constitute an argument for change. Such talk is elicited most often by weighing the pros and cons of behavioral decisions, but it may emerge at any time. Routinely, patients' expressions of future aspirations or personal values should be acknowledged and explored for areas of ambivalence and patterns of emotional avoidance.

FOSTERING ACCEPTANCE OF EMOTIONAL EXPERIENCES

Mindfulness may be defined as the practice of paying deliberate, non-judgmental attention to present moment experiences. During clinical encounters, patients can be guided mindfully to observe any emotions that may arise in the moment, providing their feelings with a name and carefully denoting the thoughts, behavioral urges, and visceral sensations that compose them. Terms such as "observing ego" or "self-as-context" (from ACT) arguably refer to this capacity, which is necessary for learning DBT skills such as distress tolerance and emotion regulation. Psychoeducation regarding the transience, physiological correlates, and effects on perception and behavior of emotional states is valuable and bears repeating. Learning to "be with" emotions and "surf" reactive urges can help patients overcome whatever emotion avoidance behaviors may be keeping them from living according to their true values.

INSTILLING HOPE AND SELF-EFFICACY

Life coaches and cheerleaders have something to teach any clinician who prescribes medication, something likely related to the effects of social synchronization on "mirror neurons" (see Praszkier 2016). Whenever and however, instilling realistic hope that a desired change is possible and that "I believe you can do this if you put your mind to it" will help to mobilize the nebulous inner resources through which individual humans realize success.

FINDING THE MIDDLE PATH: BALANCING CONFIDENTIALITY AND DISCLOSURE IN RISK ASSESSMENT

Finally, although the salience of *Sturm und Drang* (German for "storm and stress") in normal adolescence is debatable, the prevalence of dramatic turmoil among adolescent psychiatry patients is certainly high. Emotional cognition and impulsive risk taking are frequently the main reasons for a young person's referral for treatment. The "middle path" concept offered by DBT for parenting teens can also help guide clinicians, who must balance the confidentiality needed to maintain a therapeutic alliance with the need to communicate about risky behavior with parents or guardians. Aiming to be "not too tight, not too loose" in the psychiatric role can help reconcile such competing priorities when assessing imminent risk in gray areas such as substance use or self-injurious behavior. Encouraging patient self-disclosure to parents when risk is less acute is often the best-case resolution in terms of fostering autonomy and maintaining adherence to treatment.

Conclusion

The effectiveness of psychopharmacological treatment appears to be enhanced by an individual's medication adherence as well as their psychological engagement in the process of working toward meaningful goals. Motivational and process-oriented cognitive-behavioral techniques can be integrated into the process of pharmacotherapy to foster both of these. Nonjudgmentally collaborating with an individual patient to uncover his or her most meaningful functional outcomes helps to establish an empathic alliance across cultural or identity differences and to mobilize the inner resources believed to be necessary for healing. Because of adolescent developmental processes, young people in particular may benefit from the emphasis on autonomy, self-regulation, and self-efficacy that these strategies entail. Discovering "what's in it for me" can enhance treatment adherence and provide psychotherapeutic benefit through the course of routine pharmacotherapy.

References

Casey BJ, Jones RM, Hare TA: The adolescent brain. Ann N Y Acad Sci 1124:111–126, 2008 18400927

Channon SJ, Huws-Thomas MV, Rollnick S, et al: A multicenter randomized controlled trial of motivational interviewing in teenagers with diabetes. Diabetes Care 30(6):1390–1395, 2007

De Nadai AS, Karver MS, Murphy TK, et al: Common factors in pediatric psychiatry: a review of essential and adjunctive mechanisms of treatment outcome. J Child Adolesc Psychopharmacol 27(1):10–18, 2017 27128785

DiLallo JJ, Weiss G: Motivational interviewing and adolescent psychopharmacology. J Am Acad Child Adolesc Psychiatry 48(2):108–113, 2009 20040823

Frank JD: Persuasion and Healing: A Comparative Study of Psychotherapy. Baltimore, MD, Johns Hopkins University Press, 1973

Frank JD, Frank JB: Persuasion and Healing: A Comparative Study of Psychotherapy, 3rd Edition. Baltimore, MD, Johns Hopkins University Press, 1991

Goldstein TR, Krantz ML, Fersch-Podrat RK, et al: A brief motivational intervention for enhancing medication adherence for adolescents with bipolar disorder: a pilot randomized trial. J Affect Disord 265:1–9, 2020 31957686

Häge A, Weymann L, Bliznak L, et al: Non-adherence to psychotropic medication among adolescents—a systematic review of the literature. Z Kinder Jugendpsychiatr Psychother 46(1):69–78, 2018 27925499

Hamrin V, Iennaco JD: Evaluation of motivational interviewing to improve psychotropic medication adherence in adolescents. J Child Adolesc Psychopharmacol 27(2):148–159, 2017 27487472

Harris R: ACT Made Simple: An Easy-to-Read Primer on Acceptance and Commitment Therapy. Oakland, CA, New Harbinger, 2009

Hayes LL, Ciarrochi J: The Thriving Adolescent: Using Acceptance and Commitment Therapy and Positive Psychology to Help Teens Manage Emotions, Achieve Goals, and Build Connection. Oakland, CA, New Harbinger, 2015

Hayes SC, Hofmann SG: The third wave of cognitive behavioral therapy and the rise of process-based care. World Psychiatry 16(3):245–246, 2017 28941087

Hayes SC, Strosahl KD, Wilson KG: Acceptance and Commitment Therapy: The Process and Practice of Mindful Change, 2nd Edition. New York, Guilford, 2012

Linehan MM: Cognitive-Behavioral Treatment of Borderline Personality Disorder. New York, Guilford, 1993

McCauley E, Berk MS, Asarnow JR, et al: Efficacy of dialectical behavior therapy for adolescents at high risk for suicide: a randomized clinical trial. JAMA Psychiatry 75(8):777–785, 2018 29926087

Miller A, Rathaus J, Linehan M: Dialectical Behavior Therapy With Suicidal Adolescents. New York, Guilford, 2007

Miller WR, Rollnick S: Motivational Interviewing: Preparing People for Change, 2nd Edition. New York, Guilford, 2002

Miller WR, Rollnick S: Motivational Interviewing: Helping People Change. New York, Guilford, 2013

Naar A, Safren SA: Motivational Interviewing and CBT: Combining Strategies for Maximum Effectiveness (Applications of Motivational Interviewing). New York, Guilford, 2017

Praszkier R: Empathy, mirror neurons and SYNC. Mind & Society 15(1):1–25, 2016

Priebe S, Dimic S, Wildgrube C, et al: Good communication in psychiatry—a conceptual review. Eur Psychiatry 26(7):403–407, 2011 21571504

Prochaska JO, DiClemente CC: Stages and processes of self-change in smoking: toward an integrative model of change. J Consult Clin Psychol 5:390–395, 1983 6863699

Prochaska JO, DiClemente CC, Norcross JC: In search of how people change: applications to addictive behaviors. Am Psychol 47(9):1102–1114, 1992 1329589

Reisner AD: The common factors, empirically validated treatments, and recovery models of therapeutic change. Psychol Rec 55:377–399, 2005

Substance Abuse and Mental Health Services Administration: The TEDS report: age of substance use initiation among treatment admissions aged 18 to 30. Rockville, MD, Center for Behavioral Health Statistics and Quality, 2014

Zolnierek KB, DiMatteo MR: Physician communication and patient adherence to treatment: a meta-analysis. Med Care 47(8):826–834, 2009 19584762

CHAPTER | 5

PROVIDING PSYCHOEDUCATION IN PHARMACOTHERAPY

Srinivasa B. Gokarakonda, M.D., M.P.H.

Peter S. Jensen, M.D.

Psychoeducation is a frequently used concept that is included in most best practice guidelines for providers, both for mental health specialists and for primary care providers, as something that the provider must "do" for or with a patient and family in the context of providing optimal care for any mental health condition. Interestingly, however, practice guidelines are rarely explicit about how one should go about the task of psychoeducation. In fact, psychoeducation is actually a much more interesting and intricate topic than we might have assumed. Consider the following cases.

CASE EXAMPLE 1

A 9-year-old boy with a history of disruptive behaviors, inattention, and hyperactivity presented for initial evaluation. A cheerful and bright boy, his grades were mostly B's and C's. After a careful clinical diagnosis of

ADHD and school interventions were in place, the patient was started on a sustained-action psychostimulant. His mother noted no improvement in his symptoms despite further titration. Although the child complained of some initial symptoms of nausea and abdominal pain, the clinician discussed the potential benefits of daily medications and the likely short-term nature of the side effects, and both the mother and child agreed to continue medication. After five visits over several months, the mother reported that she discovered that her son was hiding his medications in various places at home. Although she thought he was taking the medications, she did not observe him actually taking them. Since the incident, she started observing the child swallow his medication daily, and from that point she reported no complaints from school or at home.

This case illustrates that even small subtleties in "psychoeducation" can make great differences in outcomes.

CASE EXAMPLE 2

An 11-year-old girl diagnosed with persistent depressive disorder, anxiety, ADHD, high-functioning autism spectrum disorder, and severe irritability and aggression was followed in an outpatient clinic. During treatment in a 30-day semi-acute inpatient facility, she was prescribed an atypical antipsychotic for aggressive behaviors, which was added to her initial regimen of a long-acting morning and short-acting afternoon psychostimulant medication. Although she responded to treatment, she gained 35 lb in 4 months. The patient's parents, divorced and often in conflict, blamed each other for the child's weight gain and unhealthy eating habits. Throughout this time, the provider provided psychoeducation about the child's newly emerging obesity accompanied by elevated triglycerides, cholesterol, and borderline elevations in HbA1c. Despite changing agents, the child gained another 20 lb. At that point, the provider decided to discontinue the second atypical agent because of the lack of meaningful long-term improvement and continued weight gain. After 11 months, during a thorough reassessment of the child's medication regimen with both parents, adherence and administration of medications were rediscussed. At that point, it was learned that the father did not know about (nor was he ensuring) the child's mid-afternoon dose of short-acting stimulant (both on weekends and during school days). The child's behavior improved significantly after both parents ensured consistent morning and afternoon medication at their respective homes and at school.

This case illustrates that "psychoeducational" needs vary both as a function of time and as a function of person.

CASE EXAMPLE 3

A 6-year-old boy presented with a history of disruptive and impulsive behaviors both at home and at school. After a thorough assessment,

ADHD (combined presentation) was diagnosed. The provider discussed all treatment modalities, recommended beginning psychostimulant medication, and made a referral for therapy. The patient's parents were divorced and were sharing custody; their son was at the mother's home on weekdays and the father's home on weekends. The parents disagreed regarding psychostimulant medication treatment, despite initial psychoeducation provided to both about its risks and benefits. Moreover, the father did not believe that his child had "a problem" and consequently refused consent to start medication at his home. The patient began psychotherapy only but continued to have disruptive behaviors and declining grades. At that point, a decision was made to start medication while the child was in the mother's home. Eventually, the provider asked the father to come in again to apprise him of the situation and further educate him on the risks and benefits of medication. Only after the child told his father that "the medication helps me" did the father consent to try a small dose of psychostimulant for a short period. After administration of the medication in both settings, the father saw dramatic improvements in the child's behavior and returned to the next appointment requesting increases in the dose to maximize the benefits.

In this situation, despite the provider's best efforts, the child delivered the most important effective and convincing "psychoeducation" to the reluctant parent.

These cases implicitly reveal the incorrect nature of simplistic assumptions about psychoeducation. To be effective, psychoeducation is intertwined with and dependent on the processes of engaging authentically with the patient and family, forming a therapeutic alliance (resulting in the family's growing trust in the provider), determining what the patient's and family's current beliefs are (including any misconceptions), and determining their understanding of relevant facts about the child's condition. In addition, effective psychoeducation may change over time with a given family, affecting, for example, what information the family needs to know now (vs. later in the course of management) and what information is needed to facilitate the family's readiness and willingness to participate in an intervention plan. Even more subtle factors can make or break the effectiveness of a psychoeducational effort, including *how* the information is imparted (e.g., verbally, by written handout, or by video or web programs, and in the case of text materials, whether the textual information is presented in paragraph form or through use of carefully prepared, brief bullet points) and how well any textual content has been vetted by other patients or families in the same socioeconomic and ethnocultural groups.

Moreover, as described in this chapter, optimal psychoeducation requires an appreciation of the importance of determining not only how the message is conveyed (e.g., bullets vs. paragraphs) but also *who* is in the best position to effectively deliver the message (i.e., the messenger). For a given patient and family, the best "messenger" might actually be someone else whom the family can more easily relate to, such as another parent or community member of similar demographic or ethnocultural background, a peer parent at a local self-help group (e.g., CHADD [Children and Adults with Attention-Deficit/Hyperactivity Disorder], NAMI [National Alliance on Mental Illness]), a nurse or a medical assistant working in the same office who might be less threatening to the patient and family, or, as seen in the third case, a child who provides "psychoeducational" information to their parent.

Thus, as the American Academy of Child and Adolescent Psychiatry Work Group on Quality Issues noted, psychoeducation is a longer-term interactive and co-constructed process (Walkup and Work Group on Quality Issues 2009). It entails an effective exchange of information between two or more parties, such that it is possible for the parties to accomplish mutually agreed-on objectives. Implicit in the work group's description is that effective psychoeducation is inextricably linked to the performance of new behaviors—in other words, *behavior change* on the part of the patient and family. What behaviors?—adhering to an agreed-on treatment plan, being comfortable raising concerns that may occur in the course of managing a condition, seeking out additional information that the family may need, and so on. Because psychoeducation is an interactive process, information exchanged may also lead to behavior change *in the provider*, such as changing a dose of medication, providing new or additional information needed by a family, working with a family to modify a treatment plan, or even adjusting how the provider communicates with a family.

Psychoeducation as Behavior Change

From a behavior change perspective, effective psychoeducation has several necessary components and preconditions, including initial patient and family engagement, building and strengthening a socially and culturally attuned therapeutic alliance, and ascertaining the preexisting beliefs and understandings held by the patient or family about the diagnosis and its treatment (both initially and over time). All are necessary elements for a treatment plan to succeed as it unfolds over time. The elements of patient engagement, the therapeutic alliance, and the psychology of pharmacotherapy are addressed in other chapters, so we will not discuss them in detail here.

Fortunately, there are two large empirical, theory-guided literatures, one related to behavior change and how it is accomplished and a second literature based on communication science (used by advertisers and experts in persuasive communications). These two literatures (Fishbein et al. 2001), assembled over seven decades, have been applied to many key patient behavior change areas in the fields of substance use, diet, exercise, AIDS, and other areas. Unfortunately, they have only rarely penetrated the fields of psychiatry and mental health, and even less the field of child and adolescent psychiatry.

BEHAVIOR CHANGE SCIENCE

Most of the behavior change models—the theory of reasoned action (Fishbein and Ajzen 1977), the theory of planned behavior (Ajzen 1991), social learning theory (Bandura 1975), and the health belief model (Janz and Becker 1984)—are only modestly different and, in fact, have three major common elements: 1) health beliefs, expectancies, and attitudes; 2) norms; and 3) self-efficacy (Fishbein et al. 2001). For educational activities to achieve their ultimate objectives (patient or parent behavior change), health care providers must take into account each of these elements when considering psychoeducational efforts with patients and families. Each factor is described briefly below.

Beliefs, Expectancies, and Attitudes

When a person anticipates adopting a new behavior (e.g., taking a medicine or engaging in psychotherapy), he or she will invariably have unspoken beliefs and expectations about what will happen if he or she performs the new behavior. These beliefs may be correct or incorrect, and they may also be either positive (beliefs that the new behavior will be advantageous for the patient) or negative (beliefs that the new behavior will lead to bad outcomes). For example, if a family has heard and believes that selective serotonin reuptake inhibitors (SSRIs) "cause" suicide and this concern is not uncovered in the exchange between the health care provider and the patient and family, this belief will decrease the likelihood that the new behavior will be adopted. On the other hand, if the patient and family have a relative who benefited greatly from an SSRI, they may believe that the medicine is more likely to help them. In addition to expectancies about the positive or negative consequences of a new behavior, parents and families may have *attitudes* about a new behavior, such as the mindset that one is a "bad" parent if their child has to take medicine or a teen who believes that if they need a psychiatric medication, it means that they must be "crazy."

Invariably, any and every new behavior has an associated set of positive (behavior-promoting) and negative (behavior-undermining) beliefs. Only in the context of a high degree of trust and a therapeutic alliance will these potentially hidden beliefs be revealed. And even if there is a high degree of trust in the relationship, other factors may make the patient and family reluctant to disclose them, such as fear of offending a doctor (whom they see as an authority figure whose judgment they do not want to question). However, they may reveal such concerns to a best friend or spouse (see subsection "Communication Science Relevant to Psychoeducation" for more discussion about the impact of differences in the "messenger" [i.e., who delivers the message]).

Norms

The second area that behavior change theories have identified as relevant to whether a person is willing and able to perform a new behavior is their personal and local norms, such as the expectations and beliefs of their family members, peers, or cultural group. For example, a parent might feel that her relatives will be critical of her for "drugging" her child. If the parent believes that some or most of the influential persons in her life have such attitudes, these norms will undermine the parent's ability and comfort with pursuing an appropriate intervention. On the other hand, if the parent becomes connected to a parent support group, in which other parents share successful experiences with their own children's treatment, these new peers may help the parent establish new norms for her behavior. In addition, the parent might feel comfortable with disclosing some worries and concerns to these other individuals, allowing incomplete understandings or misperceptions to be addressed.

Self-Efficacy

Self-efficacy refers to an individual's beliefs that he or she has the skill and necessary knowledge to accomplish a new behavior. For example, if the doctor indicates that a parent should "watch for side effects," the parent may actually feel that he does not know how to do it and as a consequence feel uncertain about whether he should proceed. The doctor must anticipate this and be prepared to coach or guide patients and families in areas where they may have low self-efficacy. This also applies to any parent- or patient-based psychotherapy: the therapist may give guidance on specific new behaviors that the parent or patient might perform, but the individual might secretly say to himself, "I can't do that" or "That really won't work for me."

Thus, behavior change research has revealed critical linkages between attitudes and beliefs, norms, and self-efficacy for a new behavior to be adopted. Likewise, for any "psychoeducation" to be useful in helping patients and families adopt a new behavior, these three factors are essential for providers to understand and address as we attempt any psychoeducational strategies.

COMMUNICATION SCIENCE RELEVANT TO PSYCHOEDUCATION

In parallel with theory-driven studies of behavior change, communication scientists have studied what constitutes effective (i.e., persuasive) communication, beginning as early as 1948 (see, e.g., Allen and Preiss 1998; Hovland et al. 1953; Katz 1957). The key determinants of communication effectiveness include 1) the source of the information (i.e., who the "messenger" is), 2) the specific characteristics of the message being communicated (the message itself), 3) the medium (or channel) by which the message is being delivered (e.g., written, verbal, internet, video), and 4) characteristics of the recipient or audience the message is intended to reach. This last factor, the audience or recipient, is largely covered under the three behavior change elements described earlier (personal beliefs and expectancies, norms, and self-efficacy), so it is not repeated here. Within communication theory, these four factors are needed to fully understand the processes by which a message is effectively presented and is adequately persuasive—that is, enabling a message to change one's personal beliefs, and ultimately, to change one's behavior.

The *source* of the information is the person or group who creates the message and delivers it to the receiver or audience. According to communication theory models, specific characteristics of the source or messenger can make that person more persuasive and credible. Expertise, trustworthiness, and ready availability of the source to the recipient have all been identified as important aspects of persuasive sources (McGinnies and Ward 1980; Wiener and Mowen 1986). Specifically, a recipient is more likely to pay attention, retain ideas, and accept a message if the messenger or source is respected, trusted, and readily available if questions arise.

The *message* is the specific information that the source is communicating and the receiver is obtaining. Messages (or psychoeducational content) may possess characteristics that make them more or less believable, such as the organization and order in which information is presented, the use of one- versus two-sided arguments (e.g., pros vs. cons of using a medication), and the actual content itself (e.g., quality of arguments, evidence). When the message is presented in a simple, tightly organized format without excessive or extraneous details, receivers are able to comprehend and attend to the message more adequately. With regard to content, messages are more persuasive and accepted if they contain several strong and high-quality arguments (Andrews and Shimp 1990). Finally, messages are more persuasive if they contain an urgent need that is serious; could affect the receiver personally; and contain a solution.

The *medium*, or channel, by which the message is delivered refers to the manner in which the message is being communicated. For parents, this means that passively reading information about the pros and cons of a specific medication via one channel (e.g., a brochure) will not be as effective for behavior change as having this information conveyed to them via multiple channels and over an extended period of time. In addition, learners vary in their preferred communication channels, so educational methods that provide content via multiple channels (e.g., brochures, parent discussion groups, web content, and repeated face-to-face discussion in individual clinical sessions) are more likely to reach individuals successfully.

Last, the *recipient* (or audience) is the person or persons receiving the information being communicated by the source. Motivation, past experience, knowledge, skills, beliefs, and expectations differ widely among families and patients, each of whom come with their own social and cultural experiences and attitudes regarding psychiatric medicines, and which can greatly influence a recipient's ability to be persuaded by a message.

Implications of Behavior Change and Communication Science Research for Psychoeducation

Given these considerations, it is not surprising that most research on psychoeducation as a stand-alone process finds that it is generally ineffective (Haynes et al. 2005; Kahana et al. 2008; Kripalani et al. 2007). When psychoeducation has been shown to be effective, it is usually a multicomponent intervention using a range of strategies—carefully prepared handouts in culturally attuned patient- and family-friendly language, interactive discussions with the opportunity to ask questions, interactions with supportive peers, web- and video-based materials, and careful tailoring of the information to each patient and family's needs.

In the same way, an effective clinician must *personalize* the psychoeducational and communication process for each family based on a thorough understanding of their attitudes, beliefs, myths, and misconceptions, as well as based on any accurate mindsets held by the patient and family members. These beliefs, attitudes, and misconceptions are likely to change over time.

In what follows below, we review the extant literature on the elements of effective psychoeducation, including what is known about the 1) impact of initial engagement, the therapeutic alliance, and trust; 2) the degree to which psychoeducational needs vary as a function of time over different periods of clinical encounters; 3) the optimal amount of information to be provided ("too much versus too little"); 4) the impact of discrepancies between socioeconomic status and authority status of the health care provider and the patient's family; and 5) the impact of child age, development, illness severity, ethnocultural factors, and other child and family characteristics. We then describe good clinical practices and strategies that we believe constitute best practices in psychoeducation. We close the chapter with a discussion of future research needs.

ENGAGEMENT, THERAPEUTIC ALLIANCE, AND TRUST

As noted earlier, in communication science, effective messages (i.e., psychoeducation) depend in part on a trustworthy messenger. Numerous studies have established the necessity of a strong therapeutic alliance, not merely for purposes of adherence to treatment regimens, but also as a factor that independently leads to improved treatment outcomes (Bosworth et al. 2018; Castro-Blanco and Karver 2010; DiLallo and Weiss 2009; Shirk et al. 2011). Many of these elements (engagement, alliance, and trust) have been subsumed under the heading "common factors" by various authors (De Nadai et al. 2017). If sufficiently carried out by the clinician (and if experienced by the patient or family), these processes will not only result in accurate empathy within the clinician but also lead to higher patient or family self-efficacy and more positive attitudes toward any recommended treatment plan and more effective psychoeducation.

Although most studies of common factors do not explicitly discuss "psychoeducation" per se, a careful perusal of the literature reveals additional elements that we can apply to psychoeducation for both psychotherapeutic and pharmacological interventions. For example, in a meta-analysis of 16 youth therapy studies of the links between alliance and outcomes, Shirk et al. (2011) found that alliance and treatment outcomes were intercorrelated. Busch and Auchincloss (2018) emphasize the importance of psychoeducation for engaging patients in both therapy and pharmacotherapy and recommend its use to help patients and families understand how medication and therapy work. As Graves et al. (2017) have noted, even younger patients require specific psychoeducational efforts (in child-friendly language) to establish an effective alliance and to promote treatment adherence.

Only if the clinician is properly skilled in generating sufficient trust and a strong therapeutic alliance (described earlier) will these potential myths and misunderstandings be revealed. When providers use open-ended questions and reflective listening, allowing frequent pauses, asking patients about what they have heard or read about the specific disorder or its treatments, and it can facilitate the patient's or family's comfort in asking questions. This allows therapist and patient to more fully discuss and clarify the issues. Yet even if the clinician has such skills, the patient or family may not reveal any misunderstandings because of other factors that hinder trust or open communication (e.g., socioeconomic or ethnocultural differences).

Specific strategies to strengthen common factors are discussed more fully in other chapters in this volume, but three approaches worth noting are described by Cheng (2007) as skills that providers need training and supervision in to become maximally effective: solution-focused interviewing, motivational interviewing, and medication interest model–related applications.

CHANGES IN PSYCHOEDUCATIONAL NEEDS OVER TIME

The timing of one's psychoeducational efforts and differences in patients' or families' psychoeducational needs over time are critical considerations. For example, Bosworth et al. (2018) report that nonadherence to treatment and patients' related psychoeducational needs vary during different treatment phases. They propose a taxonomy of time-based phases of adherence, including initiation, implementation, and discontinuation, and recommend multicomponent psychoeducational interventions to target the different phases of adherence.

For example, during a medication initiation phase (when patients are at greatest risk of actually not beginning treatment or discontinuing it early), patients may need targeted information about the risk-benefit ratios of not obtaining treatment or of common but nonserious side effects that may undermine initial treatment even though the side effects dissipate over time. Similar arguments can also apply to beginning psychotherapy, when the process may feel awkward, unfamiliar, or even ineffective to patients and families.

In similar fashion, some medication side effects may not be felt immediately but only emerge over time (e.g., weight loss on psychostimulants), so educational needs may change as treatment unfolds. Similarly, when a treatment is to be discontinued, how should the clinician prepare for this phase (e.g., discontinuing an SSRI or an atypical agent, or terminating therapy) and prepare the patient? As Iglay et al. (2015) noted, providers must thoughtfully attend to educational interventions in each of these phases, and successful psychoeducation and full engagement in treatment often depend on specific aspects of the clinical picture and the therapist-patient relationship.

WHAT PATIENTS AND FAMILIES NEED TO KNOW ("HOW MUCH IS TOO MUCH VERSUS TOO LITTLE?")

Despite universal recognition among providers about the need for psychoeducation, they face a predicament: how much is too much versus too little? Most providers discuss common side effects (e.g., nausea, vomiting, and abdominal pain for SSRIs; appetite suppression and insomnia for psychostimulants) with most patients. Based on specific needs or expressed concerns, patients may require additional information about the proposed treatment approach or outcome. With a 15-year-old adolescent female patient worried about weight changes, it may be prudent to have a more detailed discussion of the potential for weight gain/loss as a side effect of several SSRIs; a teen who is not sexually active may not necessarily benefit from or care about changes to libido, yet a year later they may.

Rather than detail all common and rare side effects, we recommend as a best practice that providers briefly discuss the most common side effects at a visit before initiating a treatment, provide a lengthier informational handout for reading in the interim (as "homework"), and then elicit questions at the next visit. This approach would also help in decreasing liability issues and provide an opportunity for the patient and family to engage and discuss the issue at the next visit.

If a provider were to discuss all the rare side effects during the initial visit, it might scare the patient and family away and disengage them from treatment. The risks and benefits of treatment and medication should be clearly discussed to avoid this situation. Psychoeducation should be targeted based on age of the patient, stage of readiness of the family, and specific situations (e.g., family history, previous history of suicide attempts, overdose and situations of overtaking, skipping doses). For example, if a patient has a personal or family history of suicide attempts, it is imperative to discuss all the possible side effects of SSRIs, including suicidal thoughts and serotonin syndrome, even though they are very rare. Another example is a patient who has a history of either overtaking or undertaking a medication (e.g., discussing Stevens-Johnson syndrome during initiation and maintenance of lamotrigine, withdrawal dyskinesia with antipsychotics). Clinicians should use their best judgment in certain difficult situations to educate and engage patients in treatments. Finally, clinicians should create a safe and comfortable environment for patients and families to discuss their issues freely.

IMPACT OF DIFFERENCES BETWEEN SOCIOECONOMIC AND AUTHORITY STATUSES

As noted earlier, communication science suggests that the clinician must recognize that although he or she may have all of the relevant psychoeducational information that the patient and family might "need to know," the family may not disclose to the clinician their worries and fears about the illness or its treatment, nor will they necessarily "believe" the psychoeducational information conveyed by the clinician to the family. The messenger may be "wrong" even if the message is "right." Unfortunately, the child mental health literature has not sufficiently examined this possibility despite decades of evidence from more general communication science studies. In our experience, we have found that some patients and families may find it easier to discuss their concerns with a nurse (or even a receptionist on the way in or out of the office) than with a doctor, who may seem unapproachable to a given patient or family or for other reasons related to the authority status of medical clinicians. For example, some cultures hold doctors in such high regard that there may be discomfort with raising any questions whatsoever.

For these reasons (to address possible mismatches between messengers and recipients), we make it a regular practice to link new patients and families to other, well-informed parents in local parent support groups (e.g., CHADD, NAMI), assigning all new parents and families to attend at least two sessions as homework. These and other organizations have strong scientific boards, so that the messages that permeate these organizations are evidence based, enabling parent leaders to serve as effective messengers in delivering the science-based messages to recipient families.

IMPACT OF CHILD/FAMILY CHARACTERISTICS ON PSYCHOEDUCATIONAL NEEDS

Although psychoeducational effects have not been examined from the perspective of the impact of age, development, or other child and family characteristics, a related lens through which we can view a child and family's psychoeducational needs is through studies of medication adherence. As Hack and Chow (2001) noted while examining treatment adherence generally, children and youth with psychiatric illness may be at greater risk for poor medication adherence than those with other medical conditions. In addition, the educational needs of children may be different from those of teens, who also differ from adults (De Nadai et al. 2017). Edgcomb and Zima (2018) conducted a systematic review of adherence in pediatric psychiatry, finding that among children with more complex (comorbid) conditions and greater illness severity, their families had greater difficulties ensuring treatment adherence. In adult populations, García et al. (2016) reviewed 38 studies of antipsychotic medication adherence in patients with schizophrenia or bipolar disorder, finding that younger age, substance abuse, poor insight, cognitive impairments, low level of education, minority status, poor therapeutic alliance, barriers to care, symptom severity, and low socioeconomic status were all independent predictors of nonadherence. Opler et al. (2004) have argued that one must also address culturally specific issues to maximize adherence. An important insight from their own experience was notably shared in the very beginning of their paper:

> [W]e came to realize that non-adherence was due primarily to differing concepts of illness, of medication, and of medication side effects between ourselves and our patients….By learning to respect and address our patients' views, we were able to offer them real treatment. In retrospect, before we came to adequately appreciate our patients' perspective and its implications, not only was our clinical expertise of little benefit, but it was, in fact, interfering with their treatment. In many cases, our initial treatment choices probably caused more rather than less distress for our patients. Fortunately, we were able to acquire culturally responsive clinical insights and to make corrections in our prescribing practices based on these insights, leading to improved medication adherence and clinical status among our patients. (p. 134)

Good Clinical Practices and Strategies

In this chapter, we have reviewed the fundamentals of psychoeducation and various factors that are vital for effective delivery of psychoeducation. We have also discussed important culturally attuned strategies and skills that clinicians should try to master for engaging with diverse patients and families in building a therapeutic relationship. In this section, we summarize a number of best practices (drawn from our own experiences as well as the existing literature) that can enhance psychoeducation delivery.

Several investigators (Kai and Crosland 2001; Stafford and Colom 2013) have described psychoeducation as "an intervention that seeks to empower patients with tools that allow them to be more active in their therapy process" (Stafford and Colom 2013, p. 12). They also suggest four core skills (communication, information flow, patient involvement in decision making process, and trust) that must be used when developing treatment plans to maximally empower families.

In our experience, we have found that patient involvement in treatment and satisfaction can be increased by providing "goodies," which might include information sheets, website linkages, and information about local community resources. Clinicians must thoroughly vet such handouts and related information (perhaps using parents and consumer advisers and avoiding pharma-sponsored materials when possible) offered to the patients and families to maximize readability and effectiveness. Relatedly, we always encourage patients and families to access parent support organizations' websites (e.g., CHADD, NAMI) and to attend several local chapter meetings or join the organizations' Facebook groups or follow them on other social media platforms (e.g., Instagram, Twitter). Such organizations uniformly provide scientifically vetted information to families, and parents with a newly diagnosed child will have the opportunity to learn from other messengers (i.e., experienced parents) to further their own "psychoeducation."

To be most effective, psychoeducation must be a continuing process— set in motion by the clinician but continuing *outside of office visits*. For example, clinicians might create a lending library of top books that a parent might be encouraged to thumb through in the office and take home and read, guided by the specific chapter homework assignments. These assignments should be discussed at the next visit. In the same vein, families also may need advice about "what to avoid"—which other books and websites have credible information versus the vast number that do not. In the same way, because families often have questions that they may forget in the midst of a visit, the clinician might proactively assign families some homework or exercises (if this term is preferred)—to write down their top three questions or concerns prior to the next visit. In our experience, assigning such homework often increases families' engagement in treatment. Although some families might think it is extra work, most believe that it shows that the clinician cares for them.

Other clinical activities that are common components of good clinical practice also can serve as psychoeducational tools. For example, if a parent or youth completes a depression rating scale, the meaning of each of the questions, how they are scored, and how they link to DSM diagnoses should be explained and discussed (American Psychiatric Association 2013). Used this way, such tools (including sleep logs, behavior logs, and so on) serve multiple educational, communication, and monitoring purposes.

Because of the ineffectiveness of stand-alone psychoeducation, to be maximally effective, clinicians must design a combination of strategies as discussed in this chapter, both inside and outside the office, to educate and empower their patients.

Future Research Needs

Our review of the extant literature on psychoeducation reveals multiple gaps in what we know versus what we need to know. First, although research has established that stand-alone psychoeducation is largely ineffective, commonly used psychoeducational strategies within child mental health settings are usually developed ad hoc and are either stand-alone or an admixture of what seems to be common sense (e.g., patient handouts, videos and websites, or allowing questions at the end of a clinical visit). But all are largely untested, and only rarely are they systematically and thoughtfully developed and tested.

In contrast, commercial companies carefully test a range of messages and even then focus on which messages are likely to be most effective with specific consumers within a zip code region. Advertisements we see on television or in printed media have been carefully developed and then screened for acceptability, believability, and impact in multiple studies or focus groups. Some companies target and vary their ads based on their knowledge of the recipients, with different versions of advertisements mailed to different zip codes, based on their knowledge of socioeconomic or ethnocultural differences across neighborhoods.

In the field of child mental health, what is ultimately needed is a series of randomized controlled trials that test different educational strategies, testing not only different messages but also different messengers and different media (Bevan Jones et al. 2018). Different areas of focus or family beliefs or myths may require separate study, such as that recommended by Bravo-Mehmedbašic and Kucukalic (2017) to reduce the impact of stigma. In the area of ADHD, one of this chapter's coauthors (P.S.J.) conducted a study consisting of five focus groups of parents of children with ADHD about to begin treatment, eliciting from them information concerning their attitudes, beliefs, and expectancies about their child taking a psychostimulant. Interestingly, whereas 17 positive beliefs were spontaneously identified by parents related to possible *benefits* of stimulant treatment, 25 *negative attitudes*, *beliefs*, and *concerns* were raised by parents about possible adverse consequences of starting a psychostimulant (Coletti et al. 2012). From these data, investigators then developed a 22-item attitudes and beliefs questionnaire, which they then administered to 131 parents with a child with newly diagnosed ADHD. The measure essentially allowed investigators and providers to proactively identify parents' attitudes and beliefs concerning stimulant medication (essentially, parents' *psychoeducational needs*) and to use the tool not only to predict future families' adherence and nonadherence with medication but also to guide clinicians' discussions and psychoeducational activities with families.

A second area in which research is needed centers on ways to better understand the means of improving trainees' skills in psychoeducation and related areas (therapeutic alliance, common factors, cultural engagement, and culturally attuned messaging). Teal and Street (2009) have enumerated some of the key skills, including active listening, attending to sociocultural aspects of the patient's illness, eliciting patients' perspectives, empowering patients and families to make decisions, and "reading" patients' verbal and nonverbal behaviors. Amazingly, they listed a total of 57 listed clinical behaviors that therapists must master to achieve maximum competence.

Conclusion

Effective psychoeducation is tightly intertwined with many of the skills and topic areas discussed in this book—patient and family engagement, active listening, therapeutic alliance formation, empathy, shared decision making, and the complex psychology of the interactions between all parties engaged in clinical encounters. From this perspective, it is a core clinical activity, simply by virtue of its close relations to these skills. Yet psychoeducation, in our view, is often treated as an easily understood, taken-for-granted activity in clinical practices. When appropriately understood, psychoeducation deserves much more attention, study, supervisory and training efforts, and research as a *core clinical activity* in its own right with its own unique demands, skills, and basic science underpinnings.

References

Ajzen I: The theory of planned behavior. Organ Behav Hum Decis Process 50(2):179–211, 1991

Allen M, Preiss RW: Persuasion: Advances Through Meta-Analysis. Cresskill, NJ, Hampton Press, 1998

American Psychiatric Association: Diagnostic and Statistical Manual of Mental Disorders, 5th Edition. Arlington, VA, American Psychiatric Publishing, 2013

Andrews JC, Shimp TA: Effects of involvement, argument strength, and source characteristics on central and peripheral processing of advertising. Psychol Mark 7(3):195–214, 1990

Bandura A: Analysis of modeling processes. School Psych Rev 4(1):4–10, 1975

Bevan Jones R, Thapar A, Stone Z, et al: Psychoeducational interventions in adolescent depression: a systematic review. Patient Educ Couns 101(5):804–816, 2018 29103882

Bosworth HB, Blalock DV, Hoyle RH, et al: The role of psychological science in efforts to improve cardiovascular medication adherence. Am Psychol 73(8):968–980, 2018 30394776

Bravo-Mehmedbašic A, Kucukalic S: Stigma of psychiatric diseases and psychiatry. Psychiatr Danub 29 (suppl 5):877–879, 2017 29283982

Busch FN, Auchincloss EL: The role of psychoeducation in psychodynamic psychotherapy. Psychodyn Psychiatry 46(1):145–163, 2018 29480786

Castro-Blanco DE, Karver MS: Elusive Alliance: Treatment Engagement Strategies With High-Risk Adolescents. Washington, DC, American Psychological Association, 2010

Cheng MK: New approaches for creating the therapeutic alliance: solution-focused interviewing, motivational interviewing, and the medication interest model. Psychiatr Clin North Am 30(2):157–166, 2007 17643833

Coletti DJ, Pappadopulos E, Katsiotas NJ, et al: Parent perspectives on the decision to initiate medication treatment of attention-deficit/hyperactivity disorder. J Child Adolesc Psychopharmacol 22(3):226–237, 2012 22537185

De Nadai AS, Karver MS, Murphy TK, et al: Common factors in pediatric psychiatry: a review of essential and adjunctive mechanisms of treatment outcome. J Child Adolesc Psychopharmacol 27(1):10–18, 2017 27128785

DiLallo JJ, Weiss G: Motivational interviewing and adolescent psychopharmacology. J Am Acad Child Adolesc Psychiatry 48(2):108–113, 2009 20040823

Edgcomb JB, Zima B: Medication adherence among children and adolescents with severe mental illness: a systematic review and meta-analysis. J Child Adolesc Psychopharmacol 28(8):508–520, 2018 30040434

Fishbein M, Ajzen I: Belief, Attitude, Intention, and Behavior: An Introduction to Theory and Research. Reading, MA, Addison-Wesley, 1977

Fishbein M, Triandis HC, Kanfer FH, et al: Factors influencing behavior and behavior change, in Handbook of Health Psychology. Edited by Baum A, Revensen TA, Singer JE. New York, Taylor & Francis, 2001, pp 3–18

García S, Martínez-Cengotitabengoa M, López-Zurbano S, et al: Adherence to antipsychotic medication in bipolar disorder and schizophrenic patients: a systematic review. J Clin Psychopharmacol 36(4):355–371, 2016 27307187

Graves TA, Tabri N, Thompson-Brenner H, et al: A meta-analysis of the relation between therapeutic alliance and treatment outcome in eating disorders. Int J Eat Disord 50(4):323–340, 2017 28152196

Hack S, Chow B: Pediatric psychotropic medication compliance: a literature review and research-based suggestions for improving treatment compliance. J Child Adolesc Psychopharmacol 11(1):59–67, 2001 11322747

Haynes RB, Yao X, Degani A, et al: Interventions for enhancing medication adherence. Cochrane Database Syst Rev 19(4):CD000011, 2005

Hovland CI, Janis IL, Kelley HH: Communication and Persuasion. New Haven, CT, Yale University Press, 1953

Iglay K, Cartier SE, Rosen VM, et al: Meta-analysis of studies examining medication adherence, persistence, and discontinuation of oral antihyperglycemic agents in type 2 diabetes. Curr Med Res Opin 31(7):1283–1296, 2015 26023805

Janz NK, Becker MH: The health belief model: a decade later. Health Educ Q 11(1):1–47, 1984 6392204

Kahana S, Drotar D, Frazier T: Meta-analysis of psychological interventions to promote adherence to treatment in pediatric chronic health conditions. J Pediatr Psychol 33(6):590–611, 2008 18192300

Kai J, Crosland A: Perspectives of people with enduring mental ill health from a community-based qualitative study. Br J Gen Pract 51(470):730–736, 2001 11593834

Katz E: The two-step flow of communication: an up-to-date report on an hypothesis. Public Opin Q 21(1):61–78, 1957

Kripalani S, Yao X, Haynes RB: Interventions to enhance medication adherence in chronic medical conditions: a systematic review. Arch Intern Med 167(6):540–550, 2007 17389285

McGinnies E, Ward CD: Better liked than right: trustworthiness and expertise as factors in credibility. Pers Soc Psychol Bull 6(3):467–472, 1980

Opler LA, Ramirez PM, Dominguez LM, et al: Rethinking medication prescribing practices in an inner-city Hispanic mental health clinic. J Psychiatr Pract 10(2):134–140, 2004 15330410

Shirk SR, Karver MS, Brown R: The alliance in child and adolescent psychotherapy. Psychotherapy (Chic) 48(1):17–24, 2011 21401270

Stafford N, Colom F: Purpose and effectiveness of psychoeducation in patients with bipolar disorder in a bipolar clinic setting. Acta Psychiatr Scand Suppl 127(442):11–18, 2013 23581788

Teal CR, Street RL: Critical elements of culturally competent communication in the medical encounter: a review and model. Soc Sci Med 68(3):533–543, 2009 19019520

Walkup J; Work Group on Quality Issues: Practice parameter on the use of psychotropic medication in children and adolescents. J Am Acad Child Adolesc Psychiatry 48(9):961–973, 2009 19692857

Wiener JL, Mowen JC: Source credibility: on the independent effects of trust and expertise, in Advances in Consumer Research. Edited by Lutz RJ. Provo, UT, Association for Consumer Research, 1986, pp 306–310

PART II

PARTNERS

CHAPTER 6

#KEEPITREAL: THE MYTH OF THE "MED CHECK" AND THE REALITIES OF THE TIME-LIMITED PHARMACOTHERAPY VISIT

Max S. Rosen, M.D.
Anne L. Glowinski, M.D., M.P.E.

The primary goal of providing routine psychiatric visits is to evaluate and promote mental health and well-being (Torrey et al. 2017). As child and adolescent psychiatrists, we have the unique goal of gaining detailed insights into young people's lives and, when appropriate, using pharmacotherapy to help alleviate psychiatric symptoms or disorders that are sources of suffering or impairment, including deviation out of the range of normative developmental trajectories. Yet the psychopharmacological revolution of the past 50 years, as well as the nuanced criteria in DSM (American Psychiatric Association 2013), which catalogues hundreds of disorders, has given rise to significant concern that psychiatry is now a specialty characterized by a lack of interest in individuals' stories and an oversimplification in service of "checklist psychiatry" (Vázquez 2014). This unfortunate view of clinical psychiatry, the increase in number of people using mental health services over the past decades, and the shortage of psychiatric care providers, as well as the decline in funding for outpatient care, have all converged toward psychiatrists too often resorting—or being relegated—to abbreviated "med check" visits (Torrey et al. 2017; Vázquez 2014).

However, as is often pointed out, given the limitations of what medications can accomplish, the most complete plan that has the best chance of leading to real-world, functional outcomes is one that is driven by a patient's culturally informed biopsychosocial information—that is, informed by a patient's culture (values, beliefs, family traditions), biology (family history; unique symptom manifestations, including comorbidities; and history of responses to medications and side effects), psychology (personality and temperament traits, cognitive styles, defense mechanisms), and social history (a patient's family, school, and neighborhood environment).[1] As such, arriving at a clear conceptualization of factors with possible impact on our patients and of the relationships of these factors to one another is critical and is an approach with the best chance of improving a patient's life. It may, in fact, involve doing something—from exercise or dietary changes, to behavioral modifications that can increase well-being, to interventions that challenge one's anxiety or depressive symptoms—other than taking a medication (Torrey et al. 2017).

This model of using "med check" appointments and thus splitting a patient's care into medication and "what's going on in my life" (Torrey et al. 2017) has unfortunately become common. This schism in outpatient psychiatric care is evidenced by survey data collected from psychotherapists and prescribing mental health clinicians. Roughly 40% of the respective patients were seeing a second professional, meaning that that proportion of patients had multiple providers to address their mental

---

[1]We acknowledge that this popular division into cultural, biological, psychological, and social factors is itself an oversimplification, because a good child psychiatrist should understand how biology can manifest as environment. For example, an adolescent's largely genetically inherited psychiatric disorder such as bipolar disorder can correlate with the same illness in a biologically related primary caretaker, such as a mother or a father, and lead directly to major social environmental changes for a child.

health concerns with therapy and medication treatment (Kalman 2015). Although this could be a sign that many patients are receiving recommended best-evidence care by combining psychotherapy and pharmacotherapy from a connected team of two different providers, all too often this instead represents fragmented care, with the act of talking to patients carved out of the psychiatrist's job. Evidently, with systemic pressures to maximize profit or sustain systems of care with limited financial resources and thus see as many patients as possible, a provider who is both the psychopharmacologist and the psychotherapist has become the exception.

Without necessarily having specialized training in evidence-based treatments such as cognitive-behavioral therapy (CBT), interpersonal therapy, dialectical behavior therapy, dyadic developmental therapy, or applied behavioral analysis (to name a few), we child and adolescent psychiatrists must extend our roles beyond just psychopharmacology if we want to be effective. We also posit that the term "med check" is not only a misnomer that simply does not exist in child and adolescent psychiatric treatment (as if patients just come to us wanting to "talk about their meds"); it is also a disservice to the nature and intention of our work with youth and families. For such time-limited visits during which the medication issues are a primary focus, we propose the term *brief pharmacotherapy visits*, which allows us to retain our role as therapists (as an inextricable part of psychopharmacology).

As we outline in this chapter, an effective pharmacotherapy appointment necessitates appreciation of many things that inform treatment and thus pharmacotherapy decisions, including the intricacies of an individual's culturally informed, biopsychosocial story. It has consistently been shown that strong therapeutic alliances between a patient and their mental health provider, as well as empathy demonstrated by the latter, lead to more positive clinical and functional outcomes (Lebowitz and Appelbaum 2019) and thus to the primary goal, cited earlier, of evaluating and promoting mental health and well-being.

We practice clinical child and adolescent psychiatry in an academic teaching clinic at Washington University in St. Louis. This setting includes primarily faculty in child and adolescent psychiatry, residents in general psychiatry, and fellows in child and adolescent psychiatry, where all providers are consistently afforded 30 minutes for pharmacotherapy appointments. We see a wide range of patients from diverse socioeconomic, ethnocultural, and geographic backgrounds, both reflecting and also transcending the immediate Greater St. Louis area demographics, because we often provide tertiary care to patients from afar, and to patients who live in child and adolescent psychiatry "deserts" (coming from several hours away). We have structured the middle of this chapter to elaborate on our "typical" patient encounter, which evolved from a combination of evidence-based practices and accumulated clinical expertise. Our usual 30-minute pharmacotherapy visits (as outlined in Table 6–1) generally follow this sequence when applicable: 1) tend to rapport, 2) obtain updates on environmental influences, 3) provide counseling on environmental influences, 4) elicit and discuss obstacles to treatment, 5) review medication efficacy and benefits and side effects, 6) make decisions and have a discussion regarding maintaining or changing course of treatment, and 7) answer any additional questions.

Each of these steps helps us to make better informed judgments and decisions with our patients and their families when selecting appropriate pharmacotherapy, clarifies what we need to recommend outside of pharmacotherapy, and enhances the therapeutic alliance while also helping patients and their families invest and collaborate in treatment, thereby improving the odds of better long-term clinical outcomes. Obviously, developmental considerations permeate child and adolescent psychiatry, so we address these next within each step.

The Brief Pharmacotherapy Visit

TEND TO RAPPORT

Child and adolescent psychiatry is not simply the practice of psychiatry as usual on "little people." Most children are predisposed to bond with warm and nurturing adults, and most adolescents are predisposed to be closed off to adults perceived as poorly attuned to them. In addition to the myriad behaviors that go into alliance building with adults (e.g., kindness, humor, active listening, validation, and trust building), an attuned child and adolescent psychiatrist knows how to discuss a young person's favorite website, Instagram follow, book, movie, or video game; how to get on the floor and build castles and imaginary worlds; how to play ball while conversing with a fidgety child; how to make a joke at the right moment; and how to avoid the joke that distracts from important content. The attuned child psychiatrist does that concomitantly with establishing rapport with the entire family accompanying the child. With families and patients seen regularly for follow-up appointments after initial evaluation and treatment planning, the goal is to tend to this rapport (and occasionally to repair it). We usually manage to parsimoniously use what the patient and family bring us to achieve this: asking a child or a parent what book they happen to have in hand, what music is flowing

---

Table 6–1. Typical sequence of steps for 30-minute brief pharmacotherapy visits

Task	Example questions or phrases
1. Tend to rapport	What is that book you are holding?
	Have you seen any new shows recently?
	What are your favorite social media sites?/ Which YouTubers are you following?
2. Obtain updates on environmental influences	How have things been at home? Any changes happening with you or your family members?
	What things have been going well for you at school? What's your favorite class/ subject? Which class gives you the most challenges? Who is the one adult you can lean on/depend on at school if you need to talk to someone?
3. Provide counseling on environmental influences	We are going to discuss changing things that (we know from our past meetings) can affect your mental health (child/ teen), or your child's mental health (if with a parent).
4. Elicit and discuss obstacles to treatment	What are your thoughts about taking a medication for your ADHD?
	Is there anything making it particularly challenging to take a medication every day?
	A lot of young people tell me that they don't think as much about having depression when they don't take their medications. Does that resonate with you?
5. Review medication efficacy and side effects	Do you believe the medication is doing anything, either good or bad?
	What do you feel this medication should or should not be doing?
6. Make decisions and have a discussion regarding maintaining or changing course of treatment	We discussed that you were planning to cut down on the sugary drinks; how is that going?
	How do you like the psychotherapist we recommended for family therapy?
7. Answer any additional questions	What other questions do you have about anything we have discussed today?

through their smart device, or if the sibling toddler sitting on a parent's knee "gets into everything." In effect, this demonstrates our genuine ongoing interest in addition to possibly enabling learning more, at every visit, about our patients and their families. If alliance building is establishing a bridge that will be a conduit for effective treatment, alliance tending is simply making sure the bridge still exists, and is done at every visit.

OBTAIN UPDATES ON ENVIRONMENTAL INFLUENCES

Overlapping with alliance tending, but also with the specific purpose of evaluating the state of potentially important influences on psychopathology symptoms and well-being, we ask for updates on family environment (How are people getting along? Are family members sick or healthy?) and school environment (How are peer relationships? Are teachers liked or disliked and why? Is school difficult or easy? What is their favorite class? Is there at least one trusted adult in school? Is our patient being bullied? Are there structural issues such as those that frequently impact our transgender patients, who may or may not always be able to use the school bathroom they would prefer, for instance?). With patients and families we know well, patterns usually emerge over time: We know that one patient is exquisitely sensitive to his parents' fighting or to his grandmother's declining health, or we know that another patient is particularly sensitive to criticism by her grandfather, and we combine open-ended questions with focused ones about common destabilizing factors.

PROVIDE COUNSELING ON ENVIRONMENTAL INFLUENCES

Here we refer to the common example of parental anxiety as an environmental influence that we encounter and discuss often. Unlike poverty, neighborhood, or current school of attendance, it is an environment that our treatment approaches can successfully target and change for the better. Parental anxiety impacts offspring anxiety symptoms (e.g., Cunningham et al. 2019) and is also highly impacted by offspring anxiety (Ahmadzadeh et al. 2019). We typically use a combination of words and drawings to illustrate why, of all the interventions we recommend, addressing parental anxiety is a priority. We recommend this as carefully and compassionately as possible, acknowledging that the topic itself can be a source of enormous guilt or denial for parents. We endeavor to remind parents that we have the common goal of helping the child they love and brought to us for expert opinion and treatment, while we summarize briefly the literature on this topic, illustrating the concepts with examples that the family has related to us or even child mental status exam changes that we are noticing in the room when a parent gets anxious. We have similar conversations regarding parental substance abuse, depression, or any other parental factor that is clearly (and believably, according to the extant literature) impacting a child's symptoms. Ideal clinical settings would fully facilitate the referral of parents who need psychiatric evaluation and treatment. As with many academic medical center clinics, we are not ideal in that respect, but we facilitate care of parents by addressing issues of stigma and the importance of treatment for themselves and their children and by providing every resource we can to facilitate entry into care for parents if needed. We also provide practical examples of what less anxious parents might do in similar situations so that new parenting habits can develop over time.

ELICIT AND DISCUSS OBSTACLES TO TREATMENT

Throughout this next subsection, we emphasize the practical importance of using much of our time with patients in assessing any potential obstacles to treatment. We first provide the evidence for expecting baseline variable rates of treatment adherence, then review patient-level barriers to treatment adherence for both children and adolescents, and finally assess the role that stigma of psychiatric illness might play in treatment adherence.

When we are treating our patients using the culturally informed biopsychosocial model, our role is to recommend treatment plans, monitor them, and edit them as needed. No treatment plan, however well conceived and constructed, can elicit expected results if not adopted by the patient and their family. Furthermore, within the limitations of our era, the best treatments may or may not work well enough even if scrupulously applied, and they rarely are. Many aspects of the psychopathology we treat as mental health providers are often familial and can impact motivation, emotional regulation, and cognition in one or more family members, all of whom can affect patient treatment adherence. Additionally, we know that psychiatric disorders we treat in child mental health, such as ADHD, are often highly comorbid with other psychiatric disorders (Sun et al. 2019), which may further complicate and interfere with treatment plans in one form or another, as when a medication to treat inattention exacerbates anxiety or a medication to treat depression in a patient with autism spectrum disorder increases aggression. Finally, the stigma associated with a psychiatric illness treated with psychopharmacology exceeds the stigma of psychiatric illness itself (Hinshaw 2010), a common but often underexplored or misunderstood factor in nonadherence to medications, especially in adolescents, who already struggle with identity and norms. As such, it is important to discuss new and ongoing obstacles to treatment plans during the appointment.

When adherence is being discussed, it is important to first note the terminology used (Hack and Chow 2001; Kyngas et al. 2000; Muzina et al. 2011). To physicians, *compliance* often refers to "the extent to which a person's behavior (in terms of taking medication, following diets, or executing life-style changes) coincides with medical or health advice" (Kyngas et al. 2000). *Compliance* is also a word that implies a submission of the patient to the plan. By using the term *adherence* instead, the importance of the therapeutic alliance developed by the physician with the patient to collectively enact a treatment plan is underscored (Hack and Chow 2001; Kyngas et al. 2000; Muzina et al. 2011). This rapport building and development of the therapeutic alliance takes time, both within a session and longitudinally over the course of treatment (Pappadopulos et al. 2009). Adherence thus appropriately places the onus on the physician to optimize the treatment plan, not only in selecting the most appropriate medication but also in building a structural environment in which this treatment plan can be enacted.

We take the time here to discuss the importance of compassionately evaluating adherence to a treatment plan because we know that reported rates of adherence are extremely variable, from as low as 10% to as high as 90% (Hack and Chow 2001; Nagae et al. 2015; Townsend et al. 2009). Nonadherence is a pervasive issue and is better studied in adult psychiatric patients than in child and adolescent psychiatric patients, with approximately half of adult patients discontinuing a new antidepressant within 3 months (Muzina et al. 2011). We know less about the epidemiology of nonadherence in pediatric patients. In a review of the pediatric psychopharmacology literature, Hack and Chow (2001) found that the only peer-reviewed articles assessing adherence focused on ADHD medications. Within that literature, adherence ranged from 35% when only teachers and parents were asked, to 91% when the patients themselves provided reports. Ultimately, they concluded that adherence to psychiatric medications is similar to, but slightly worse than, adherence to nonpsychiatric medications. Swanson (2003) similarly found highly variable rates of stimulant nonadherence, in the range of 20% to 65%.

Adult studies have identified nonadherence as being strongly associated with relapse in adults affected by severe mental illness (Townsend et al. 2009). With this knowledge in hand, we need to devote much of our initial appointment, and then continually in follow-up visits, to addressing questions and concerns from the patient and their family that may signal ambivalence to treatment and herald nonadherence. Lack of adherence to prescribed medication—and thus the likely inefficacy of treatment—often leads to increased suffering (Pappadopulos et al. 2009), burden, and health care costs, as well as further therapeutic interventions (Niemeyer et al. 2018). Although a dearth of systematic evidence in pediatric psychopharmacology prevents us from citing a study involving children, a study of adults (Niemeyer et al. 2018) concluded that explicit instructions on expected duration of treatment and side effects reduced selective serotonin reuptake inhibitor discontinuation and that patients with three or more follow-up visits were more likely to continue the initially prescribed antidepressant medication. Furthermore, whereas shorter and more infrequent doctor appointments correlate with poorer adherence, those that are long enough to allow for questions and answers improve adherence and outcomes (Hack and Chow 2001).

Several studies have looked at patient-level factors that can precipitate nonadherence. Swanson (2003) determined that children and adolescents are reluctant to take medications, often because of social stigma. Nagae et al. (2015) found several factors that decreased medication adherence, leading to more severe psychiatric symptoms, declining academic performance, and familial stress. These factors included presence of comorbidity, adverse reactions to medications, the social stigma relating to psychotropic medications and "needing" a medication, and family struggles (Nagae et al. 2015). Additionally, Hack and Chow (2001) took time to explore this phenomenon in adolescents, noting additional mediators of adherence, including adolescent desire for separation, individuation, and control. The study highlighted important issues, including familial dysfunction with poor parent-child communication, as well as parents who are dissatisfied with their physicians, as leading to less adherence.

Finally, Niemeyer et al. (2018) explored the cross-disorder factors that influence adherence in adolescent patients. Those who were not completely adherent were more likely to report lack of ability to improve symptoms on their own, constricted physician-patient communication, limited trust in their physician, limited family knowledge about the adolescent's disorder, and negative change of attitude toward medication because of adverse effects. Townsend et al. (2009) also agree that certain unique developmental concerns arise with adolescents, to the point that when adapting their adherence measurement tool, the Drug Attitude Inventory, to the adolescent population, they needed to create additional items reflecting autonomy concerns, diagnostic characteristics, treatment length, and side effect profiles specifically relevant to the adolescent experience (especially weight gain) (Townsend et al. 2009). Finally, Kyngas et al. (2000) comment on the specifically difficult conundrum of the unique experience of an adolescent coping with a chronic illness. Although those authors discuss how this may relate to nonpsychiatric chronic illnesses, such as asthma and diabetes, the implications for a chronic illness such as depression and anxiety remain: there is a negative sense from the adolescent of being different and sensing shame. Thus, a higher risk than in adults of stigma-related social withdrawal exists at an age when being different is viewed with great ambivalence, and this interacts negatively with psychiatric illnesses that already predispose to isolation (Kyngas et al. 2000). Similarly, when the clinician is discussing common adolescent topics such as substance use with an anxious or depressed adolescent, it is important to address the risks of destabilizing the patient's psychiatric illnesses. Clearly, this stage of development relates to autonomy, experimentation, and individuation, all of which are important to validate when adherence to a treatment plan is being considered.

Patients and families also can have concerns over safety and long-term effects of treatment, concerns about unpleasant effects associated with treatment, attitudes toward medication, or unfavorable socioeconomic factors in the way of affording medication (Swanson 2003). Additional factors may be involved. In a 3-year longitudinal study of children with ADHD, the significant moderators of adherence included younger age (presumably less adolescent individuation and more cooperation with parents) and fewer symptoms at school. However, response to treatment at 12 months was not a mediator of stimulant adherence, indicating that we as mental health providers must avoid believing the falsehood that if the medications we prescribe help, they will necessarily be taken.

Although we have discussed understanding and assessing adherence, it is important to emphasize the energy it takes within a given appointment to improve medication adherence. Hack and Chow (2001) support this notion and strongly recommend scheduling enough time for office visits so that patients and their families can be actively engaged in building a treatment plan, and not simply be passive recipients, to improve the treatment alliance. Because studies have shown that only 50% of a doctor's instructions are recalled immediately after a visit (Hack and Chow 2001), we take the time to provide written instructions and explanations of the medication regimen and make any other recommendations such as websites for resources, psychotherapy information, or support group numbers. Additionally, it is extremely useful to give patients sufficient time by themselves and (at a certain age) to ask them their views on medications and what effects (both positive and negative) they think medications are causing and for any other insights they may have. Only by gathering this information, as well as psychosocial information to ensure timing of the dosages, cost of the medication, and prior experiences with medication, can the mental health provider construct a treatment plan with the highest odds of success for the particular patient.

Relatedly, we recommend frank discussion of mental illness stigma with peri- and postpubertal patients. Our understanding of mental illness has come a long way toward a recent trend over the past few decades favoring primarily biomedical explanations (Lebowitz and Appelbaum 2019). Studies have remained conflicted on the effects of using a biomedical explanation describing psychiatric disorders as brain-based illnesses. Although some studies have found that biomedical explanations produce lower feelings of helplessness than do cognitive-behavioral explanations (Lebowitz and Appelbaum 2019), other studies have found that the more that is attributed to genetics and biochemical causes, the longer patients expect to be psychiatrically ill, which engenders a sense of determinism and immutability (Lebowitz and Appelbaum 2019; Ojio et al. 2019).

Overall, however, we have seen that by spending time to provide a culturally informed biopsychosocial explanation of mental illness—how it is based in genetics and neuroconnectivity but also influenced by cultural norms, psychological traits, and social situations—we can provide, with most of the patients we see, models of psychopathology in which patients and their families will experience themselves not as passive enactors of defective genomes or nature but rather as important participants in influencing nature to move themselves or their families toward less suffering and impairment. This can take time because symptom exacerbations are difficult to endure and sometimes lead families and patients to question the heuristic models we offer. We often have to patiently repeat and re-explain these models to justify why the family collaboration with our recommended plan is critical to success.

REVIEW MEDICATION EFFICACY AND SIDE EFFECTS

Medication Efficacy

Another major aspect of our patient appointment is reviewing the evidence for or against a particular treatment option if we are starting or changing a treatment plan, or alerting the patient to identified change patterns we observe over time. Regarding the former, to build toward informed consent, we use the strength of evidence-based medicine when available and explain its limitations. Explaining, for example, the superiority of combination treatment with fluoxetine and CBT over either as monotherapy in achieving depression remission (Kennard et al. 2006), and then explaining why this particular trial may or may not apply to the patient's given circumstance, takes time but is important in emphasizing the science of psychiatry. Also, if there is a dearth of data on treatment plans we are suggesting, we make that very explicit. In general, we emphasize optimism about a given treatment plan (Frank 1984) but are practical about the risk of medication nonefficacy or insurmountable side effects. This is also part of alliance building: The offer of hope in things to come can also include an explicit discussion of possible failure before the failure occurs, and having such a discussion can increase the trust that our patients and their families have in us. If they interpret us as guaranteeing treatment efficacy, we risk damaging that trust. Although the field of child and adolescent psychiatry has engaged in research into methods such as pharmacogenetics to predict treatment outcome, we do not currently possess the tools to predict which specific treatment will work best for an individual patient (Wehry et al. 2018). Finally, it has been demonstrated that parental knowledge and opinion play significant roles in the family's decision to enroll in treatment (Corkum et al. 1999). Thus, engaging parents early in order to attend to the dual alliance (to both patient and parent) in pharmacotherapy is crucially important (Joshi 2006), and providing the evidence for efficacy can start that initial process of buy-in.

In addition to providing cohort-level data on efficacy of certain treatment plans, we find it extremely valuable to make explicit the individual-level changes we observe in the given patient. We believe it is very important to carve out time to discuss how macroscopic-level evidence may apply—or not—to the patient's individual situation. We have found that pointing out how the patient's specific demographic and psychological attributes—age, ethnocultural context, socioeconomic status, psychiatric comorbidity—need to be taken into account helps to build alliance, allay concerns, and strengthen adherence. Although it is often easy for a patient and their family to get bogged down by the daily struggles of psychiatric illness, we point out that from our vantage point as providers who receive interval updates from many families, it is often easier to take a bigger-picture point of view. Hack and Chow (2001) highlighted that mothers' recognition of improvement in their children's symptoms after visiting psychiatrists can also lead to improving children's medication adherence (Hack and Chow 2001). Even strategies such as showcasing responses from measurement forms, such as the Screen for Child Anxiety Related Disorders (SCARED), completed before and after treatment as a way to demonstrate objective, tangible changes, can be extremely valuable. Explaining study sample– and individual-level efficacy is thus an important strategy in maintaining the alliance and improving the odds of successful treatment.

Benefits and Side Effects

When we start to consider a certain pharmacological treatment plan, we believe it is critical to start gaining informed assent from the patient in addition to the required consent from the caregiver. Although there is no universal guideline to assess for decision-making capabilities of adolescents (Garanito and Zaher-Rutherford 2019), we still find it important to include the pediatric patient in this process, allowing for exceptions in cases of developmental limitations (e.g., a very young child or a severely cognitively disabled child). In obtaining consent from the family, we discuss the risks of treating, and, just as important, the risks of not treating, a patient pharmacologically, the benefits, alternatives to treatment, and side effects of treatments. Obtaining assent from a minor, we believe, is just as important so we can assess the understanding by the individual patient of the implications of their psychopathology and the potential benefits of resulting treatment (Koelch and Fegert 2010; Unguru et al. 2008). We want to know what the symptoms mean to the patient: Why does he or she have them? Where do the symptoms come from, and what causes them? As discussed earlier, the child or adolescent is the most important agent determining adherence, especially as he or she gets older.

The psychopharmacology we deploy most commonly as mental health clinicians ranges in its side effects from relatively benign gastrointestinal side effects (Cousins and Goodyer 2015) to more severe side effects, including seizures (Schwasinger-Schmidt and Macaluso 2019), Stevens-Johnson syndrome (Wang et al. 2015), and suicidality (Sharma et al. 2016). Additionally, the mean number of televised antidepressant commercials seen per year by U.S. adults is 85 (Lebowitz and Appelbaum 2019). Therefore, part of the time of our appointments includes dispelling myths, as well as more accurately putting risks and benefits into clinically meaningful perspectives. Finally, chronic medications and polypharmacy are becoming more common and prevalent (Feinstein et al. 2019), and thus, evaluating for medication interactions, as well as considering possible ways to reduce polypharmacy, is crucial. All of these steps serve to further strengthen the treatment alliance, assuage concerns, and allow clinicians to assess the true concerns of a patient instead of those perceived by the parent or the prescriber.

MAKE DECISIONS AND HAVE A DISCUSSION ABOUT MAINTAINING OR CHANGING COURSE OF TREATMENT

Finally, our appointments end with joint decision making (Halpern 2018; Hubner et al. 2018; Kon 2010), when choosing whether to maintain or change the course of treatment. First, we use the information gathered from updates to the patient's story, including new medical conditions, new medications, new or ongoing barriers to adherence, and perception of psychopathology. While we elicit updates from the patient individually before asking for observations from the caregiver, we also use our mental status exam to determine integral changes in the child or adolescent's understanding, affect, cognition, or behavior. Weighing all these factors with each visit as part of the assessment of children and adolescents (King et al. 1997) is crucial in incrementally developing an individualized treatment plan. By building on each of the previous steps, we can make our case for any new proposed treatment options while also developing and maintaining rapport with the family and patient and gaining buy-in. Although changes to the initial plan often occur, these factors allow physician, patient, and family to make a collective decision about staying on course versus adopting a new course of treatment.

ANSWER ADDITIONAL QUESTIONS

Before concluding our session, it is imperative to answer any additional questions our patient and their family may have. This helps to tie in previous steps of rapport building and tending, as well as joint decision-making. If necessary, we will also utilize documentation of the answers to their questions and treatment plans, as above, in order to close the loop of communication and provide clear instructions.

Discussion and Areas for Future Research

As noted previously, the realities of the "med check" appointment often exist to ensure that scheduling needs and reimbursement targets are met (Ghaemi et al. 2018). However, child and adolescent patients and their families benefit most from longer and more comprehensive appointments. We structure our follow-up appointments as 30-minute "brief pharmacotherapy visits" that permit us to conduct a more humanistic approach to both the science and the art of psychopharmacology. The time spent with patients and their families, often with complex psychosocial stories, helps us to develop and nurture a therapeutic relationship and tailor more individualized treatment plans, as well as present them in ways that are more likely to register. Although we do not practice strict, manualized psychotherapy, the information we glean from our encounters often plays a large role in informing medication selection and adjustment. In many cases, too, this approach avoids unnecessary dose titrations or polypharmacy if we can contextualize a patient's reported decompensation, for example.

Much research is needed in this area. From an academic standpoint, much of the work done thus far on medication adherence comes from adult populations. Youth populations (including children, teens, and transition-age youth) deserve to be the focus of further research to see how development, caretaker factors, psychoeducation, and many other variables affect adherence and response to treatment.

Although the field of psychiatry—and of psychopharmacology specifically—has taken great steps forward, we must remember a quote from William Osler:

> Diagnosis, not drugging, is our chief weapon of offence. Lack of systematic personal training in the methods of the recognition of disease leads to the misapplication of remedies, to long courses of treatment when treatment is useless, and so directly to that lack of confidence in our methods which is apt to place us in the eyes of the public on a level with empirics and quacks." (Ghaemi 2008, p. 192)

TAKE-AWAY POINTS

- Brief pharmacotherapy visits as short as 30 minutes can allow for a thorough reassessment of several factors, which can lead to improvement in patient well-being. It is important to use a culturally informed biopsychosocial formulation—one that accounts for the patient's cultural context and genetic, psychological, and environmental factors—to craft and adjust a treatment plan with the best chance of acceptability to both patient and family.

- The evaluation of a patient's adherence to a treatment plan and of the barriers influencing this adherence requires time and finesse. This evaluation is most effective when done in the context of a fully developed therapeutic alliance, not only with the patient but also with the parents or other caregivers.

- The term "med check" is oversimplified and inaccurate because it does not capture the elements of the most effective treatment planning approaches; a more meaningful and relevant term is "brief pharmacotherapy visit" because this more aptly describes the time-limited, focused, and therapeutic nature of both the art and science of child and adolescent psychopharmacology.

References

Ahmadzadeh YI, Eley TC, Leve LD, et al: Anxiety in the family: a genetically informed analysis of transactional associations between mother, father and child anxiety symptoms. J Child Psychol Psychiatry 60(12):1269–1277, 2019 31106427

American Psychiatric Association: Diagnostic and Statistical Manual of Mental Disorders, 4th Edition. Washington, DC, American Psychiatric Association, 1994

American Psychiatric Association: Diagnostic and Statistical Manual of Mental Disorders, 5th Edition. Arlington, VA, American Psychiatric Association, 2013

Corkum P, Rimer P, Schachar R: Parental knowledge of attention-deficit hyperactivity disorder and opinions of treatment options: impact on enrollment and adherence to a 12-month treatment trial. Can J Psychiatry 44(10):1043–1048, 1999 10637684

Cousins L, Goodyer IM: Antidepressants and the adolescent brain. J Psychopharmacol 29(5):545–555, 2015 25744620

Cunningham AM, Walker DM, Nestler EJ: Paternal transgenerational epigenetic mechanisms mediating stress phenotypes of offspring. Eur J Neurosci 53(1):271–280, 2019

Feinstein JA, Hall M, Antoon JW, et al: Chronic medication use in children insured by Medicaid: a multistate retrospective cohort study. Pediatrics 143(4):e20183397, 2019 30914443

Frank J: Interview with Jerome Frank, Ph.D., M.D. Exploring concepts of influence, persuasion, and healing. J Psychosoc Nurs Ment Health Serv 22(9):32–34, 36–37, 1984 6567665

Garanito MP, Zaher-Rutherford VL: Adolescent patients and the clinical decision about their health. Rev Paul Pediatr 37(4):503–509, 2019 31241694

Ghaemi SN: Toward a Hippocratic psychopharmacology. Can J Psychiatry 53(3):189–196, 2008 18441665

Ghaemi SN, Glick ID, Ellison JM: A commentary on existential psychopharmacologic clinical practice: advocating a humanistic approach to the "med check." J Clin Psychiatry 79(4):1–2, 2018 29701934

Hack S, Chow B: Pediatric psychotropic medication compliance: a literature review and research-based suggestions for improving treatment compliance. J Child Adolesc Psychopharmacol 11(1):59–67, 2001 11322747

Halpern J: Creating the safety and respect necessary for "shared" decision-making. Pediatrics 142 (suppl 3):S163–S169, 2018 30385623

Hinshaw SP: The Mark of Shame: Stigma of Mental Illness and an Agenda for Change. New York, Oxford University Press, 2010

Hubner LM, Feldman HM, Huffman LC: Parent communication prompt to increase shared decision-making: a new intervention approach. Front Pediatr 6:60, 2018 29616204

Joshi SV: Teamwork: the therapeutic alliance in pediatric pharmacotherapy. Child Adolesc Psychiatr Clin N Am 15(1):239–262, 2006 16321733

Kalman TP: A failure to communicate: psychiatry's split-care experience. Lancet Psychiatry 2(11):e28, 2015 26544752

Kennard B, Silva S, Vitiello B, et al: Remission and residual symptoms after short-term treatment in the Treatment of Adolescents with Depression Study (TADS). J Am Acad Child Adolesc Psychiatry 45(12):1404–1411, 2006 17135985

King RA: Practice parameters for the psychiatric assessment of children and adolescents. J Am Acad Child Adolesc Psychiatry 36(10, suppl):4S–20S, 1997 9606102

Koelch M, Fegert JM: Ethics in child and adolescent psychiatric care: an international perspective. Int Rev Psychiatry 22(3):258–266, 2010 20528655

Kon AA: The shared decision-making continuum. JAMA 304(8):903–904, 2010 20736477

Kyngas HA, Kroll T, Duffy ME: Compliance in adolescents with chronic diseases: a review. J Adolesc Health 26(6):379–388, 2000 10822178

Lebowitz MS, Appelbaum PS: Biomedical explanations of psychopathology and their implications for attitudes and beliefs about mental disorders. Annu Rev Clin Psychol 15:555–577, 2019 30444641

Muzina DJ, Malone DA, Bhandari I, et al: Rate of non-adherence prior to upward dose titration in previously stable antidepressant users. J Affect Disord 130(1–2):46–52, 2011 20950862

Nagae M, Nakane H, Honda S, et al: Factors affecting medication adherence in children receiving outpatient pharmacotherapy and parental adherence. J Child Adolesc Psychiatr Nurs 28(2):109–117, 2015 25989262

Niemeyer L, Schumm L, Mechler K, et al: "When I stop my medication, everything goes wrong": content analysis of interviews with adolescent patients treated with psychotropic medication. J Child Adolesc Psychopharmacol 28(9):655–662, 2018 30148662

Ojio Y, Yamaguchi S, Ohta K, et al: Effects of biomedical messages and expert-recommended messages on reducing mental health-related stigma: a randomised controlled trial. Epidemiol Psychiatr Sci 29:e74, 2019 31753045

Pappadopulos E, Jensen PS, Chait AR, et al: Medication adherence in the MTA: saliva methylphenidate samples versus parent report and mediating effect of concomitant behavioral treatment. J Am Acad Child Adolesc Psychiatry 48(5):501–510, 2009 19307987

Schwasinger-Schmidt TE, Macaluso M: Other antidepressants. Handb Exp Pharmacol 250:325–355, 2019 30194544

Sharma T, Guski LS, Freund N, Gøtzsche PC: Suicidality and aggression during antidepressant treatment: systematic review and meta-analyses based on clinical study reports. BMJ 352:i65, 2016 26819231

Sun S, Kuja-Halkola R, Faraone SV, et al: Association of psychiatric comorbidity with the risk of premature death among children and adults with attention-deficit/hyperactivity disorder. JAMA Psychiatry 76(11):1141–1149, 2019 31389973

Swanson J: Compliance with stimulants for attention-deficit/hyperactivity disorder: issues and approaches for improvement. CNS Drugs 17(2):117–131, 2003 12521359

Torrey WC, Griesemer I, Carpenter-Song EA: Beyond "med management." Psychiatr Serv 68(6):618–620, 2017 28245703

Townsend L, Floersch J, Findling RL: Adolescent attitudes toward psychiatric medication: the utility of the Drug Attitude Inventory. J Child Psychol Psychiatry 50(12):1523–1531, 2009 19686336

Unguru Y, Coppes MJ, Kamani N: Rethinking pediatric assent: from requirement to ideal. Pediatr Clin North Am 55(1):211–222, 2008 18242322

Vázquez GH: The impact of psychopharmacology on contemporary clinical psychiatry. Can J Psychiatry 59(8):412–416, 2014 25161065

Wang XQ, Xiong J, Xu WH, et al: Risk of a lamotrigine-related skin rash: current meta-analysis and postmarketing cohort analysis. Seizure 25:52–61, 2015 25645637

Wehry AM, Ramsey L, Dulemba SE, et al: Pharmacogenomic testing in child and adolescent psychiatry: an evidence-based review. Curr Probl Pediatr Adolesc Health Care 48(2):40–49, 2018 29325731

CHAPTER 7

PHARMACOTHERAPY OR PSYCHOPHARMACOTHERAPY

When Therapist and Pharmacologist Are Different People—or the Same Person

Mari Kurahashi, M.D., M.P.H.

Elizabeth Reichert, Ph.D.

Nithya Mani, M.D.

David S. Hong, M.D.

Mental health issues in children and adolescents are highly prevalent, and the demand for specialized psychiatric services continues to steadily increase. From a systems perspective, there are comprehensive challenges in meeting this critical clinical need within the context of limited resources and the supply of trained clinicians. As a result, various models of care have been developed to adapt to these demands, reflecting the changing face of child and adolescent psychiatric practice. These include, in ambulatory care settings, the integrated treatment model, in which both psychotherapy and pharmacotherapy are administered by a single provider, contrasting with a "split treatment" or interdisciplinary model, in which psychiatric care is divided among a team of clinical providers, with the most common iteration comprising a psychiatrist managing pharmacotherapy in conjunction with a therapist delivering psychotherapy. Although other chapters in this book address the various aspects of alliance, transference, and meaning of medication inherent to the psychology of pharmacotherapy, these themes take on an added degree of complexity when we explicitly consider the dual roles of these clinical functions within the clinician-patient relationship, particularly when these provider roles are filled by different people. The additional complexities and contrast between these models are explored within this chapter.

To provide a historical context, the current delivery of child and adolescent psychiatric care reflects an ongoing evolution in psychiatric practice. For the first half of the twentieth century, the predominant model of treatment for "neurotic" conditions that did not require institutionalization was centered on Freudian approaches to psychoanalysis, conducted primarily by psychiatrists (Reidbord 2014). When psychotropic medications were first widely introduced in the 1950s, there was a significant concern that psychopharmacology would act to suppress symptomatology, potentially interfering with access to psychic conflict and preventing resolution of underlying psychodynamic causes of psychiatric conditions. Later, in the 1960s and 1970s, behavioral therapists similarly voiced concerns that pharmacological relief of symptoms would prevent acquisition of new behaviors (Koenig et al. 2013). Nevertheless, meprobamate, a tranquilizer marketed as an "emotional aspirin," became the best-selling drug in America within 1 year of its introduction in 1955, while Valium, which was introduced in 1963, became the most commonly prescribed medication from 1964 to 1982 (Groopman 2019), reflecting the rapid establishment of psychopharmacology as a mainstay of psychiatric treatment. Randomized clinical trials subsequently enacted since the 1980s provided empirical support that pharmacotherapy could be efficacious for patients with a range of psychiatric conditions. Many of these studies demonstrated additional efficacy when using combined treatment with psychotherapy and pharmacotherapy, leading to wider acceptance of combined treatment by the 1990s.

Today, combined treatment is often the consensus recommendation for most moderate to severe psychiatric conditions, including in psychiatric disorders in youth, ranging from depression and anxiety to obsessive-compulsive disorder. Data from the U.S. Centers for Disease Control and Prevention indicate that 7.5% of children ages 6–17 years received a prescription medication for emotional or behavioral difficulties over a 6-month period (Howie et al. 2014) and about 4% of adolescents ages 12–17 years received some form of nonmedication mental health services in that period (Jones et al. 2014), broadly defined as counseling services across school, clinic, emergency, and inpatient settings. These staggering numbers indicate the degree to which combined treatment has impacted utilization of youth psychiatry services. Over the past years, the split treatment model has increasingly become the standard model for delivery of combined treatment. It has been posited that this shift has been driven in large part by managed care companies citing the economic benefits of this arrangement, though limited evidence contrasting economic measures of split versus integrated treatment has not identified a clear benefit of one delivery system relative to the other. Other contributing factors may also include the relative shortage of child and adolescent psychiatrists to meet demand for services and evolving standards in child and adolescent psychiatry fellowship training to fully master pharmacotherapy and psychotherapy competencies, among others.

Overall, the increase in split treatment delivery has understandably resulted in robust discussion around implementation and efficacy, as well as ongoing relevant concerns reflecting the aforementioned long-standing themes regarding the psychology of aligning pharmacotherapeutic and psychotherapeutic principles across both models (Miklowitz and Gitlin 2014). The few studies on the topic suggest that split treatment approaches are similar to integrated treatment with regard to patient satisfaction and treatment adherence (Baruch and Annunziato 2017; Jacobs 2005). However, each context presents unique clinical challenges, particularly with respect to navigating the psychology of psychopharmacology within each context.

Developmental Considerations

The sparse literature examining integrated and split treatment models is limited to the study of adult populations. Although some principles from adult practice may simply be extrapolated to child and adolescent psychiatric practice, a number of unique needs also warrant separate consideration. Indeed, childhood and adolescence represent stages of rapid cognitive, emotional, and behavioral maturation, with a large impact on treatment factors. When one is considering differences between integrated and split treatment in youth, developmental considerations play a more central role. As an example, the cognitive stage of a child may influence the selection of a therapy modality, particularly when considering the degree of psychoeducation needed for both therapeutic and psychopharmacological interventions. Additionally, the manner in which younger children integrate their understanding of illness into their sense of self may further affect how split or integrated treatment modalities are delivered, as well as the potential benefit of one modality over the other. In contrast, more developed cognitive maturation may allow adolescents to navigate integrated or split treatment models with greater agency, given their understanding of the differing treatment modalities and prescriber-therapist roles. In fact, it is not uncommon in child and adolescent psychiatry for youth to be referred for psychiatric care by parents without a full understanding of the presenting problem or need for treatment. In many cases, engagement in either treatment model is often their first exposure to mental health intervention, with only limited understanding of the roles of the psychiatrist or therapist, requiring thoughtfulness in how treatment is implemented.

Developmental differences impact core aspects of treatment, including alliance, engagement, and symptom reporting, which may manifest in integrated and split treatment models differently. As an example, one major developmental task of adolescence is individuation: In an integrated setting, this may lead to rejection of treatment recommendations in an integrated format if the adolescent feels the provider and parents are overly aligned. However, in a split treatment approach, the adolescent may align more with the provider she believes her parents are less inclined to support, complicating delivery of care. Indeed, psychiatric care in youth extends beyond the identified patient and necessarily encompasses the entire family system. As such, parents and children may provide a different narration of symptoms and have different perceptions of privacy and confidentiality, which may also impact treatment planning and selection. This paradigm extends further into the systems in which youth interact and where symptoms manifest, which often include school environments. For both integrated and split treatment providers, these factors represent additional challenges regarding coordination of care and management of information flow. In integrated care, communicating with parents and schools may be more straightforward, but a split treatment model may require additional layers of coordination to ensure the highest delivery of care.

Implications for Treatment

The totality of these factors should be considered in both integrated and split treatment models. Unsurprisingly, a review of the literature comparing these treatment modalities in adult psychiatric practice indicates that a primary predictor of satisfaction, regardless of treatment model, is therapeutic alliance (Goldman et al. 1998). It would be reasonable to infer that these principles are similarly relevant in working with youth. Here, we further explore themes of alliance and transference and countertransference as they pertain to psychopharmacotherapy (integrated) and pharmacotherapy (split) treatment models in child and adolescent psychiatry.

ALLIANCE

Decades of research have established that the strength of the therapeutic alliance between patient and clinician has a profound impact on outcomes in both psychotherapeutic and psychopharmacological treatment modalities (Krupnick et al. 1996). This confirmation of the importance of the therapeutic alliance can be traced back to Freudian theories of transference, in which unconscious feelings toward primary caregivers were projected onto the therapist and were thought of as a negative therapeutic interference. Freud then expanded the idea of the relationship between the patient and therapist to include an understanding of the potential benefits of an attachment between the therapist and patient. Subsequent psychological theories made a distinction between transference and therapeutic alliance, in which *alliance* is defined as a reality-based collaboration between patient and therapist rather than projections from childhood experiences (Greenson 1965). Rogers (1951) defined the active components in the therapeutic relationship to include empathy, congruence, and unconditional positive regard with an emphasis on the therapist's active role in the relationship, which was important in client-centered therapy. Strong (1968) emphasized the patient's confidence in the therapist's competence and adherence as an important factor in the therapist's being able to influence the patient enough to elicit change. Bordin (1979) elaborated on the definition of the therapeutic alliance so it could be applicable to any therapeutic approach by naming the three core elements that make up the therapeutic alliance: agreement on the treatment goals, agreement on the tasks, and the development of a personal bond between the clinician and patient that was based on reciprocal positive feelings.

Integrated Treatment

Keeping these core principles of alliance in mind, there are potential advantages to achieving these benchmarks within an integrated model (Figure 7–1). These include less complexity in establishment of treatment

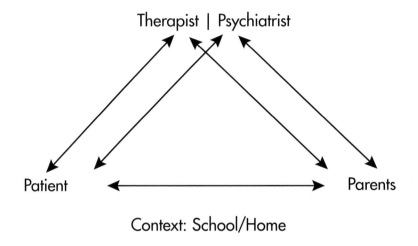

Figure 7–1.   Integrated treatment model.

goals and reaching consensus within the child-family-provider system with regard to the treatment process. The integration of both psychotherapy and pharmacotherapy within the same provider largely reduces logistical and psychological obstacles in initial formation of the alliance and may moderate subsequent stresses on that bond during treatment. One consideration is that increased visits with the same provider may influence clinical outcomes: meta-analyses have indicated that increased frequency of visits with a clinician improves treatment outcomes in psychotherapy (Falkenström et al. 2016) and medication management (Rutherford et al. 2014). Although higher frequency of visits may be achieved in both integrated and split treatment paradigms, the impact of accomplishing treatment goals with a single provider, rather than multiple providers, merits future consideration.

CASE EXAMPLE

A 15-year-old adolescent has seen multiple therapists and psychiatrists from the age of 11 years for the treatment of depression and anxiety. She and her parents are frustrated by her limited symptom relief over the years. They were recently referred by a family friend to a psychiatrist who specializes in treatment of anxiety and depression, including extensive experience with psychotherapy. The parents and teen are thoughtful and engaged in treatment during the intake process. When discussing past psychiatric treatment, they relay challenges with prior providers, including their most recent experience of receiving conflicting recommendations from their therapist and psychiatrist, leading to confusion about the treatment process and prompting them to present for a second opinion and possible transfer of care.

Split Treatment

In the split treatment model (Figure 7–2), a series of therapeutic relationships are cultivated: therapist-patient, psychiatrist-patient, therapist-psychiatrist. Busch and Gould (1993) refer to this as the "therapeutic triangle." In each relationship, the development of a strong therapeutic alliance or "triadic therapeutic alliance" is targeted (Kahn 1991). Goin (2001) equates this to the parent-child relationship, emphasizing the importance of mutual respect and communication between providers, with the shared goal of providing adequate care and concern for the child. Within the context of child and adolescent psychiatry, this model should be extended to further include parents as another member of the therapeutic system. The multiple directions of communication required in this treatment approach may inadvertently increase the complexity of providing any treatment because of increased dimensions of interpersonal dynamics between both providers, the family, and the identified patient. As such, the development of a robust therapeutic alliance is of equal importance within split treatment and necessarily includes both clinical providers and patient, as well as the parent or other caregiver. Although the core components of alignment and congruence, empathic understanding, and unconditional acceptance of the patient's experience are unchanged, these factors must now be implemented in a balanced way across multiple clinical providers. A critical aspect of maintaining these principles in split treatment is the necessity of clear role definitions across all aspects of treatment delivery, from engagement in care through to termination.

Various factors may impact the strength of the triadic (or tetradic) alliance, leading to differing degrees of rapport across relationships. Variability in visit frequency and the content of sessions have the potential to influence alliances within this structure. Cultivating a shared respect between providers and between the patient and each provider and maintaining clear lines of communication can substantially support the strength of the triadic alliance. When challenges arise in either relationship that lead to rupture in therapeutic alliance, the split model may minimize the impact on the patient because the alliance with the other provider may not be impacted, thereby providing a measure of resilience in the care delivery system. An example within the context of split treatment is when a patient disagrees with a medication-related recommendation from his psychiatrist, which may impact his relationship with the psy-

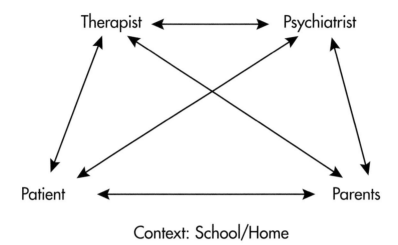

Figure 7–2.   Split treatment model.

chiatrist but not the therapist. Alternatively, when patients experience a dramatic shift in symptoms after starting medication, they may feel less connected or motivated to engage with their therapists. Additionally, the split model can offer professional and emotional support within the treatment system, particularly between providers, which in turn may improve clinical outcomes for patients and families when the therapist-psychiatrist relationship is synergistic—and may negatively impact care when it is antagonistic. Mutual respect and a collaborative stance are key to facilitating the alliance between providers. Especially with high-acuity cases, interdisciplinary care can help to alleviate the burden on a single provider, facilitate increases in visit frequency, and allow enactment of multiple clinical strategies simultaneously. Adequate transfer of important information may also help with monitoring treatment progress while evaluating risk factors that may impact the treatment planning and timing of both pharmacological and psychotherapeutic interventions— for example, when choosing which medication to prescribe or deciding when to begin behavioral exposures within therapy. There is robust evidence for the efficacy of combined psychotherapy and medication treatment compared with medication treatment alone in a number of psychiatric conditions in youth, and there is no evidence to suggest that pharmacotherapy undermines psychotherapy efficacy (Gitlin and Miklowitz 2016). Furthermore, when two providers are involved, each is able to devote the entire session toward the patient's therapeutic goals specific to the type of appointment, perhaps allowing fewer distractions and more focus on each treatment modality. This can alleviate the potential burden of balancing dual functions in psychopharmacotherapy (integrated treatment) and allow each provider to concentrate more fully on one particular set of goals.

CASE EXAMPLE

An outgoing 16-year-old adolescent with ADHD was seeing a psychiatrist for treatment with psychostimulants, which appeared to have a positive effect on his symptoms of inattention. The teen and his parents respected the psychiatrist's expertise and knowledge of psychiatric medications yet also felt intimidated at times by a singular focus on pharmacological aspects of the treatment plan. The mother observed certain features in her son's behavior that made her wonder if he struggled with anxiety as she did herself, and she made an appointment with a psychologist. The teen quickly established rapport in the therapy setting and together with the therapist determined he experienced generalized anxiety. The psychologist and psychiatrist often shared patients in a split treatment model and communicated via e-mail about their shared patients on a monthly basis with the patients' permission. The providers' mutual formulation indicated the presence of anxiety before psychostimulant treatment, with a worsening at higher doses. Together with the family, it was decided to incorporate cognitive-behavioral therapy into treatment to address anxiety symptoms while trying a lower dose of psychostimulant for ADHD.

TRANSFERENCE, COUNTERTRANSFERENCE, AND TRIANGULATION

Integrated Treatment

An important psychological process that can occur in an integrated model is the transference of the patient and family toward the clinician and his or her dual roles in psychopharmacotherapy. There can be complexity in the patient and family's transference toward the duality of the clinician's roles and the related psychological meaning embedded in the different treatments being provided. When both treatments are administered by the same provider, a conflicted perception or experience of one treatment may similarly negatively impact the experience of the other treatment modality, as well as overall transference toward the provider, such as changing perceptions of the clinician's competency or regard for the patient. An additional focus in integrated treatment is managing potential confusion about the biological and psychosocial focus of two different treatment modalities. On the other hand, positive transference may be leveraged to reinforce adherence to the parallel treatment recommendations (e.g., the practice of taking medication daily that is prescribed by the therapist may serve as a reminder to practice therapeutic goals as well). In these ways, integrated models may facilitate psychopharmacotherapy through a synergistic approach to both medication and therapy goals. Additionally, from a psychodynamic perspective, a therapist prescribing medication can be thought of as a transitional object for the patient, which may help the patient to internalize aspects of the therapy to further augment the treatment.

Not only is it necessary to be aware of the patient's perspective, but it is also important to be mindful of the clinician's experience. When one provider is filling both roles, it may be difficult to balance both the pharmacotherapy and psychotherapy agendas. Although the overall treatment goals may be the same, the therapeutic actions and agendas may vary, as well as the patient and family's responses. This may include managing countertransference toward patient and family behaviors around adherence and expectations around treatment priorities. The duality of roles should also be considered in the provider's own level of comfort in shifting from psychotherapeutic interventions to medication management. In some instances, this transition can feel abrupt, similar to ending a session on time or discussing any other logistic concerns.

Split Treatment

The opportunity for the patient and family to engage in two therapeutic relationships–one with the therapist and one with the prescriber—may also impact transference. Two providers may offer patients additional infrastructure to receive treatment when implemented effectively. With therapy visits typically occurring weekly and medication appointments having a more flexible follow-up schedule, patients may have weeks when they see more than one provider in 1 week, thereby providing an additional degree of support or a boost in treatment progress when needed. Furthermore, there is the potential to cover more ground in each session because each provider is able to target their respective therapeutic goals as part of the larger treatment plan.

However, the process of triangulation, or splitting, within the therapeutic triangle is a more common risk in the split treatment model. Patients and caregivers can triangulate between providers, and providers themselves have the potential to inadvertently contribute to this triangulation. Splitting is a common defense mechanism in which an individual struggles with integrating the positive and negative qualities of himself or herself or another person in a cohesive, realistic manner, which may result in idealization of one clinician and devaluation of the other. At the same time, even within an integrated model, splitting can occur in other dimensions of the therapeutic triangle, such as when a child splits the clinician and caregiver, caregivers split the clinician and child, and so on. Competition, lack of respect, misalignment of goals, and poor communication can intensify risk for triangulation (Goin 2001). This commonly occurs when the therapist and prescriber differ in their therapeutic approach and overarching treatment goals are misaligned, providing challenges to effective interdisciplinary care that forms the core of effective split treatment. A competitive (not collaborative) relationship may ultimately result in incompatible efforts toward implementing a shared treatment plan.

Additionally, when patients choose to share different information with their respective providers, the risk for triangulation increases. Although common and at times unavoidable, patterns of unequal communication can form quickly. Providers can further contribute to this dynamic when competition is high. Similarly, patients can idealize one provider and undermine the interventions of the other. For instance, unrealistic expectations about the impact medication may have on one's symptoms can contribute to low motivation and engagement in psychotherapy interventions. Providers can feel devalued when they experience their patient as aligning more with the other provider. Additionally, it is common for treatment to be initiated between a patient and one provider before moving toward a collaborative treatment model (e.g., initiating therapy with a psychologist and then adding a psychiatrist to the treatment team). To reduce the propensity for splitting, providers must be sensitive to the previously established provider-patient relationship while balancing the importance of a "fresh perspective."

Transference and countertransference can also occur between two providers. In some cases, a power differential may exist in which one provider holds a more senior role (e.g., clinical director versus clinical staff), or the prescriber may be viewed as the "real doctor" with respect to the type of degree (e.g., M.D. or D.O. vs. Ph.D., Psy.D., M.F.T., L.C.S.W., or other counseling degree/credential), presenting unique challenges that may potentially diminish the likelihood of collaboration and important communication. This can further jeopardize the trust the patient establishes with each provider, leading to greater alignment with one provider than the other. Differing patterns of communication between providers may also increase the risk for splitting. Providers may differ in degree of reciprocity of sharing information (Gitlin and Miklowitz 2016). The therapist, for example, may regularly share updates on the patient's treatment progress and goals, whereas the prescriber may be less inclined to reciprocate, such as failing to share recent medication changes. On the other hand, the prescriber may think the therapist is demanding too much time for collaboration or sharing too many details. An inherent difference in therapist versus prescriber caseloads can contribute to this differential and is one of several factors that should be considered in monitoring countertransference in this relationship.

CASE EXAMPLE

A 15-year-old adolescent with a history of generalized anxiety disorder, major depression, and complicated family dynamics was reluctant to consider medication at his initial therapy intake. He began attending weekly psychotherapy sessions and eventually engaged in discussions with his therapist about the potential utility of medications. After more than 1 year of therapy, he met with a psychiatrist and agreed to add medication to his treatment plan. He experienced some symptom relief with pharmacotherapy; however, his perfectionistic tendencies contributed to a desire to "please" his psychiatrist by presenting a more positive view of his symptoms and family circumstances than what he was truly experiencing. Limited contact with his psychiatrist maintained this dynamic. This behavior resulted in his psychiatrist receiving a more positive review of the patient's functioning, whereas the therapist was often faced with a more negative report. Additionally, the patient's parent was frequently critical of providers when symptoms worsened. Although both providers made efforts to engage in regular communication and shared treatment goals, a sense of competition between providers emerged over the necessary steps to achieve clinical improvement.

Practical Applications and Strategies

Translation of these principles to clinical practice is aimed to improve clinical outcomes when combined treatment (either integrated or split model) is indicated. Although there are currently no specific guidelines for integrated treatment, some clinical recommendations around consultative models may be applicable to both integrated and split treatment modalities (American Psychiatric Association 2009). Among many variations of practical implementation, several components may be of particular relevance to clinicians and are discussed next.

REGULAR AND ROUTINE COMMUNICATION

Communication across various members in the therapeutic triangle supports alliance and positive development of transference and countertransference. With respect to communication with patients and families, clear messaging is important in both treatment modalities. This conversation can be done as part of setting the frame of treatment to help the patient better understand the shifts in treatment modalities. Also, specific to split treatment, providing an agreed-upon cadence between providers to discuss the different issues associated with medication management and psychotherapy enhances clinical outcomes. Coordination of clinical care between providers allows improved clinical outcomes, reduces burden on patients and families, and aligns treatment goals. Unfortunately, practice surveys indicate routine communication is often lacking in clinical treatment (Avena and Kalman 2010; Kalman et al. 2012). Communication with schools and educators is a routine aspect of child psychiatric care: although both providers in a split treatment model will likely obtain collateral information in an intake process, ongoing communication with parties outside of the immediate therapeutic frame should be coordinated. To support this foundation, particularly within the split treatment framework, we recommend the following:

1. Early in treatment, establish a mode of communication between providers that incorporates consent of the patient and family and maintains compliance standards for sensitive information.
2. Determine a cadence of communication between providers, establishing regularity of meetings appropriate for clinical severity and agreeing which scenarios would entail additional communication between intervals. This may prove particularly difficult when providers have to coordinate with those with whom they do not have a previously established relationship.
3. For child and adolescent psychiatry, provide ongoing discussion and sharing of information from relevant collateral sources. This may include teachers, caregivers, and other individuals in the patient's life. For a further discussion of the alliance among providers, parents, and teachers, see Chapter 9 ("The Pharmacotherapeutic Alliance in School Mental Health") of this book.

RESPECT AND COUNTERTRANSFERENCE

There is the potential for one provider to diminish the value of the other provider's interventions, which can interfere with treatment. For example, a therapist may indicate unequivocal recommendations for a particular medication, or a psychiatrist may insist on a particular approach to therapy. In either case, the other provider's efforts are undermined. To manage these dynamics, we recommend the following:

1. Increase the youth's and parents' understanding of provider roles in the treatment system. Brief pharmacotherapy visits and psychotherapy have different cadences with regard to duration of individual appointments, frequency of contact, and so on that are optimal for efficacious delivery of the indicated treatment. A patient-centered approach orients the patient and family to the scope of each provider's function in an interdisciplinary team, allowing a provider to serve a specific role and simultaneously establish boundaries of care delivery that best serve the patient or family.
2. Affirm other providers' expertise, role, and alliance with the family. Recognize potential countertransference within a therapeutic triad, which may reflect power differentials with respect to degree, rank, age, seniority, or gender.
3. Implement strategies to manage countertransference around these domains. Develop an ongoing network of providers with prior positive experiences in shared clinical acumen and effective communication practices. Engage in frequent, structured, and open conversations when establishing new relationships with peer providers.

RESOLVING CONFLICT

Alignment of diagnostic and treatment goals is critical when there is disagreement in the therapeutic triangle (i.e., when there is a competitive rather than a collaborative relationship between providers). In most cases, a conflictual dynamic between providers needs to be resolved for patients to progress to symptom remission. In order to manage these issues, it is recommended that providers

1. Communicate frequently in order to achieve consensus on a collaborative framework.
2. Engage in proactive rather than reactive discussions.
3. Elicit help from neutral parties as necessary or refer the patient or family for consultation.

CASE EXAMPLE

A 17-year-old with a history of generalized anxiety and panic disorder decided to pursue a "medication consultation" on recommendation from his therapist of 8 months. Regular coordination of care was established between providers in an effort to remain aligned on treatment goals and monitor response to medication and progress. The patient reported some positive impact with a selective serotonin reuptake inhibitor and remained in weekly exposure and response prevention therapy.

After several months of treatment, the patient reported continued impairment from panic attacks to his psychiatrist, resulting in an as-needed prescription for benzodiazepines. Because of a lapse in communication, the psychiatrist did not share this change to the treatment plan with the therapist. A few weeks later, the patient experienced immediate relief after taking the medication. Furious with his therapist, the patient threatened to quit therapy at his next appointment, stating, "How do you expect me to keep practicing 'exposures' when this makes me feel so much better?" Feeling undermined, the therapist initiated a call to review the treatment plan, leading the psychiatrist to acknowledge the oversight and then facilitate a fruitful discussion realigning treatment recommendations to identify a strategy, with the goal of reducing reliance on as-needed medications and building his ability to tolerate somatic triggers, which ultimately reduced the patient's panic attacks and worry.

Conclusion

Both integrated treatment from one clinician (psychopharmacotherapy) and split treatment across two clinicians (psychotherapy and medication management) can be efficacious in the delivery of combined treatments and share many common characteristics. Particularly with more than one provider involved, care must be taken to appropriately facilitate comprehensive and coordinated treatment. Early and proactive consideration of alliance principles, transference, countertransference, and conflict within treatment settings allows for productive delivery of mental health care to families. Further research is needed in this important domain exploring how these models can be best implemented, with a specific focus on pediatric populations.

References

American Psychiatric Association: Guidelines for psychiatrists in consultative, supervisory or collaborative relationships with nonphysician clinicians, 2009. Available at: www.psychiatry.org/psychiatrists/search-directories-databases/library-and-archive/resource-documents. Accessed December 1, 2019.

Avena J, Kalman T: Do psychotherapists speak to psychopharmacologists? A survey of practicing clinicians. J Am Acad Psychoanal Dyn Psychiatry 38(4):675–683, 2010 21171905

Baruch RL, Annunziato RA: Outcomes of combined treatment: evaluating split versus integrated treatment for depression. Prof Psychol Res Pr 48(5):361–368, 2017

Bordin ES: The generalizability of the psychoanalytic concept of the working alliance. Psychotherapy (Chic) 16:252–260, 1979

Busch FN, Gould E: Treatment by a psychotherapist and a psychopharmacologist: transference and countertransference issues. Hosp Community Psychiatry 44(8):772–774, 1993 8375839

Falkenström F, Josefsson A, Berggren T, Holmqvist R: How much therapy is enough? Comparing dose-effect and good-enough models in two different settings. Psychotherapy (Chic) 53(1):130–139, 2016 26928273

Gitlin MJ, Miklowitz DJ: Split treatment: recommendations for optimal use in the care of psychiatric patients. Ann Clin Psychiatry 28(2):132–137, 2016

Goin MK: Split treatment: the psychotherapy role of the prescribing psychiatrist. Psychiatr Serv 52(5):605–606, 609, 2001 11331793

Goldman W, McCulloch J, Cuffel B, et al: Outpatient utilization patterns of integrated and split psychotherapy and pharmacotherapy for depression. Psychiatr Serv 49(4):477–482, 1998 9550237

Greenson RR: The working alliance and the transference neurosis. Psychoanal Q 34:155–181, 1965 14302976

Groopman J: The troubled history of psychiatry. The New Yorker, May 29, 2019. Available at: www.newyorker.com/magazine/2019/05/27/the-troubled-history-of-psychiatry. Accessed December 1, 2019.

Howie LD, Pastor PN, Lukacs S: Use of medication prescribed for emotional or behavioral difficulties among children aged 6–17 years in the United States, 2011–2012. NCHS Data Brief 148. Atlanta, GA, Centers for Disease Control and Prevention, 2014. Available at: www.cdc.gov/nchs/products/databriefs/db148.htm. Accessed December 1, 2019.

Jacobs JT: Treatment of depressive disorders in split versus integrated therapy and comparisons of prescriptive practices of psychiatrists and advanced practice registered nurses. Arch Psychiatr Nurs 19(6):256–263, 2005 16308125

Jones LI, Pastor PN, Simon AE, Reuben CA: Use of selected nonmedication mental health services by adolescent boys and girls with serious emotional or behavioral difficulties: United States, 2010–2012. NCHS Data Brief 163, 2014. Available at: www.cdc.gov/nchs/products/databriefs/db163.htm. Accessed December 1, 2019.

Kahn DA: Medication consultation and split treatment during psychotherapy. J Am Acad Psychoanal 19(1):84–98, 1991 1676395

Kalman TP, Kalman VN, Granet R: Do psychopharmacologists speak to psychotherapists? A survey of practicing clinicians. Psychodyn Psychiatry 40(2):275–285, 2012 23006119

Koenig A, Friedman E, Thase M: Integrating psychopharmacology and psychotherapy in mood disorders, in Integrating Psychotherapy and Psychopharmacology. Edited by Reis de Oliveira I, Schwartz T, Stahl SM. New York, Routledge, 2013, pp 66–86

Krupnick JL, Sotsky SM, Simmens S, et al: The role of the therapeutic alliance in psychotherapy and pharmacotherapy outcome: findings in the National Institute of Mental Health Treatment of Depression Collaborative Research Program. J Consult Clin Psychol 64(3):532–539, 1996 8698947

Miklowitz DJ, Gitlin MJ: Clinician's Guide to Bipolar Disorder: Integrating Pharmacology and Psychotherapy. New York, Guilford, 2014

Reidbord S: A brief history of psychiatry. Psychology Today, 2014. Available at: www.psychologytoday.com/us/blog/sacramento-street-psychiatry/201410/brief-history-psychiatry. Accessed January 15, 2020.

Rogers CR: Client-Centered Therapy. Boston, MA, Houghton Mifflin, 1951

Rutherford BR, Tandler J, Brown PJ, et al: Clinic visits in late-life depression trials: effects on signal detection and therapeutic outcome. Am J Geriatr Psychiatry 22(12):1452–1461, 2014 24200597

Strong SR: Counseling: an interpersonal influence process. J Couns Psychol 51:81–92, 1968

CHAPTER 8

THE PHARMACOTHERAPEUTIC ROLE OF THE PEDIATRICIAN, ADVANCED PRACTICE CLINICIAN, AND OTHER PRIMARY CARE PROVIDERS

Katherine M. Ort, M.D.
Amy Heneghan, M.D.

Mental health conditions are among the most common childhood illnesses. Approximately one in five children have symptoms that meet diagnostic criteria for a mental health disorder, and many more struggle with functional problems related to their emotional health (Perou et al. 2013). However, only about 20% of children are treated by a medical professional

(Kataoka et al. 2002). Of the youth who do seek care, many are seen by their primary care provider (PCP), who may be a pediatrician, family practitioner, or advanced practice clinician, rather than by a psychiatrist. In fact, there are more pediatric outpatient visits to PCPs for mental health care than visits to psychiatrists. Pediatricians prescribe approximately 50% of all psychotropic medications in the United States. Furthermore, children and teens seeing PCPs are more often prescribed psychotropic medications than those seeing psychiatrists (Anderson et al. 2015).

PCPs are uniquely positioned to treat patients with mental health conditions, given their longitudinal relationships with patients and their families. The role that PCPs have in providing mental health care has been described as "the primary care advantage," which encompasses the PCP's developmental mindset and their role on the front line of children's health care (Foy and American Academy of Pediatrics Task Force on Mental Health 2010). PCPs have the privilege of seeing patients and their families over the long term, sometimes since birth, enabling them to develop trusting therapeutic relationships. In addition, PCPs often have a unique and deep understanding of a family's functioning, culture, and values system. Given that they see patients regularly for routine health care maintenance, they have the opportunity to educate patients and provide anticipatory guidance for mental health issues. Support and regular care in primary care offices can help prevent escalation of mental health concerns. Furthermore, PCPs routinely screen their patients (including for mental health conditions such as depression) and can intervene quickly if issues emerge (Foy et al. 2019).

In 2009, the American Academy of Pediatrics (AAP) released a policy statement, updated in 2019, that provides guidelines for PCPs treating mental health conditions. These mental health competencies include the expectations that pediatricians have foundational communication skills, the capacity to incorporate mental health content and tools into health promotion and primary and secondary preventive care, skills in the psychosocial assessment and care of youth with mental health conditions, knowledge and skills in evidence-based psychosocial therapy and psychopharmacological therapy, skills to function as a team member and comanager with mental health specialists, and a commitment to embrace mental health practice as integral to pediatric care (Foy et al. 2019). Several toolkits and training programs also exist to assist pediatric PCPs in their efforts to improve their comfort and effectiveness in treating children and adolescents with mental health disorders in their practices (American Academy of Pediatrics 2010). The AAP (American Academy of Pediatrics 2010) and The REACH Institute have model toolkits that can be accessed online (The Reach Institute 2018).

Challenges

Despite these and similar guidelines, studies suggest that PCPs identify only 25% of mental health conditions in children. Data show that as of 2013, only 57% of pediatricians were consistently treating patients diagnosed with ADHD, and less than 25% were treating patients diagnosed with any other mental health condition, such as anxiety or depression (Wissow et al. 2016). The reasons for this are manyfold. There remains a large stigma toward mental health, and even when asked, children and their parents may not disclose mental health concerns to their PCPs. When PCPs do identify concerns, they may feel poorly equipped, trained, supported, or reimbursed to manage mental health concerns in primary care. In 2004 and 2013, the AAP completed a survey of PCPs in identifying barriers to providing care to patients with mental health concerns. Fewer barriers were identified in 2013; however, the majority of those surveyed still reported they had inadequate training, a lack of confidence, and limited time to manage mental health concerns (Horwitz et al. 2015).

EDUCATION

PCPs continue to believe that they are not adequately trained to provide mental health care to children and adolescents. According to AAP surveys, 66% of pediatricians reported lack of training in treating children with mental health concerns, and 58% reported they lacked confidence (Horwitz et al. 2015). A different survey done by the AAP in 2007 revealed that although approximately 90% of graduating pediatric residents had completed a rotation in developmental and behavioral pediatrics, fewer than half rated their competency as "very good" or "excellent" (Horwitz et al. 2010). In another study, pediatricians reported a high degree of comfort with prescribing psychostimulants for ADHD, a relatively high degree of comfort prescribing selective serotonin reuptake inhibitors (SSRIs), and a lack of comfort prescribing other classes of psychotropic medications without consultation (Horwitz et al. 2015).

TIME

The structure of the primary care clinic contributes to barriers in providing psychopharmacological treatment. In primary care settings, follow-up appointments are typically brief, often no more than 20 minutes; in contrast, mental health visits are usually 30- to 60-minute sessions, with a defined and protected start and end time (Wissow et al. 2016). If a PCP identifies a mental health concern during a health care maintenance visit, there may be other competing demands. Taking time to do a thorough screening and obtain a detailed history from both the patient and the caregiver within a short time frame may be challenging, and having a thoughtful, balanced discussion of risks and benefits of potential treatments may be untenable in a single visit. With busy and overbooked schedules, it is also challenging to have a patient return in a timely fashion with good continuity. Patients may need to be seen by covering providers when they return, which hurts continuity and rapport (Horwitz et al. 2015).

AVAILABILITY OF SUPPORTIVE MENTAL HEALTH RESOURCES

Even when mental health concerns are identified, especially when they are severe, accessing consultation and having access to appropriate referrals may be challenging. Wait times to see providers in the community can be long, and PCPs may not have access to appropriate and timely consultation to facilitate appropriate treatment in the interim. Additionally, many PCPs lack staff in their practices who can facilitate mental health referrals or provide care to their patients. Many PCPs also have concerns about the adequacy of community resources in serving their patients (Horwitz et al. 2007; Rushton et al. 2004). Furthermore, even when patients are referred, one study showed that only 40% of families follow through on a mental health referral made in primary care (Rushton et al. 2002).

COMORBIDITIES AND COMPLEXITIES OF DIAGNOSIS

One study showed that 80% of pediatricians believed they were responsible for identifying mental health problems in their patients. Seventy percent believed that they were responsible for treating ADHD, yet less than a third believed they were responsible for managing other mental health concerns, such as anxiety, depression, or substance use (Stein et al. 2008). Underlying comorbidities complicate managing these diagnoses. Furthermore, following through on more complex mental health diagnoses, such as bipolar disorder or psychosis, may be outside the comfort zone and perceived competency of many PCPs.

REIMBURSEMENT

Reimbursement also represents a significant challenge. Billing structures may not correlate with the standard office visit regimen, which often requires multiple visits and time spent gathering collateral information from other providers. For example, in one study, half of pediatricians reported that they felt that insurers limited reimbursements for assessment and management of patients with ADHD (Rushton et al. 2004).

Developmental Considerations

INFANTS AND PRESCHOOL CHILDREN

Signs of an underlying mental health disorder in young children can be quite varied. These patients often require diagnostic assessment from a mental health professional with specialized training in early childhood or from a developmental and behavioral pediatrician. Therefore, it remains consistent that PCPs are more comfortable managing medication for older children, ages 12–18 years (Mayne et al. 2016). As described previously, lack of access to appropriate consultation and referral sources contributes to caution when prescribing medication, particularly for younger children (Cheung et al. 2018). Furthermore, in this age group, the American Academy of Child and Adolescent Psychiatry guidelines recommend psychosocial therapies as a trial first, and PCPs are generally less familiar with these treatment modalities (Wolraich et al. 2019). In young children, the primary role of the PCP is to provide appropriate education to families and to facilitate referrals for formal diagnostic assessment and therapy, as indicated for children identified with mental health disorders. Moreover, the PCP will continue to provide the family with ongoing support and encouragement.

PCPs also provide support to mothers when they present for their early newborn visits. In many practices, PCPs screen mothers for postpartum depression (PPD); however, it may be variable how comfortable pediatricians feel in managing PPD when there is a positive screen result. One study showed that nearly half of all pediatricians had little to no knowledge of PPD and underestimated its incidence in their practice (Horwitz et al. 2007).

SCHOOL-AGE CHILDREN AND ADOLESCENTS

"Addressing Mental Health Concerns in Primary Care" is a toolkit that was developed by the AAP to help PCPs manage the most common mental health problems in children and adolescents, with clear guidelines for pediatricians for identifying and managing common mental health concerns, including depression, anxious and avoidant behaviors, impulsivity and inattention, disruptive behavior and aggression, substance use, and learning challenges (American Academy of Pediatrics 2010). Pharmacotherapy in primary care is more likely to occur if there is mild to moderate impairment, especially given available treatment guidelines that indicate use of medications with well-established safety profiles, such as psychostimulants and SSRIs (Riddle 2015).

Despite increased comfort in managing medication for older adolescents, confidentiality concerns come up when PCPs are considering prescribing psychotropic medication for teenagers. It is standard practice that during yearly health maintenance visits, the PCP meets with the teen alone for at least part of the visit. If an adolescent discloses a mental health issue and there is no safety concern, then it is not required that the parent be informed, even if it may be recommended. This presents a barrier to prescribing medications to teenagers, who may not want their parents included in these discussions, given that parents will need to give consent for medication treatment to begin. It is especially important to build a strong therapeutic alliance with teenagers and provide guidance for involving a parent in their care. It is also important to set clear boundaries for safety, namely that clinicians must inform a parent if a patient is suicidal.

Implications for Treatment

The attitude of the PCP, who is often the first point of contact when a family seeks help, can have implications for disclosure of information as well as follow-through on treatment recommendations. Even when PCPs do identify a need for a referral to psychiatric care, patients may face barriers such as lack of available mental health providers in the area, insurance issues, and long wait times, or they may not want to see psychiatrists because of bias and prefer to see their PCPs. Families and patients may be reluctant or not ready to engage in therapy and may prefer that their PCPs initiate or oversee treatment. Furthermore, some patients may have urgent psychiatric issues and cannot wait to see a mental health provider. In these cases, it is important for PCPs to have appropriate skills in place. PCPs must not only understand the pharmacology of medications used in treatment but also partner with families to help them accept the need for treatment and ensure that families follow through on recommendations for treatment, which may include therapy, psychotropic medication treatment, coordinating with community resources, or any combination of these modalities. The PCP is essential to shaping a family's experience of mental health care.

THERAPEUTIC ALLIANCE

Therapeutic alliance has been shown to be the strongest predictor of favorable treatment outcome when it comes to psychotherapy. Given that PCPs have often had significant longitudinal relationships with patients and their families, they are uniquely poised to provide this type of care, even in time-limited settings (Wissow et al. 2010). Studies on interview style show that communication skills such as questioning about psychosocial issues, making supportive statements, and listening attentively can increase the likelihood of a patient disclosing sensitive information (Wissow et al. 2008a). In the PCP's office, treatment can begin immediately when a patient presents with a mental health concern, even when the diagnosis may be uncertain. PCPs can provide optimism and hope and help build positive expectancies for treatment. Even without engagement in formal psychotherapy, understanding families' experience of their problems can promote change (Wissow et al. 2008a).

ENGAGEMENT

Training PCPs in communication as it relates to engagement has been shown to be a key to success in improving children's mental health symptoms and reducing impairments in carrying out daily social, home, and school functions. Though crucially important, these concepts are not new. Milton Senn (1948) strongly encouraged the pediatrician to embrace their psychosocial roles of engagement, presence, and witnessing:

> The question that may be asked is, "How does a physician instill confidence in a patient and maintain rapport?" The primary requisite in the development of a therapeutic physician-patient relationship lies in the ability of the physician, first, to be aware of the feelings that the patient brings and, second, to be able to accept them whatever their nature. Actually, in order to help the patient it is neither necessary nor desirable in every instance to offer anything more than the opportunity for the establishment of a relationship. In the beginning of treatment the physician is an observer, interested in his patient and particularly the feelings that he brings with him. The important thing is not whether these feelings are positive or negative but rather how the pediatrician is able to allow the patient to experience them in the time spent with him. Once the patient has had the experience of being accepted, he begins to develop trust in the physician. It may be said that the therapeutic situation has

been established when the patient has succeeded in identifying the physician as a reliable and trustworthy person. (pp. 147–148)

Furthermore, given the significant relationships PCPs have with parents, the ability to engage them has also been shown to reduce parent mental health issues, which in turn improves their children's well-being. Even brief provider communication training can have a positive impact on mental health care delivery (Wissow et al. 2008b).

BRIEF INTERVENTIONS

When a patient presents with a mental health concern, the first step is to establish that there is no imminent threat to safety. After that is established, the PCP can assess next steps without rush, including assessing the need for pharmacotherapy. Next steps may include gathering more collateral information from the child's school or other medical providers, using secondary screening tools, having a family create a diary of problem behaviors, and facilitating referral of a family member to help them address their own mental health needs (Foy et al. 2019). Active listening and active support can strongly influence outcomes. Short interventions, even less than 10–15 minutes, may also be implemented in practice. Wissow et al. (2008b) studied brief interventions that may be accessible to PCPs and that can be used to improve patients' functioning or prevent escalation while awaiting higher levels of care. Simple skills, such as relaxation techniques or challenging negative thoughts, can be taught in the PCP's office.

THE COMMON ELEMENTS APPROACH

For every mental health disorder, evidence-based practices and factors from these treatments can be implemented by the PCP. This is often called the "common elements" or "common factors" approach. These techniques can help diverse and large groups of people rather than specific individuals with specific diagnoses. The underlying principle is that an individual does not need to have an official diagnosis or participate in a specific treatment, but rather, common elements of different treatment modalities can be used to help patients with their specific challenges, and this can, in turn, improve outcomes. For example, this could include using exposures for anxiety or avoidant behaviors. For attention and hyperactivity problems, this could include tangible rewards, parent praise, parent monitoring, time-out, and commands or limit setting. For depression, this might include psychoeducation, cognitive or coping skills, or problem-solving skills (Wissow et al. 2008a). For PCPs, these common factors can play a large and important role even without considering other interventions such as referral to a child and adolescent psychiatrist. In the adult literature, it has been well studied that good physician communication enhances depression treatment. In youth, research has now shown the importance of common factors for outcomes. One review showed that "relationship factors" (the ability to build a therapeutic relationship) and "direct influence skills" (explaining processes, focusing on practical concerns, and addressing barriers to treatment) had the strongest impacts on clinical outcomes (Wissow et al. 2008a).

As part of this theory, it is critical to assess a patient's perceptions of mental health concerns and perceptions of treatment and services. Given that many patients and their families may not see primary care as the place to seek mental health treatment, information may not be divulged without prompting. Additionally, given how significant parental mental health issues influence their children's own mental health, treatment by pediatricians may need to be targeted toward parents. This may include encouraging parents to participate in family therapy or even to seek their own mental health treatment.

Practical Applications and Strategies

PCPs have opportunities to provide pharmacotherapy for their patients. The next sections list principles that PCPs need to consider when managing or comanaging patients with mental health concerns—in particular, when prescribing psychotropic medications.

CREATE THE BEST SETTING

Because pediatric examination rooms may not always be conducive to having sensitive conversations, the PCP should always try to sit at the patient's eye level, which can be facilitated by having a chair that has an adjustable height or having a smaller chair in the room to sit with the child at their level. Having toys in the room can keep the child occupied when the PCP is talking with parents, as well as give the PCP something to make conversation about or use as a tool in explaining things, or simply give the child something to fidget with if they feel anxious. Finally, to avoid or eliminate interruptions, a sign can be placed on the door to indicate a sensitive conversation is in progress and that one should interrupt only in case of emergency.

CREATE A SENSE OF TIME LIMIT AS WELL AS TIMELESSNESS

Eugene Beresin describes the concept of providing an atmosphere of *time-lessness in a time-limited setting* (Kaye et al. 2002). He emphasizes that it is indeed important for children and families to understand the time limit of a visit, to allow them to get all their concerns heard and set priorities during a visit. At the same time, it is important for children and families to believe that the provider is giving them his or her full and undivided attention. Placing a clock behind the child and his or her family can help facilitate timekeeping without obtrusiveness. Providing families a notice when the appointment is nearing a close to wrap things up and identifying next steps with a clear plan to deal with unaddressed concerns at a future visit can help families feel heard and attended to.

REMEMBER THE DUAL RELATIONSHIP

Pediatric visits are unique in that the provider must manage their role in caring for both the patient and the parent. Parents are ultimately the ones who make the final medical-legal decisions, and they often administer or supervise treatment at home. However, it is equally important to include the child in the intervention, develop rapport, and obtain the child's input for treatment. It is crucial for the pediatric clinician to navigate this dual relationship thoughtfully. (For further discussion on this topic, see Joshi 2006.)

CASE EXAMPLE: JACKIE, 11 YEARS OLD

Jackie and her mother present to their PCP for a follow-up on behavioral issues. Jackie has been recently diagnosed with ADHD, combined type, based on reports from parents and teachers. The PCP recommends a trial of a psychostimulant to help manage symptoms of hyperactivity and impulsivity that have been getting Jackie into frequent trouble. Jackie's mother is on board with medication; however, Jackie thinks she is being punished and is refusing to take the medication. Jackie and her mother are at an impasse.

Even in a brief visit, it is important to get Jackie's perspective and help her feel heard and understood. The PCP, parent, and Jackie must work to develop a shared goal, such as helping her see how the medication might help her improve something that matters to her or enable her to achieve a goal or earn a desired reward. Minimizing shame and stigma and focusing on Jackie's agency are critical. It is also important to convey the concept of a team that is in place to support her. Finally, the PCP should remind Jackie and her mother that the medication is one of many tools to help Jackie succeed.

In challenging interactions with parents, aligning over the care and best interests of the child can go a long way. It can be helpful to validate the parent's own experience of the child. For example, in the case of Jackie, the parents may feel personally victimized by their child's behavior. It can be helpful to allow the parents space to express these feelings and to validate that reaction. At the same time, providing parents with an alternative perspective on their child's behavior and drawing on their unique strengths and challenges can help parents tolerate difficult behavior. Importantly, one should also draw on and highlight parents' own unique strengths. Encouraging parents to get their own support is often needed.

SET APPROPRIATE EXPECTATIONS

PCPs should inquire about both the parents' and child's concerns and expectations regarding treatment. This is particularly important when it comes to trials of psychotropic medications, many of which take weeks to months to get to the full intended effects, unlike many other pediatric medications. Additionally, many psychotropic medications have unique side effects, such as emotional, behavioral, and physical appearance changes, and it is important for parents to be aware of these changes and to provide appropriate anticipatory guidance. At the same time, it is critical for parents to treat these medications in the same way they would treat a standard medication, such as an antibiotic, for their child and not relay unnecessary fear to the child (but instead discuss their concerns with the PCP).

PAY ATTENTION

Beresin also describes the importance of closely observing both the family and child in the room, paying attention to both verbal and nonverbal communication. PCPs must monitor their own reactions as well (Kaye et al. 2002). In psychiatry, as in pediatrics, awareness of countertransference is of crucial importance in the relationship between provider and patient as well. It is completely natural to have strong emotional reactions to certain patients or challenging parents, and being aware of these reactions can help prevent these feelings from hindering the carrying out of appropriate treatment plans.

PROVIDE PSYCHOEDUCATION

When PCPs are providing psychoeducation about psychotropic medications, it is important to elicit the family and child's prior knowledge. It is important to be aware of education level, developmental level, and cultural considerations when providing language about diagnosis and treatment options. It is also important to normalize questions and even to "get ahead" of questions by providing common concerns and reassurance for things other families have raised. When the PCP is providing anticipatory guidance, it is helpful to discuss psychotropic medications in a similar manner as any other pediatric medication.

CASE EXAMPLE: ADAM, 7 YEARS OLD

Adam is a boy with a diagnosis of generalized anxiety disorder, which has been impacting his ability to pay attention in school and spend time with friends. His worries are often expressed somatically, and he has been seen frequently by his PCP for headaches and abdominal pain. Because Adam is unwilling to engage in any form of psychotherapy, his PCP has recommended a trial of sertraline for anxiety. His mother is concerned about possible side effects of the medication because she previously tried an SSRI for herself and was unable to tolerate it because of severe nausea.

In this case, it may be helpful for the PCP to meet separately with the mother when providing anticipatory guidance regarding side effects. Point out to the mother that although she experienced side effects herself, children often react differently. Parents should be counseled to view psychiatric medications in the same way as any other medicine and to feel confident that their children will alert them if there is something significant to be concerned about.

COMMUNICATE AND LISTEN

PCPs should strive to be present and attentive and to be good listeners. Both children and their parents need to be given space to share their perspectives. Using open-ended questions that are followed by more specific questions when needed, such as gathering side effect details or timelines, can be crucial in building a strong treatment alliance. It is important not to insist that someone talk. Even with a longitudinal, trusting relationship, many children may be uncomfortable shifting from more comfortable topics such as school or interests to more sensitive topics such as mood issues or anxiety. Clear, direct language can facilitate a child's response. However, if the child does not feel comfortable addressing these things right away, it is important to be patient and provide an open, trusting space for the child to share when ready.

RESPECT CONFIDENTIALITY WITH ADOLESCENTS

Adolescents need privacy and time alone with the PCP. This can be framed to both adolescents and their families as an opportunity for the adolescents to start taking ownership of their own health as they move toward independence and adulthood. Of course, general confidentiality rules apply, and it is important for adolescents to understand that what they disclose will not be shared with their parents unless there is an imminent safety concern. However, when it comes to prescribing psychotropic medications, parents do retain legal rights to consent to medication. This can be challenging when an adolescent discloses mood or anxiety concerns or if an adolescent is engaging in behaviors that do not rise to the level of reportable behavior but are risky nonetheless. In these cases, it is important to continually revisit the discussion of confidentiality with adolescents as it relates to their treatment. Most important, PCPs need to help facilitate conversations between adolescents and their parents when needed but not necessarily mandated.

CASE EXAMPLE: LESLIE, 17 YEARS OLD

Leslie is seen by her PCP for a routine well check. When the PCP meets with her privately, she discloses that she has been feeling depressed and anxious for the past few months. She endorses frequent marijuana use because she believes this is the only thing that helps her get to sleep and alleviate anxiety. She denies active or passive suicidality. The PCP discusses the possibility of a trial of therapy and medication; however, Leslie states she does not want her mother to know what has been going on because she feels her mother "doesn't believe in mental health" and does not want to discuss this with her. Prior to this visit, her mother sent the PCP a message stating she wanted drug testing on Leslie because her grades had dropped, and she had "smelled something" in Leslie's room.

Understanding Leslie's hesitation in discussing her mental health with her mother and listening to understand her mother's concerns create a good starting point. Given that there is no imminent danger, the PCP is not required to disclose any information to Leslie's mother. It is important, however, to help Leslie find a way to share at least some information with her mother to facilitate treatment. It can be helpful for the PCP to play a role in advocating for the teen (and even facilitating a parent-teen discussion when Leslie is ready). Until that time, the PCP can provide guidance on what would be disclosed to the parent.

COLLABORATE WITH OTHER PROVIDERS

In cases in which PCPs may need to use medications that they may not be comfortable prescribing (e.g., antipsychotics, mood stabilizers), PCPs and mental health professionals can comanage care. *Comanagement* is defined as "collaborative and coordinated care that is conceptualized, planned, delivered, and evaluated by 2 or more health care providers" (Stille 2009). Skills in collaborating with providers are an important part of training and enable PCPs to help provide continuity and facilitate care when cases are complicated or when adolescents transition to adulthood.

USE THE COMMON ELEMENTS APPROACH

The following HELP mnemonic, developed by the AAP Task Force on Mental Health, is a useful way to see how aspects of the "common elements" or "common factors" approach can be used in primary care settings (Foy and American Academy of Pediatrics Task Force on Mental Health 2010).

- Hope: Hope can help both with family coping and with setting expectations for treatment. By focusing on patient and family's strengths, the PCP can increase hopefulness and help families start to take actionable steps toward well-being.
- Empathy: The PCP can demonstrate empathy by listening to the child and family, validating their experiences and concerns in a culturally informed and sensitive manner, and celebrating successes and positive progress with the child and their family.
- Language and loyalty: In helping a child and family, the PCP can use his or her own language (rather than clinical terms) to reflect back to them their concerns. Loyalty can be communicated by expressing one's willingness to tackle the problem together as a team and one's commitment to continue to work together now and in the future.
- Permission, partnership, and plan: Prior to asking sensitive questions, the PCP should ask the child and family's permission. Additionally, the PCP should ask permission before providing suggestions for next steps for the family to take if they do not ask for suggestions. The PCP should partner with the child and family to identify barriers to treatment. Troubleshooting ahead of time can lead to improved adherence, help identify resistance, and develop acceptance of the treat-

ment plan. Working with the family on next steps, and in particular, a first achievable step, can be instrumental in helping empower families and improve readiness to take action.

EMPLOY BRIEF INTERVENTIONS

Despite time pressures inherent in primary care practices, many brief interventions can be mastered and delivered by PCPs. These include self-regulation techniques (e.g., deep breathing and progressive muscle relaxation), behavioral management interventions (e.g., time-outs, reward charts), and positive parenting interventions (e.g., developing parent-child "special time" scheduled for 5–10 minutes per day). A summary table of common elements in evidence-based practice amenable to primary care is available from the AAP (American Academy of Pediatrics 2010).

Discussion and Areas for Future Research

Given the unique position of PCPs on the front lines of providing mental health care to children and their families, it is critically important for mental health to be incorporated into training models.

A variety of integrated and collaborative care models have been developed. Some research has shown that co-located care (e.g., when other mental health specialists are embedded in pediatric practices) can enhance comfort. Surveys of pediatric residents report increased confidence in treating a patient with mental health concerns when they have enhanced mental health services in their clinics (McLaurin-Jiang et al. 2020). Further research is needed on the impact of these models on prescribing habits, as well as the different models of care.

Finally, more research is needed on the use of evidence-based psychotherapy in primary care. A nice starting point is Clabby's article on adapting cognitive-behavioral techniques for primary care settings, which provides practical tips and sample scripts for the PCP to use (Clabby 2006).

TAKE-AWAY POINTS

- Primary care providers (PCPs) are at the front lines of mental health treatment and have unique opportunities to make a difference given their trusting, longitudinal relationships with children and their families.

- The supportive and ongoing care provided in primary care offices can help prevent escalation of early mental health concerns.

- Despite perceived and real barriers, including clinic and time constraints, there are opportunities for PCPs to have meaningful therapeutic interactions with patients and their families and to improve mental health care.

- Small adjustments to clinical practice can have a large impact, without significantly increasing time spent.

- Integrated and collaborative care models can be helpful in increasing comfort and practice.

- More training is needed for PCPs in mental health and collaborative models.

References

American Academy of Pediatrics: Addressing Mental Health Concerns in Primary Care: A Clinician's Toolkit. Elk Grove Village, IL, American Academy of Pediatrics, 2010

Anderson LE, Chen ML, Perrin JM, Van Cleave J: Outpatient visits and medication prescribing for US children with mental health conditions. Pediatrics 136(5):e1178–e1185, 2015 26459647

Cheung AH, Zuckerbrot RA, Jensen PS, et al: Guidelines for Adolescent Depression in Primary Care (GLAD-PC): part II. Treatment and ongoing management. Pediatrics 141(3):e20174082, 2018 29483201

Clabby JF: Helping depressed adolescents: a menu of cognitive-behavioral procedures for primary care. Prim Care Companion J Clin Psychiatry 8(3):131–141, 2006 16912815

Foy JM; American Academy of Pediatrics Task Force on Mental Health: Enhancing pediatric mental health care: report from the American Academy of Pediatrics Task Force on Mental Health. Introduction. Pediatrics 125 (suppl 3):S69–S74, 2010 20519564

Foy JM, Green CM, Earls MF: Mental health competencies for pediatric practice. Pediatrics 144(5):e20192757, 2019 31636143

Horwitz SM, Kelleher KJ, Stein RE, et al: Barriers to the identification and management of psychosocial issues in children and maternal depression. Pediatrics 119(1):e208–e218, 2007 17200245

Horwitz SM, Caspary G, Storfer-Isser A, et al: Is developmental and behavioral pediatrics training related to perceived responsibility for treating mental health problems? Acad Pediatr 10(4):252–259, 2010 20554260

Horwitz SM, Storfer-Isser A, Kerker BD, et al: Barriers to the identification and management of psychosocial problems: changes from 2004 to 2013. Acad Pediatr 15(6):613–620, 2015 26409303

Joshi SV: Teamwork: the therapeutic alliance in pediatric pharmacotherapy. Child Adolesc Psychiatr Clin N Am 15(1):239–262, 2006 16321733

Kataoka SH, Zhang L, Wells KB: Unmet need for mental health care among U.S. children: variation by ethnicity and insurance status. Am J Psychiatry 159(9):1548–1555, 2002 12202276

Kaye D, Montgomery ME, Munson SW: Child and Adolescent Mental Health Core Handbooks in Pediatrics. Philadelphia, PA, Lippincott Williams & Wilkins, 2002

Mayne SL, Ross ME, Song L, et al: Variations in mental health diagnosis and prescribing across pediatric primary care practices. Pediatrics 137(5):e20152974, 2016 27244791

McLaurin-Jiang S, Cohen GM, Brown CL, et al: Integrated mental health training relates to pediatric residents' confidence with child mental health disorders. Acad Psychiatry 44(3):299–304, 2020 31965516

Perou R, Bitsko RH, Blumberg SJ, et al: Mental health surveillance among children—United States, 2005–2011. MMWR Suppl 62(2):1–35, 2013 23677130

Riddle MA (ed): Pediatric Psychopharmacology for Primary Care. Elk Grove Village, IL, American Academy of Pediatrics, 2015

Rushton J, Bruckman D, Kelleher K: Primary care referral of children with psychosocial problems. Arch Pediatr Adolesc Med 156(6):592–598, 2002 12038893

Rushton JL, Fant KE, Clark SJ: Use of practice guidelines in the primary care of children with attention-deficit/hyperactivity disorder. Pediatrics 114(1):e23–e28, 2004 15231969

Senn MJ: The psychotherapeutic role of the pediatrician. Pediatrics 2(3):147–153, 1948 18876571

Stein RE, Horwitz SM, Storfer-Isser A, et al: Do pediatricians think they are responsible for identification and management of child mental health problems? Results of the AAP periodic survey. Ambul Pediatr 8(1):11–17, 2008 18191776

Stille CJ: Communication, comanagement, and collaborative care for children and youth with special healthcare needs. Pediatr Ann 38(9):498–504, 2009 19772236

The Reach Institute: Guidelines for Adolescent Depression in Primary Care (GLAD-PC) Toolkit. 2018. Available at: https://www.thereachinstitute.org/guidelines-for-adolescent-depression-primary-care. Accessed July 20, 2021.

Wissow L, Anthony B, Brown J, et al: A common factors approach to improving the mental health capacity of pediatric primary care. Adm Policy Ment Health 35(4):305–318, 2008a 18543097

Wissow LS, Gadomski A, Roter D, et al: Improving child and parent mental health in primary care: a cluster-randomized trial of communication skills training. Pediatrics 121(2):266–275, 2008b 18245417

Wissow LS, Brown JD, Krupnick J: Therapeutic alliance in pediatric primary care: preliminary evidence for a relationship with physician communication style and mothers' satisfaction. J Dev Behav Pediatr 31(2):83–91, 2010 20110822

Wissow LS, van Ginneken N, Chandna J, Rahman A: Integrating children's mental health into primary care. Pediatr Clin North Am 63(1):97–113, 2016 26613691

Wolraich ML, Hagan JF Jr, Allan C, et al: Clinical practice guideline for the diagnosis, evaluation, and treatment of attention-deficit/hyperactivity disorder in children and adolescents. Pediatrics 144(4):e20192528, 2019

PART III

SETTINGS

CHAPTER 9

THE PHARMACOTHERAPEUTIC ALLIANCE IN SCHOOL MENTAL HEALTH

Andrew Connor, D.O.
Shashank V. Joshi, M.D.

Psychopharmacotherapy in the School Context

The child mental health prescriber (pharmacotherapist) is merely one participant in the complex and interconnected world of children, teens, and young adults. Many other influences can determine the efficacy of medication beyond the writing of a prescription, which, if not acknowledged, can humble the most knowledgeable pharmacotherapist. Even if a drug has been extensively studied and proven to be a reliable intervention, it may be no match for a child assigning an inauspicious meaning to the medication or a teenager refusing to take it at all because of fears of untoward social embarrassment. Some of the most significant of these influences, both helpful and not, exist within the youth's school-based communities.

In the context of school mental health, "medicating a child" is full of potential implications regarding patient autonomy and confidentiality, the impact of benefits and side effects on learning and cognition, parental rights, and physician beneficence. This task must be approached thoughtfully. The prescriber (pharmacotherapist) is often the person with ultimate diagnostic and treatment authority despite sometimes limited direct contact with the patient. This situation is aggravated by the time constraints of modern pharmacotherapy encounters. Because the "offer" of any treatment to patients is much more than a neutral act (Joshi et al. 2004), prescribing medications for children and adolescents requires that special attention be paid to communication styles and messages, particularly in the school setting. Do the clinician's language and affect convey hope and confidence in things to come (Winer and Andriukaitis 1989)? Does the prescription signal the end of the interview or the beginning of an alliance (Blackwell 1973)?

As we write this chapter, the COVID-19 pandemic has abruptly and profoundly reminded us of the impact academic systems have on how we access students and families, and they access us in turn. A salient example is the prominent (nearly ubiquitous) use of telehealth visits as of Spring 2020. Many schools were skillfully adept at converting to remote learning modalities for general education when COVID-19 led to nearly 100% virtual classrooms but often lagged in offering comprehensive special education accommodations, including access to mental health resources. It became apparent that not all school districts or families were able to access technological privileges equally, highlighting important cultural and socioeconomic disparities. Pragmatically, as school consultants in psychiatry, we have had to reconsider what constitutes best practice, including consideration for school assessments without in-class observations and an increased reliance on parental "homeschooling" observations.

When the direct (virtual) access that the pharmacotherapist has to the patient is being considered, there are obvious time constraints to the now common 30-minute visit that at most would occur weekly or monthly. By contrast, teachers and other adults within the academic system have an immense access advantage. According to data from the American Time Use Survey, the average U.S. teen spends 6.5 hours each weekday on education-related activities. Although half of all teens who experience moderate to severe mental health issues have an onset of symptoms before age 14 years, two-thirds of these children never access mental health care (Cama et al. 2020). Thus, it makes sense to develop models of care delivery that expand treatment access for children and adolescents by recruiting and supporting the relationships within their school communities.

This is not a new concept. Research supports that implementing treatments within the school systems can be an effective and lasting strategy for advancing both medical and mental health endeavors. A large-scale and widely distributed intervention model looking at recruiting school nurses to improve children's access to asthma symptom screening and medication adherence showed consistent and significant reductions in presentations to the emergency department for exacerbations (Salazar et al. 2018). Investing in school-based screening and implementation of brief cognitive-behavioral therapy for trauma in schools (Stein et al. 2003) showed improvements in multiple measures, including significant reductions in depression and PTSD symptoms and reduction in overall functional impairment. In fact, Rones and Hoagwood (2000) were confident in declaring that schools have taken on a major therapeutic role and predicted that they would remain the nation's largest provider of mental health services. So, what does this mean for child and adolescent pharmacotherapists hoping to bridge the obvious gap in access for mental health treatment? It should represent an opportunity to create meaningful interventions in school-based settings.

The skilled pharmacotherapist will be required to familiarize themselves with foundational concepts for interfacing with school communities, always remembering the social and cultural context of a student, their family, the community, and the larger society. As Lin and colleagues (2001) described, "[P]harmacotherapy is fundamentally a process of social transaction, and its outcome is determined by contextual factors impinging on the patient, [family], and the clinician by forces that powerfully shape their interactions." Clinicians in turn should acknowledge "that [they] are just as malleable, consciously and unconsciously, by their sociocultural environment and prevailing ideologies." Lin et al. invite us *to struggle against* certain prevailing notions of modern pharmacotherapy, which can undermine effectiveness. These notions include that 1) the therapeutic effects of medications are determined exclusively by their biologic properties, 2) the patient is a passive recipient of the prescription and will be fully adherent with instructions, and 3) psychiatric and medical treatments represent (or are supposed to be) the only sources of care available and used by the patient. Culture influences the same areas that are central to mental health, such as behavioral expectations and tolerance, language, emotion, attention, attachment, traumatic experiences, conduct, personality, motivation, limit setting, and other aspects of parenting in general. Cultural context plays an important role not only in structuring the environment in which children with emotional and behavioral disorders function but also in the way such children are understood and treated (Lin et al. 2001). Furthermore, school-based mental health interventions are permeated by substantial cultural and socioeconomic implications. Schools are as diverse as the students they teach and can be a sort of "salad bowl" filled with children of various cultural backgrounds and economic status (we prefer the salad bowl metaphor over "melting pot"). In each consultation, there are key treatment implications rooted in both school and family cultural elements, from parents of historically disadvantaged or minority communities suspicious of the mental health system, to language concerns resulting in barriers to health literacy, to immigrant perspectives on education goals within the U.S. academic system (Owusu 2016). Further expounding on this concept, Dell and colleagues (2008) remind us that

> [d]espite perceptions by the general public—and sadly, even many clinicians—to the contrary, the act of prescribing psychotropic medications is one of tremendous [potential] psychodynamic significance to children, adolescents, families, and caregivers. Particularly in the cultural context of every patient, we must not only "uncover and appreciate the attributions given to medication," but we must also realize that without attention to this, we will have an incomplete picture of the underlying psychopathology, the real-life contexts that matter to the patient, and that affect and are affected by [their] neuropsychiatric issues, issues that influence adherence to all recommended treatments and treatment response. Furthermore, even the briefest of encounters with a prescribing physician [may] carry [significant meaning] and psychotherapeutic weight. (p. 6)

According to Bostic and Rauch (1999), there are three core subjects that school consultants—and in our case, pharmacotherapists—should be mindful of when navigating the school community. These are the "three R's" of school consultation:

- *Relationships.* Approach the consultant-consultee relationship with the school from a position of empathy as key to accessing the system. Fostering the relationships is accomplished by providing validation and cultivating respect for everyone on the team and building bridges to recruit more support inside and outside of the school system.
- *Recognition.* Recognize that system challenges are multifaceted, which may not be wholly evident at first. Taking time to understand the child's motives, school's motives, and parents' motives, and helping the involved parties see each other differently can be crucial to

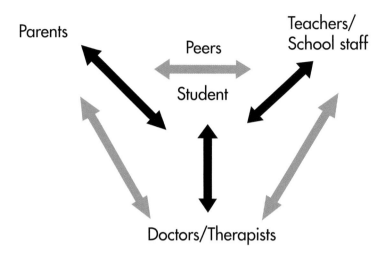

Figure 9–1. Primary therapeutic relationships and the supporting alliance.

Source. Adapted from Feinstein et al. 2009.

help the system get "unstuck." To that end, we should clarify that they were all originating from a place of good intent and trace back to where perhaps things started to diverge from that initial place.
- *Response.* Mobilize a response by empowering the consultee with a new understanding of the challenges, teaching new skills, or providing expert services.

Joshi and colleagues (2015b) have highlighted that for a school-based clinician or school consultant who provides pharmacotherapy on site, each face-time contact with administration is an opportunity to improve the school system and its response to those in greatest need and to strengthen the system as a whole. In line with the three R's, the consultant strengthens the relationships of professionals allied around students, parents, and the greater school community, building bridges among them. This partnership among parents, staff, and therapists for school mental health has been termed the "supporting alliance in school mental health" (Feinstein et al. 2009). This term, illustrated in Figure 9–1, aptly describes the key relationships in the child's school life that should be identified and fostered. The authors venture beyond the primary relationships of the child-teacher, child-doctor, or child-parent dyads and instead give attention to the secondary relationships surrounding the student, including the parent-teacher, teacher-doctor, and doctor-teacher dynamics. In this alliance, the doctor or therapist was initially identified more generally to include any mental health provider; however, we will emphasize the role of the doctor or therapist as the pharmacotherapist and focus on the implications of medication interventions in schools.

Parents, school therapists, and teachers act as the eyes and ears for the pharmacotherapist outside of the time constraints of the office visit. These trusted adults are an invaluable reservoir of observational data within the school environment. In this sense, it is helpful to appreciate that the teachers and school therapists are also on the front line for screening for early mental health concerns (Joshi et al. 2015b; von der Embse et al. 2018). One study looking at teachers' perspectives and their role in student mental health promotion showed that large numbers of teachers identify strongly as "gatekeepers," meaning they are often the first to identify problems and, if necessary, refer to mental health professionals. However, in that same study, the authors identified numerous interprofessional barriers between mental health providers and teachers, particularly when an attempt is being made to carry out more complex interventions. Examples listed include challenges related to communication and confidentiality between professionals, time constraints and scheduling difficulties, contextual presence and understanding, cross-systems contact, school leadership, and teacher competence in mental health (Ekornes 2015). The doctor who works with the teacher or school nurse to find ways for a student to take medication (e.g., coming up with a signal or giving the student an errand to run at just the right time) optimizes adherence. Once-daily preparations have further improved adherence while diminishing risks of patient embarrassment or humiliation at being publicly "reminded" to take medication (Joshi 2006). Table 9–1 provides other suggestions to optimize the alliance between a pharmacotherapist and school personnel.

The supporting alliance concept aids in the creation of a unified effort to guide therapeutic interactions by fostering key relationships. Potential pitfalls are also worth attending to, including *drain* (the relationships that bestow a nonproductive tax on time or energy), *distortion* (the strength of one part of the supporting alliance overtakes the role of the other), and *cooptation* (one participant takes on or adopts the role of another).

When the supporting alliance paradigm is used fully, these interprofessional challenges can be overcome. For example, guided by the three R's, one pharmacotherapist described an elevation in overall interprofessional cohesion and work satisfaction by mobilizing the supporting alliance effectively: "Our team's work focuses on the relationships that need to be cultivated and fostered, the recognition of human motivation

---

Table 9–1. Recommendations for establishing an effective working alliance with school staff in pediatric pharmacotherapy

---

The pharmacotherapist should strive to

Ensure that case formulation always precedes the prescription.

Emote a real sense of understanding in all communications with teachers and other school staff.

Involve the patient in the decision-making process, especially in the case of adolescents.

Assess the understanding of the mental illness and the meaning of medication for the patient and family.

Nurture all professional relationships necessary to sustain the child's health (parents, family members, other therapists, teachers, primary care providers).

Visit consumer websites often; help families connect to appropriate support groups; help teachers learn about what to expect from a medication intervention.

Identify references and books to help patients and school staff obtain useful, accurate understanding about mental health disorders.

When the subject of pharmacotherapy emerges, pause and listen to the patient's, parents', and teachers' associations and responses to the word *medication*.

For families and youth, provide a small number of choices of medications whenever possible, so that past associations with a particular product do not derail treatment; remain mindful that any change, including improvement, may be threatening to the patient and family.

Respect the patient's and family's right to informed consent and need to know about common side effects, without burdening them with so much information that they become overwhelmed

Practice the three C's of good pharmacotherapy:

1. Collaboration (with therapists, teachers, other providers)
2. Conscientiousness (of the evidence base, the standard of practice, the specific sociocultural needs of the patient and family)
3. Communication (return telephone calls and e-mails promptly from school staff, be available between sessions for quick questions, document so that others can follow the pharmacotherapy reasoning if they participate in this patient's care)

Remember that all actions have potential meanings for patients and families, from the pens used to write prescriptions (eschewing those with drug names or pharma logos), to the language employed to explain about mental illness, to the way the pharmacotherapist provides realistic hope for the future.

Source. Adapted from Joshi 2006.

during an important or sensitive time, and the responses to challenges. For us as the academic partner, each 'face-time contact' with administration was an opportunity to improve the school ethos and its response to not only those in greatest need but also the system as a whole" (Joshi et al. 2015b, p. 170).

A parent's role in the supporting alliance cannot be overstated. Each parent or caregiver comes with their own perspective (informed by past experiences and current attitude), and consideration of the parent's perspective does not stop simply at the issues directly related to the child or teen, but also includes the interactions with other members of the alliance. Parents may or may not share the same short- and long-term therapeutic goals of the school. Likewise, schools may be under significant pressures of their own in terms of resource constraints, expected time frames, and hopes of managing behaviors within the immediate academic setting. A case example is illustrative:

> The parents of a 7-year-old boy with disruptive behaviors in second grade were reluctant to agree to a referral to the school mental health team because the father felt his son might "have to take meds, and we want to avoid that. The last thing he needs is to look and feel medicated while his brain is still growing." It was later revealed that this parent had experienced trauma and loss and had been misdiagnosed as having ADHD when the correct diagnosis was PTSD. The teacher communicated this information to the school mental health team, and the pharmacotherapist was able to approach the issue of assessment, diagnosis, and treatment with more sensitivity and attunement to the parents' concerns. A positive outcome was the result of this open communication stream.

In schools, culture influences important areas that are central to mental health, such as behavioral expectations and tolerance, language, emotion, attention, attachment, traumatic experiences, conduct, personality, motivation, limit setting, and other aspects of teaching in general. Cultural context plays an important role not only in the way the school environment in which youth with emotional and behavioral disorders function is structured but also in the way such children and teens are understood and treated. Teachers play a crucial role in promoting the overall health and academic engagement of their students, in addition to their social and emotional learning and development (Franklin et al. 2012). Table 9–2 provides strategies to address the point made by McCullough and Quinlan (2016):

> Without a more direct focus on teacher well-being, the proposed strategies for promoting youth happiness may be futile, especially if the adults with whom they interact with most during the school day feel emotion-

---

Table 9–2. Strategies psychiatrists can implement to help prevent compassion fatigue and burnout among school staff

---

1. Develop productive working relationships with leaders and administrators in any district one works with. These can take up to a year or more to develop solidly, and are important when recommending systemic changes to promote teacher/staff well-being.

2. Help staff to:

   Maintain good boundaries between personal and professional life.

   Invest in activities and relationships to increase meaningful engagement and joy.

   Practice good and consistent self-care; attend to proper sleep habits, good nutrition, and moderate regular exercise.

   Improve self-awareness, interpersonal effectiveness and assertiveness, time management, and organizational skills.

   Diversify work to include administrative and leadership roles, in addition to teaching tasks.

   Engage in regular supervision and peer support, and cultivate meaningful work relationships.

   Take regular time off/vacations (if possible) at appropriately spaced intervals.

Source.   Adapted from Derenne 2018.

ally exhausted and overworked. Accordingly, Hills and Robinson (2010) emphasized that "teachers need to be the first to put on their oxygen masks prior to supporting their students' social and emotional [well-being]." (p. 104)

As parents engage with schools to advocate for accommodations for their children with mental health conditions, it is crucially important for them to know what their rights and resources are (Joshi et al. 2019). In the United States, the main laws of relevance are the Individuals with Disabilities Education Act (IDEA) and Section 504 of the Rehabilitation Act of 1973. A useful site that summarizes relevant information is https://www.understood.org/en/school-learning/special-services/504-plan/the-difference-between-ieps-and-504-plans. Building teacher self-efficacy and versatility is a big part of what a pharmacotherapist can do to cultivate a teacher's partnership. An example of a research-proven program to enhance teacher self-efficacy in engaging with high-risk students is the Kognito: At Risk for Educators Program (https://kognito.com/products/at-risk-for-high-school-educators) (Similar programs have been created for elementary and middle school teachers.) This program features interactive role-play simulations that build awareness, knowledge, and skills about mental health and suicide prevention, preparing school educators to recognize and intervene with students in psychological distress and, if needed, connect them with support services (Joshi and Jassim 2019; Joshi et al. 2015a).

Several chapters in this book have highlighted how a strong therapeutic alliance lays the foundation upon which positive outcomes in mental health treatment generally, and psychopharmacology specifically, are built. Culturally attuned pharmacotherapists should be mindful of not only the target symptoms but also the context and settings in which they occur. In addition to the psychiatrist's office, these principles apply in other treatment settings, such as that of the primary care provider, the school-based health center, or the school clinic, where psychotropic medicines are often prescribed for youth (Malik et al. 2010). In school-based pediatric psychopharmacology specifically, several alliance relationships must be acknowledged and nurtured. Prescribing clinicians should strive to include not only the patient and parent or guardian in the working alliance paradigms of goal identification, task consolidation, and therapeutic bond establishment, but when appropriate, selected members of the school team as well (Joshi 2006). Research reviews have shown that knowledge of the psychological factors and developmental implications present when medicines are prescribed improves therapeutic outcomes (Joshi 2006; Pruett et al. 2010). The following case vignette illustrates how cultural attunement by the pharmacotherapist helped a teenager and family in need of multimodal interventions (individual psychotherapy, pharmacotherapy, family therapy, school engagement) continue to participate in all forms of treatment, despite wishes to withdraw from care:

> Jodie was a 16-year-old second-generation Filipina American who lived in a household with four younger siblings and both parents. Several youth from her high school had died by suicide in the previous year, and among the victims was Jodie's best friend. School staff members were concerned about Jodie's recent English journal entries and withdrawn behavior and asked that the school's mental health team consult with her and her family to assess for depression and self-harm potential. After consent was obtained, the team was able to quickly gain the patient's and family's trust by doing the following:
>
> They began the consultation by calling the family and outlining the specific steps in consultation, assuring them that although the process would start at school, it would continue in whatever context the family felt most comfortable. In their case, it was the home.
>
> A home visit was conducted after the leader of the team, a child and adolescent psychiatrist, met with the teen at school that afternoon for initial assessment. The doctor met the teen and parents together briefly and

then asked to meet the parents alone for about 30 minutes to gain their trust and engage them in a culturally focused way. Being mindful of the potential for stigma, their potential fears about whether contact with the team might affect her chances to go to the best college, the psychiatrist selectively use a medical model ("Jodie [Jodie's brain] needs to be healthy enough to learn, and right now her brain is hurting. She is not able to think clearly and learn in the ways she is used to.") to allow the family to conceptualize Jodie's need for treatment using a more familiar paradigm.

The psychiatrist highlighted the need to work closely with the school counselor and recommended that family therapy be started to address dysfunctional patterns and to learn new parenting and coping strategies for the mood swings Jodie was experiencing. After a couple of sessions with Jodie and meetings with involved school staff, a diagnosis of major depressive disorder and posttraumatic stress traits was made. After full discussion of possible interventions, the psychiatrist recommended to the patient and family that they should consider starting psychotherapy with a colleague, and also consider a low dose of selective serotonin reuptake inhibitor (SSRI) as part of an overall treatment plan for depression. He was mindful of the potentially good response at lower doses in some patients of Asian ancestry and that this patient had been tried on medicine in the past, with the teen and family stopping treatment because "she was so sleepy and couldn't do her schoolwork." The psychiatrist also supported the teen and family request to continue the omega fatty acid (OFA) supplement because they believed this was important to her overall functioning, and the psychiatrist believed it was at least doing no harm and may have carried some meaning. (Jodie's close friend who had died had ADHD and depression, and was nonadherent with the prescribed OFAs, stimulant, and SSRI. Jodie believed she could honor the memory of her friend by trying to take the medicine as prescribed.)

The supporting alliance among doctor, parents, family therapist, schoolteacher, and guidance counselor was facilitated by the psychiatrist actively endorsing the role of the school in supporting Jodie and highlighting their role on the team as the "watchful clinical eyes" during the school day. Jodie responded well to a low-dose SSRI and standard-dose OFA in conjunction with interpersonal therapy (IPT), family therapy, and regular mental health checkups with the school counselor. The psychiatrist continued to see her monthly and had brief phone meetings with the IPT therapist weekly for the first 6 weeks.

The parents, although tempted many times to withdraw from this intensity of treatment, kept encouraging Jodie and supporting her continued participation "because the doctor talked to us about the brain and potential benefits to her learning (in addition to her mood) and asked us to make sure she attends (and we participate where needed) all these meetings, and also because he said the treatment may not last forever—it will depend on how she responds."

Pruett and colleagues (2010) remind us that, particularly with teens, attuned child and adolescent clinicians need to remain alert to changes in the meaning of medication to patients as they navigate the new developmental terrain of adolescence. The dramatic changes in bodily preoccupation, impulsive discharge, and mood lability that occur with puberty may cast any agent that in the past may have affected weight (gain or loss), endocrine function (galactorrhea), skin appearance (acne), genital arousal or dysfunction, or mood itself into an entirely different light. What might have been acceptable effects before are now intolerable because they emerge during, or simply exacerbate, already exquisitely sensitive developmental tasks. This is made even more complex by the fact that nearly all "side" effects, from extrapyramidal symptoms to nausea, are generally less well tolerated in child and adolescent populations to begin with (Joshi et al. 2019).

Leston Havens cautioned that to many patients, the doctor's trustworthiness and decency are not givens, and mental illness in particular is often a delicate subject (Havens 2000). He described three "psychological analgesics" that may facilitate the approach to painful topics in therapy (as described below; Joshi 2006). For pharmacotherapists, these analgesics might be "prescribed" for difficult matters, such as when presenting the need to take psychotropic medication to patients and families.

1. *Protect self-esteem.* The patient has been potentially affected by having to come to a psychiatrist, and the parent may feel guilty for a perception of having caused the illness through bad parenting, poor gene contribution, or both.
2. *Emote a measure of understanding and acceptance.* When this measure is successful, the patient's problem is grasped intellectually, and the patient's and family's predicament is understood from their point of view.
3. *Provide a sense of future.* Many families have experienced frustration and failure in attempting to find solutions and may have lost hope. Discussion about expectations for treatment that still acknowledges fears or even hopelessness may still preserve opportunities for change: "It may seem hopeless to you *for now…*"

School-Based Manifestations of Psychiatric Conditions

It is useful to consider how the pharmacotherapist can advocate on behalf of a student to maximize the chance of feeling understood in school settings when challenges arise. Adolescents with mood disorders, for example, are at high risk for school problems, including poor attendance, underachievement, and dropping out. Particularly in the midst of a ma-

---

Table 9–3. Common problems for youth caused by treatment of a mood disorder

---

Medication side effects

Side effects of medications can range from nuisances to significant challenges in getting through the school day.

Some side effects are very embarrassing (e.g., lithium treatment leading to bladder accidents); others may be uncomfortable (e.g., feeling thirsty, having dry mouth, or being dizzy and nauseated).

Medication titrations can be associated with headaches or sleepiness that can further interfere with schoolwork.

Other problems associated with treatment

Once-daily dosing is ideal but may not always be possible.

If a student takes their medication during the school day, there may be challenges around school nurse availability, stigma regarding the need to leave class for medicine, or logistical challenges if a parent needs to obtain an "extra medication bottle" for school.

Leaving school activities for therapy or other appointments can cause a student who is already struggling to have even more problems.

Source. Adapted from Fristad and Goldberg Arnold 2004; Joshi and Jassim 2019.

jor mood episode, these students can find it hard to pay attention, think clearly, solve problems, recall information, engage in group learning activities, and sit still—let alone follow classroom rules (Evans and Andrews 2005). Mood disorders can cause at least three types of problems for youth in school settings: 1) those caused by the core symptoms themselves (e.g., difficulty concentrating), 2) those caused by secondary factors (e.g., peer issues), and 3) those associated with the treatment itself (e.g., medication side effects) (Table 9–3) or life inconveniences associated with treatment (e.g., needing to take medications during the school day or missing school activities to attend therapy appointments). Youth with mood conditions often struggle with learning issues, and educators would do well to be aware of the additional layers of impaired concentration, reduced motivation, and emotional upheavals that the mood disorder can create (Fristad and Goldberg Arnold 2004; Joshi and Jassim 2019).

For young children, the pharmacotherapist can use play to more fully understand what the child struggles with and potentially improve the outcomes of pharmacotherapy by enhancing adherence. The act of taking medication is full of meaning for children (and this meaning may not always be obvious to adults). A pharmacotherapist is distinctively posi-

---

Table 9–4. Children's thinking about medication

Physical properties of the medication itself

Liquid, tablet, capsule, or injectable forms may each carry different meanings	Liquid is for "babies," injections are "punishment," and so on
Size	The bigger the pill (or its milligram value), the bigger the problem, or vice versa
Labeling and printing	Personalized associations to imprinted numbers or letters
Color	Associations with candy or poison
Timing of the dosage	
Frequency	More frequency, more trouble, or conversely, more help
Morning or afternoon	Morning for school, afternoon for sleeping or dreaming troubles
During school	Concern about stigma
Self or parent administered	Self is good and mature, whereas parent is now doctor's agent

---

Source.   Adapted from Pruett et al. 2010.

tioned to explore the meaning of medication as it applies to the classroom setting. As summarized in Table 9–4, some of the magical properties that are commonly given to various aspects of medications include such features as the physical properties, timing of administration, who is administering the medication, and where and when medications are given.

As pharmacotherapists, we are likely to encounter a spectrum of attitudes and beliefs related to "medicating" various behavioral problems or psychiatric issues, particularly for prepubertal children. What is the specific role for a pharmacotherapist within the supporting alliance if not to address medication questions? This role, although often considered to be teaching and knowing how to "fix problems" using medications, may in fact be the opposite and more accurately thought of as when to recognize that medication is not the solution (Fanton and Gleason 2009). We ultimately want to caution against trying to "medicate away an issue" that cannot be solved with medication because this could erode the essential trust and morale in the supporting alliance. As child and adolescent psychiatrists, pediatricians, school nurses, nurse practitioners, and other clinicians, we should embrace our roles as promoters of mental health and well-being (in addition to performing our duties as trained specialists who assess and treat mental health problems and clinical disorders) (Rettew et al. 2019).

As children grow older and progress through middle school and into high school and later approach graduation, parents and teachers experience a dramatic shift in their students' worldviews. Students experience waves of internal and external pressures, not least of all making choices about how to support themselves as an independent adult in the eyes of the community. Students with mental health concerns impacting their education have another layer of complexity when preparing for their lives after the structure of high school expires. They need to work with their parents, therapists, and teachers in coming up with a successful plan, which may or may not mean independently managing their mental health treatments. Unique supports or scenarios around continued services may be needed, including parents considering legal conservatorship or therapeutic or vocational training for their graduates. Table 9–5 describes some of these challenges, and a deeper discussion regarding the specific needs of transition-age youth is covered elsewhere in this book (see Chapter 12, "Alliance Issues to Consider in Pharmacotherapy With Transition-Age Youth").

Conclusion

In this chapter, we have attempted to describe some of the key roles of trusted adults within the youth's school life that can play a prominent part in facilitating pharmacotherapeutic interventions—namely, parents, teachers, and prescribers. Even between these seemingly straightforward relationships within the child's school community, the interpersonal dynamics can be quite nuanced. As aptly described by Bostic and Rauch (1999), "The school consultant should always consider where new relationships can occur, both within and beyond the current system" (p. 340).

TAKE-AWAY POINTS

- For clinicians caring for youth with mental health conditions, it is crucial to understand educational settings as fully as possible. Teachers and other school staff engage with affected youth on an almost daily basis, and they are key partners to help both clinicians and parents comprehend the social, educational, and cultural context where psychiatric symptoms may manifest.

Table 9–5. Special challenges in managing mood conditions during school transitions

---

Elementary to middle school

Level of responsibility and independence increase.

Relationship changes (family and school) toward greater independence, but students still need guidance and support.

Stress levels can increase because of transitions in layout of school and need to navigate new physical, personal, and social terrain.

Levels of cognition, reasoning, and planning are higher.

Child is moving away from a strictly self-centered view of the world.

Expectations from parents and teachers shift toward more independence.

Adults need to focus on identifying and documenting learning disabilities and mental health conditions.

Some students start using social media and cell phones.

Puberty and sexuality can accelerate in fourth or fifth grade for some children (body changes and body image issues).

Bullying and internet safety need to be attended to.

Parents or guardians should request a school team meeting to assess whether a 504 Plan or Individualized Education Program (IEP) for specific accommodations is needed.

Middle school to high school

Transition to independence is even greater compared with the transition from elementary to middle school.

Parents need to stay engaged and supportive without being overbearing.

Academic demands increase.

Students are expected to take on more ownership of both academics and behavior.

Learning disabilities can become more evident as academic demands increase.

Potential concerns about social pressures and cultural and social identity arise.

Sleep quality and consistency becomes a greater focus for parents, mental health professionals, and the community (e.g., advocating for later school start times).

Social media use increases. (Knowing the pitfalls becomes important for youth; need for internet safety is crucial.)

Puberty and sexuality become more relevant (body changes and body image concerns).

Exposure to bullying, drugs, alcohol, and cyberbullying may increase.

Learning disabilities and mental health conditions and 504 Plans or IEPs must be updated and documented.

Table 9–5. Special challenges in managing mood conditions during school transitions *(continued)*

High school to post–high school and college

Individuals must take ownership of their own future.

Young adults need to learn to recognize mental health issues with greater independence and be open to work with trusted adults to find the best "fit" for college or work setting after graduation.

Parents must keep lines of communication open and plan for emergencies as teenagers evolve into the transition-age youth group (18–25 years old).

Academic demands increase.

The emerging young adult must complete the following tasks:

Visiting colleges and asking the right questions to help determine the best fit

Transferring and updating medical records

Preparing for ACT, SAT, college applications, and 4-year plan

Parents and counselors must ensure that students with disabilities have the necessary documentation for standardized tests and college.

Students need to update documented learning disabilities and mental health disorders and connect with college resource officers.

Individuals need to know the signs of emotional distress to seek help early (being aware of age at onset for certain disorders).

Young adults should recognize that the risks of depression and anxiety are higher as new life transitions occur (moving away from friends and community).

Source. Adapted from Joshi and Jassim 2019.

- Several interventions have been developed to help affected youth gain better access to the school curriculum despite their psychiatric symptoms.

- Careful attention should be paid to the supporting alliance among parents, teachers, and clinicians so that members of each of these groups can be resources to best support one another in their goals to support students.

- Prescribing should be informed by the child's developmental stage. Children think about and apply meaning to medications that adults may not consider, and this meaning is important to children.

- Skilled prescribers have knowledge of the education laws specific to their areas of practice and use them to the patients' advantage.

- Future research will examine how additional complex relationships related to school communities can impact students' mental health treatment, including how future educational and treatment settings (using remote technology) may impact care delivery models.

References

Blackwell B: Drug therapy: patient compliance. N Engl J Med 289(5):249–252, 1973 4713764

Bostic JQ, Rauch PK: The 3 R's of school consultation. J Am Acad Child Adolesc Psychiatry 38(3):339–341, 1999 10087697

Cama S, Knee A, Sarvet B: Impact of child psychiatry access programs on mental health care in pediatric primary care: measuring the parent experience. Psychiatr Serv 71(1):43–48, 2020 31551042

Dell ML, Vaughan BS, Kratochvil CJ: Ethics and the prescription pad. Child Adolesc Psychiatr Clin N Am 17(1):93–111, 2008 18036481

Derenne J: The range of postsecondary options and thinking about the differences between high school and college, in Promoting Safe and Effective Transitions to College for Youth With Mental Health Conditions. Edited by Martel A, Derenne J, Leebens P. New York, Springer, 2018, pp 29–36

Ekornes S: Teacher perspectives on their role and the challenges of interprofessional collaboration in mental health promotion. School Ment Health 7(3):193–211, 2015

Evans DW, Andrews LW: If Your Adolescent Has Depression or Bipolar Disorder: An Essential Resource for Parents. New York, Oxford University Press, 2005

Fanton J, Gleason M: Psychopharmacology and preschoolers: a critical review of current conditions. Child Adolesc Psychiatr Clin N Am 18(3):753–771, 2009

Feinstein NR, Fielding K, Udvari-Solner A, Joshi SV: The supporting alliance in child and adolescent treatment: enhancing collaboration among therapists, parents, and teachers. Am J Psychother 63(4):319–344, 2009 20131741

Franklin CGS, Kim JS, Ryan TN, et al: Teacher involvement in school mental health interventions: a systematic review. Child Youth Serv Rev 34(5):973–982, 2012

Fristad M, Goldberg Arnold JS: Raising a Moody Child: How to Cope With Depression and Bipolar Disorder. New York, Guilford, 2004

Havens L: Forming effective relationships, in The Real World Guide to Psychotherapy Practice. Edited by Havens L, Sabo A. Cambridge, MA, Harvard University Press, 2000, pp 17–33

Hills KJ, Robinson A: Enhancing teacher well-being: put on your oxygen masks! Communique 39:1–17, 2010

Joshi SV: Teamwork: the therapeutic alliance in pediatric pharmacotherapy. Child Adolesc Psychiatr Clin N Am 15(1):239–262, 2006 16321733

Joshi SV, Jassim N: School-based interventions for pediatric-onset mood disorders, in Clinical Handbook for the Diagnosis and Treatment of Pediatric Mood Disorders. Edited by Singh MK. Washington, DC, American Psychiatric Association Publishing, 2019, pp 457–483

Joshi SV, Khanzode L, Steiner H: Psychological aspects of pediatric medication management, in Handbook of Mental Health Interventions in Children and Adolescents: An Integrated Developmental Approach. Edited by Steiner H. San Francisco, CA, Jossey-Bass, 2004, pp 465–481

Joshi SV, Hartley SN, Kessler M, Barstead M: School-based suicide prevention: content, process, and the role of trusted adults and peers. Child Adolesc Psychiatr Clin N Am 24(2):353–370, 2015a 25773329

Joshi SV, Ijadi-Maghsoodi R, Merrell SE, et al: Shared learning in community-academic partnerships: addressing the needs of schools, in Partnerships for Mental Health: Narratives of Community and Academic Collaboration. Edited by Roberts LW, Reicherter D, Adelsheim S, Joshi SV. Cham, Switzerland, Springer International Publishing, 2015b, pp 163–178

Joshi SV, Jassim N, Mani N: Youth depression in school settings: assessment, interventions, and prevention. Child Adolesc Psychiatr Clin N Am 28(3):349–362, 2019 31076113

Lin K-M, Smith MW, Ortiz V: Culture and psychopharmacology. Psychiatr Clin North Am 24(3):523–538, 2001 11593861

Malik M, Lake J, Lawson WB, Joshi SV: Culturally adapted pharmacotherapy and the integrative formulation. Child Adolesc Psychiatr Clin N Am 19(4):791–814, 2010 21056347

McCullough M, Quinlan D: Universal strategies for promoting student happiness, in Promoting Student Happiness: Positive Psychology Interventions in Schools. Edited by Suldo SM. New York, Guilford, 2016, pp 103–121

Owusu Y: Combined psychotherapy with psychopharmacology, in Psychotherapy for Immigrant Youth. Edited by Patel S, Reicherter D. Philadelphia, PA, Springer, 2016, pp 109–126

Pruett K, Joshi SV, Martin A: Thinking about prescribing: the psychology of psychopharmacology, in Pediatric Psychopharmacology: Principles and Practice, 2nd Edition. Edited by Martin A, Scahill L, Kratochvil C. New York, Oxford University Press, 2010, pp 422–433

Rettew DC, Satz I, Joshi SV: Teaching well-being: from kindergarten to child psychiatry fellowship programs. Child Adolesc Psychiatr Clin N Am 28(2):267–280, 2019 30832957

Rones M, Hoagwood K: School-based mental health services: a research review. Clin Child Fam Psychol Rev 3(4):223–241, 2000 11225738

Salazar G, Tarwala G, Reznik M: School-based supervised therapy programs to improve asthma outcomes: current perspectives. J Asthma Allergy 11:205–215, 2018 30214248

Stein BD, Jaycox LH, Kataoka SH, et al: A mental health intervention for schoolchildren exposed to violence: a randomized controlled trial. JAMA 290(5):603–611, 2003 12902363

von der Embse NP, Kilgus SP, Eklund K, et al: Training teachers to facilitate early identification of mental and behavioral health risks. School Psych Rev 47(4):372–384, 2018

Winer J, Andriukaitis S: Interpersonal aspects of initiating pharmacotherapy: how to avoid becoming the patient's feared negative other. Psychiatr Ann 19(6):318–323, 1989

CHAPTER 10

WHEN TIME IS TIGHT AND STAKES ARE HIGH

Pharmacotherapy, Alliances, and the Inpatient Unit

Andrea Tabuenca, Ph.D.

Jung Won Kim, M.D.

Shih Yee-Marie Tan Gipson, M.D.

In recent years, the increasing frequency and severity of child and adolescent psychiatric issues and a relative paucity of high-acuity outpatient mental health services have combined to increase the utilization of inpatient "locked unit" psychiatric beds. This has resulted in busier and more acute inpatient settings and, in many cases, prolonged wait times in the emergency department for bed availability (Teich et al. 2018). Along with an increase in the incidence of suicidality among adolescents and young adults in the United States, there are reports of younger children with suicidal ideation requiring hospitalization (Twenge et al. 2019). In this context, pharmacotherapeutic interventions and optimizations must be carried out quickly, without neglecting the critically important task of rapport building and establishment of therapeutic alliances with patients and their families. In this chapter we explore approaches to the modern inpatient psychiatric evaluation, provide a structure for initiating pharmacotherapy, and discuss the various considerations that affect decision making during psychiatric hospitalization from the psychiatric team's perspective.

Evaluation in the Inpatient Psychiatric Setting

For each patient admitted to a psychiatric inpatient unit, a comprehensive assessment that emphasizes acute risk and safety is essential. As in the outpatient setting, components of a comprehensive inpatient evaluation include understanding the presenting problem and history of the present illness in a focused manner; the psychiatric review of systems; review of the patient's psychiatric history and trauma exposures; review of psychiatric and nonpsychiatric medications and allergies; nonpsychiatric medical history; developmental history; family psychiatric history; social and educational history; family legal involvement; protective agency involvement; and any history of substance use. The treatment team's goal is to gather information to understand any factors that may directly contribute to the patient's current state of acute distress. Factors that are concomitant to the admission must be explored in depth; these factors include psychosocial stressors, family dynamic issues, and current educational supports that could impact efficacy and engagement in treatment recommendations. This process allows providers to identify modifiable risk factors that can be targeted during the inpatient stay, ultimately improving treatment outcomes.

During the assessment and formulation phase, it is important to understand the precipitating and exacerbating factors that contributed to a psychiatric crisis. Identifying modifiable and unmodifiable risks will help inform target goals for risk reduction during the hospitalization. Because admissions can be short, focus should be placed on the most impactful modifiable risks (e.g., reduction strategies for potential means of harm in the home and school) and on creating a safety communication plan with a patient's family and support network to promote early intervention during acute distress. In some cases, caregivers may not be aware of a patient's suicidal ideation or other unsafe urges, so caregiver education often needs to take place concurrently with safety planning. Knowledge of these barriers can inform brief family interventions, such as parental coaching and psychoeducation around supportive responses that encourage help-seeking behaviors from the child or adolescent. Addressing these issues can promote greater efficacy of medication interventions by minimizing compounding factors affecting a patient's symptoms. A full treatment plan will include not only pharmacotherapeutic and therapy recommendations but also a culturally informed biopsychosocial assessment, "four P's" case formulation (predisposing, precipitating, perpetuating, and present factors), and an explicit list of modifiable and unmodifiable risks (Winters et al. 2007).

Initiation of Treatment and Treatment Planning

STRENGTHENING THE THERAPEUTIC ALLIANCE AND PROVIDING COLLABORATIVE PSYCHOEDUCATION AS A PATH TOWARD TREATMENT ADHERENCE

The quality of the therapeutic alliance formed between the patient and the team not only fosters the perceived helpfulness of an admission among a patient and their family, but also influences adherence to medication during acute hospitalization (Blanz and Schmidt 2000; Day et al. 2005). In a meta-analysis of the role of therapeutic relationships in pharmacological treatment outcomes, Totura et al. (2018) emphasized a need to focus on communication skills that enhance the therapeutic alliance. The task of engaging adolescents in treatment comes with unique challenges related to their developmental needs and stage. Developmental tasks related to individuation often include a frustrating tug-of-war between growth toward autonomy and expectations for compliance with authority figures. In this dynamic developmental context, clinicians can optimize rapport by creating a relationship based on authenticity and mutual respect and by balancing family involvement with teen confidentiality (Bolton Oetzel and Scherer 2003; Joshi 2006). These challenges are often amplified by the stressors of the inpatient unit, where relatively brief admissions limit the time available for building the trusting relationship that is so central to effective management. Adolescents in crisis are often experiencing a host of concurrent psychosocial stressors, which, if ineffectively managed, may perpetuate a sense of hopelessness in finding help and relief. Anxious and depressive symptoms often manifest as irritability and frustration. This can be misperceived by members of the treatment team as a patient being "closed off," adversarial, or confrontational. These perceptions may result in transference or countertransference that impacts the quality of collaborative communication between the patient and provider and subsequently reduces adherence to treatment recommendations (Joshi 2006).

Motivational interviewing (MI) emphasizes nonconfrontational communication strategies and has been shown to be effective in short-term treatment settings such as inpatient units (Colby et al. 2012). MI can be especially effective in reducing ambivalence about treatment in adolescents because options are presented in a collaborative and nonauthoritarian manner (DiLallo and Weiss 2009). Rather than providing treatment directives, this approach fosters adolescent autonomy by exploring the patient's own treatment goals and providing psychoeducation on the pathways available to meet those goals. Within an MI framework, the provider supports precontemplative adolescents by providing empathy and validation of their perspectives as experientially true while empowering them to realize that they are in control of treatment plans. Treatment goals must be mutually understood by the patient, family, and provider for a strong alliance to be formed across team members (Joshi 2006). This allows the provider to take a collaborative role as an educator who works with the patient to identify the tasks necessary to achieve their desired outcomes.

A strong therapeutic alliance also makes it possible to better assess potential barriers to medication adherence, whether related to the stigma associated with taking psychotropic medication, any personal meaning a patient has ascribed to being on medication, or the patient's assessment of how medication may or may not affect him or her. Some patients may suspect that medication implies an intrinsic psychological failure or a damaged sense of self. Others may anticipate that medication leads to a "zombie effect" or a perpetually altered and inauthentic state of "being a different person." Without proper exploration of how these concerns conflict or align with the patient's treatment goals and the intended therapeutic effects of medication, adherence to the intervention is threatened (Joshi 2006). Even in the compressed time frame of an inpatient hospitalization, the prescriber must take time to understand the patient's attributions and expectations while approaching psychoeducation collaboratively from a mindset of teammates seeking pathways toward a shared treatment goal (Joshi 2006).

Parent or guardian involvement in the psychiatric care of minors is legally necessary for consent to treatment, but early engagement and alliance building with caregivers is also central to fostering medical adherence (Ingoldsby 2010; Joshi 2006). The therapeutic alliance must be extended to include a patient's family, who may themselves have concerns about the implications of medication on their child's future health and well-being. In addition to receiving adequate psychoeducation on the potential risks and benefits of recommended medication, parents can engage in collaborative coaching regarding how medications are discussed with their child. After an inpatient hospitalization, parents are often left with the complex task of reducing access to means for harm in the home. This commonly involves locking up all medications and dispensing each dose with close supervision, thereby promoting a context of frequent communication about medication between the caregiver and child. Providing positive comments or praise that emphasizes adherence as a demonstration of a child's commitment to self-care may reinforce adherent behaviors (Joshi 2006). Conversely, commentary that primarily attributes symptom improvement to the medication (e.g., "You're doing better; you must be taking your meds") minimizes the child's self-efficacy in managing their health and thus may be detrimental to long-term adherence (Joshi 2006). Coaching parents on the importance of such helpful and unhelpful language can promote empowerment in the effective support of their child's mental health.

Although some patients are psychotropic medication naive upon admission, others will have an outpatient psychiatric provider who has managed past medication trials and will continue to provide longitudinal care after hospital discharge. Carefully exploring the patient's alliance with any established outpatient provider is a particularly helpful tool toward extending that alliance to the inpatient setting. Families may feel more confident in recommendations provided if they know that care is being closely coordinated with any therapist, psychiatrist, or primary care physician with whom they have a long-standing and trusted relationship. Open communication with outpatient providers also facilitates a warm handoff in transitioning care after discharge, allowing supportive treatment to continue more seamlessly.

STARTING MEDICATIONS ON AN INPATIENT UNIT

Children, adolescents, and transition-age youth who are admitted to locked inpatient units are typically considered to be of potential harm to themselves or a harm to others or are in some way unable to function safely in settings such as at home or school because of psychiatric concerns. Most locked units have a psychiatrist or psychiatric nurse practitioner on staff as part of a multidisciplinary team to evaluate the patients' daily progress to monitor medications or consider medication initiation.

Providing information and education to the patient and family helps build a platform for informed consent. Although emergency medications may be needed during hospitalization, it is imperative to discuss the goal of initiating medication with the patient and family as part of the consenting process. Because of the prevailing stigma around psychotropic medication, many parents and patients are hesitant to take medication for the first time while hospitalized. Fear and stigma may complicate patient and caregiver decision making when they are presented with a provider's recommendation to initiate psychotropic medications. Understanding each caregiver's role in supporting the patient is critical in treatment. When there are disagreements among legal guardians, the team must ensure all parties receive appropriate and adequate information regarding the recommendation to make an informed decision. If an indicated treatment would largely benefit the patient and disagreement is present, it is important to review the legal authority of the guardians regarding decision-making rights. Although the provider should take care to not fracture a family dynamic or further disturb it, treating the patient is the highest consideration, no less so when a psychiatric condition is life threatening. In emergency cases, providers may consult with their ethics and legal counsel on the process of informed consent because it may vary across states and between caregivers. Special considerations exist for medical providers when there are significant concerns of imminent harm to the patient or others, such as in cases of catatonia or when command auditory hallucinations are present. In such cases, emergent intervention with medications may be necessary before an extensive discussion with the family.

At the time of this writing, most hospitalizations for children and adolescents last between 3 and 10 days. Often, within this relatively brief period, not all of a given patient's symptoms will resolve. The paradigm then is one of multimodal crisis stabilization, in which a patient's safety is prioritized while laying the groundwork for further outpatient progress.

Inpatient initiation of medications, with the close monitoring intrinsic to these units, can enable the clinician to titrate to therapeutic dosages at an accelerated pace. Typically, a patient will have their vital signs evaluated at least daily while in the hospital. This can inform any acute changes from titration of medication and allow for quicker titration compared with the outpatient setting. Advanced laboratory testing and imaging are more readily available to the clinician in this setting. For severely ill patients, especially patients with mania or severe psychosis, monitoring for response and improvement of symptoms daily in an inpatient unit also allows for families to receive feedback and updates quickly. However, the relative brevity of inpatient psychiatric admission means that often there is insufficient time to achieve optimal dosing. Thus, this work must be taken up by an outpatient colleague, depending on the community resources available to the patient. When discussing the start of medication in various settings, it is important to discuss these considerations with the family to help them make the most informed decision.

When medication is being initiated, it is also important to discuss with family the targeted symptoms and expected effects while in the hospital and beyond. This discussion can allow for realistic expectations while in the hospital and promote hope for medication adherence for the intended duration. When appropriate, reviewing the evidence base available with family can be helpful to best promote a full understanding and buy-in to a specific approach.

Generally, we advise against starting a medication or making significant medication changes on the day of discharge because of concerns over lack of ability to monitor its effects. For the same reason, inpatient clinicians should avoid recommending or guiding further medication changes over the phone after a patient has been discharged from their service, because the care team has a reduced ability to make changes or intervene with any changes in the patient's condition except for recommending a visit to the emergency department or hospital. These considerations underscore the importance of having a warm handoff with a provider in the next setting of care at the time of discharge from the inpatient unit.

CONSIDERING MEDICATIONS IN CONJUNCTION WITH LEVELS OF CARE AND DISCHARGE PLANNING

In some cases, a patient may require a step-down level of care, such as residential care or an intensive outpatient treatment program. In the United States, available levels of care, including long- and short-term residential placements, partial hospitalization day programs, intensive outpatient day programs, and close outpatient clinic follow-up, can vary from state to state and may further depend on a patient's insurance provider. In these scenarios, medication initiation, titration, and other longitudinal therapeutic considerations should take this into account. Depending on a patient's discharge plan, consideration of medications approaching discharge from the hospital should be done early and in a deliberate fashion because facilities have different policies and management criteria. Careful planning and consideration of levels of care allow for a smoother transition and increased success in treatment plans.

Regardless of whether a patient is taking medication or not, we encourage a warm handoff with the provider at the next level of care, which can help smooth the transition. Communicating the rationale behind medications as well as ongoing recommendations of titrations or medication changes to the family and outpatient provider facilitates unimpeded continuity of the treatment course. At the time of discharge, most psychiatric units provide prescriptions to support a patient during the transitional period between hospital discharge and establishment or reestablishment with an outpatient treatment setting, generally on the order of 2–4 weeks. This duration is, of course, informed by the specifics of each case and provider level of comfort, but it is important to provide an appropriate amount of medication to "bridge" a patient until their next scheduled appointment. We therefore also strongly encourage that patients have a known and confirmed outpatient post-hospitalization appointment before discharge or step-down. Again, it is our recommendation to providers that if a refill is needed after discharge, the request be rerouted to the outpatient provider. Under certain circumstances, including when there is a lack of resources or care, some providers provide a second prescription, but this must be done with caution. When a patient is readmitted to the hospital, a review of the medication plan in conjunction with the safety plan and step-down levels of care should be considered to further mitigate the presenting risks.

Discussion of Guiding Principles

UNDERSTANDING THE HISTORY AND RECOGNIZING STIGMA

When mental illness and inpatient psychiatric hospitalization are being discussed, it is important to reflect on the history of psychiatric inpatient units and media portrayals over time. A basic understanding of this history helps ground and identify potential stigma and hesitance about initiating medication and gives a context for the child's hospitalization. Historically, psychiatric inpatient admissions were long, often 1 year or more in duration, with a patient's time within these facilities often characterized by long-term psychotherapy. This changed in the 1980s when the payment structure to hospitals and physicians changed at federal and state levels (Lave and Frank 1988). In addition to having possibly inaccurate expectations of interminable admissions, inconsistent psychotherapy practices, and forced medication administration, many patients and families may approach their first hospitalization with an outsize and unwarranted fear of invasive interventions such as the use of restraints and electroconvulsive therapy, both commonly and often luridly depicted in popular media. Frequently, a tour of the unit and discussion of patient and family rights and the overall treatment approach can help with an understanding of the hospitalization course and put their minds at ease regarding their care (Valenkamp et al. 2014). This also helps build rapport and trust in the treatment team to provide the necessary therapeutic interventions, from individual to family treatments. It is also important to educate early regarding the advancements in brain science and psychopharmacology that aid our understanding of psychopathology, especially in youth depression, anxiety, bipolar disorder, psychosis, and obsessive-compulsive disorder.

A typical inpatient psychiatric unit staffing structure may include a psychiatrist, a psychiatric nurse practitioner or physician assistant, psychologist, social worker, milieu counselors, recreational therapists, occupational therapists, and psychiatric nursing staff. Psychiatric teaching hospitals within academic institutions are generally also staffed in part by trainees, including fellows, residents, medical students, nursing students, and allied health students. Although the team structure was similar in the past, patients historically received significant amounts of psychotherapy from psychiatrists or psychologists. It is important to introduce the members of the staff and their role as part of the orientation to a hospitalization. Although a psychiatrist or psychiatric nurse practitioner is part of the treatment team, it is important to reassure families that their role is not solely focused on medication management.

Because of stigma around mental illness and a misperception that its symptoms are largely in control of an individual, some families can be hesitant to start medications. Part of psychoeducation for the family and patient includes the idea that a psychiatric illness is a medical illness. It is useful to highlight that symptoms can be exacerbated by environmental factors and stressors, and that there is evidence about brain pathology and dysfunction in many mental health conditions, which can be treated in combination with medication and therapy. Some families may consider that being in therapy in the hospital will help uncover the root cause of a patient's presentation or illness. We encourage a focus on safety planning and dialectical behavior therapy–based coping and well-being interventions, and we use a combination of psychotherapy modalities to aid the process of stabilization for discharge. Cognitive-based approaches have become particularly common, and these have been successfully adapted to inpatient settings and their associated lengths of stay (Katz and Cox 2002).

UNDERSTANDING THE IMPORTANCE OF NONPHARMACOLOGICAL THERAPEUTIC INTERVENTIONS ON THE INPATIENT UNIT

Initiation and optimization of psychotropic medication regimens cannot be the sole achievement of an inpatient hospitalization. Other critical tasks within these brief admissions include identifying and addressing acute psychosocial stressors, including understanding a patient's cultural background and its impact on their self-construct and family dynamic. By virtue of their admission, patients are physically removed from some of the social issues, familial stressors, and psychological demands that often contribute to psychiatric crises. This serves as an immediate intervention and allows time for stabilization and safety planning. Safety planning can be conducted as a brief yet comprehensive intervention that emphasizes both crisis prevention and effective crisis management. Stanley and Brown (2012, p. 258) describe the basic components of a safety plan created through the Safety Planning Intervention, deemed a best practice by the American Foundation for Suicide Prevention. These components include "(a) recognizing warning signs of an impending suicidal crisis; (b) employing internal coping strategies; (c) utilizing social contacts and social settings as a means of distraction from suicidal thoughts; (d) utilizing family members or friends to help resolve the crisis; (e) contacting mental health professionals or agencies; and (f) restricting access to lethal means."

Support should be provided for patients to explore and plan for each of these components. Creating a written document that outlines the details of a patient's individualized plan allows the patient to return home with an accessible reminder of how to manage escalating distress. Moreover, written plans can be reviewed with family members, who are encouraged to identify their own strategies for supporting the patient in enacting this plan. We have adapted the safety plan template developed by Stanley and Brown (2008) and utilized tools from evidence-based psychotherapy such as the feelings/fear thermometer in creating the Stoplight Safety Plan (SSP). This plan is created with the patient and reviewed in detail with the custodial parents/guardians several times during the hospital admission and is a critical component of discharge planning. This not only gives agency and responsibility to the adolescent patient, but also helps them regain their sense of agency and self-efficacy so crucial to their psychosocial development. Figure 10–1 provides an example of how an SSP is developed and utilized. A specific example of a Stoplight Safety Plan is given in Figure 10–2.

10 **Describe the RED ZONE:**
Thoughts: Prompt for specific thoughts that contribute directly to SI such as thoughts about self/others and the future. Facilitate patient in identifying any distortions that could benefit from therapeutic support.
Feelings: Prompt for specific emotional reactions that could benefit from adaptive coping strategies that patients can learn during hospitalization, such as DBT skills for distress tolerance. Address these in coping plan.
Actions: Prompt for any maladaptive actions that serve to link distressing emotions with suicidal behaviors such as isolating/shutting others out, continuing to engage in unproductive discussions, and seeking immediate relief in ways that exacerbate the issue at hand. Address these in coping plan.

9
> *Description Checklist:*
> __ *Cues that define this zone are specific, and maladaptive cues are highlighted*
> __ *Frequency/length of time typically spent in this zone is listed*

Coping plan:
— **I communicate that I am in this zone by (what words will you use?):**
Prompt for specific words that allow helpers to distinguish this zone from others. If verbal communication is too difficult, explore nonverbal strategies for communicating unsafe urges (e.g., writing/texting/code words).

8 — **Others can respond to me by (what can they say and do?):**
Support patient in considering the types of behaviors they might expect from parents after communicating unsafe urges. Identify which of these contribute to communication avoidance, and help the patient explore appropriate alternatives that parents/helpers can be coached in. If the plan includes giving space, identify the location and time length for providing space. Define what helper check-ins look like (verbal/nonverbal, numerical) and check-in frequency. Determine threshold for calling 911 or going to the hospital.

7
> *Communication Checklist:*
> __ *Language chosen is specific enough that family will understand patient's distress*
> *and be able to distinguish this communication from communication in other zones.*
> __*If plan includes nonverbal communication, ensure alternative communication*
> *strategies are practical and can be clearly understood by others (e.g., use of color*
> *codes or numbers on scale).*
> __ *Plan addresses modifications needed for different environments (school vs. home).*
> __ *Backup plans are in place, including access to other trusted adults, therapist,*
> *suicide hotlines.*
> __ *Specific behaviors or triggers that could exacerbate patient's distress in this zone*
> *were explored and alternatives identified.*
> __ *If plan includes taking space, a "safe space" plan is established (i.e., location is*
> *accessible to parent/helper by line of sight or frequent check-ins).*

— **I can use the following coping skills:**
Provide psychoeducation regarding coping tools that are most relevant to the thoughts, feelings, and actions described for this zone. Prompt for patient to identify tools that have previously benefited them and are easily accessible. Remain alert to patient describing tools which they may consider helpful in theory but could be triggering in practice (e.g., reaching out to peers who share SI, accessing social media, isolating excessively). Support patient in identifying alternative behaviors that meet these needs in a safe manner (e.g., reaching out to a safe peer, writing a letter, going through a photo album). Ensure that all strategies are safe for this zone, taking patient history into account (e.g., going for a walk alone may be high risk and require supervision). Provide psychoeducation to parents/helpers regarding how chosen tools address modifiable risk factors in this zone, and help parents brainstorm how they may reduce barriers to accessing these tools.

> *Coping Checklist:*
> __ *Specific coping strategies are identified with barriers to accessing these strategies*
> *problem-solved.*
> __ *Explored a variety of tools, including somatic skills (ice, hot shower, breathing,*
> *scents, food) cognitive skills (thought stopping, accessing wise mind, using*
> *comparisons, positive journaling), and behavioral skills (distraction via activities,*
> *accessing pets, exercise, etc.).*
> __ *Psychoeducation was provided regarding any maladaptive coping skills that patient*
> *included, and plan for ways to avoid these has been included (e.g., avoiding*
> *excessive isolation, avoiding accessing social media if triggering).*
> __ *Included PRN medication plan if appropriate*

— **It is important to go to the hospital or call 911 when:**

Review and highlight the patient's commitment to safe communication and behaviors outlined above. Identify concrete indicators for when 911 will be called or patient should be taken to the hospital for further evaluation.

> *Safety and Supervision Checklist:*
> __ *Reviewed the "safe space" plan, including patient's commitment to remain in*
> *designated location and respond to parent/helper check ins.*
> __*Reviewed threshold for calling 911 or visiting the hospital. Included verbal and*
> *behavioral cues that will alert family to take these actions (e.g., stating suicidal*
> *intent, preventing supervision, attempting to access means for harm).*

Figure 10-1. Stoplight Safety Plan template with prompts.

(continued on pages 188–189)

Describe the YELLOW ZONE:
Thoughts: Prompt for thinking patterns that place patient at risk for continuing to escalate toward the red zone.
Feelings: Prompt for feelings that can serve as cues/alerts that they are in the yellow zone and need to take action.
Actions: Prompt for actions are common within this zone. Support patient in identifying specific triggers that place them at risk for escalating to the red zone. Prompt for common behaviors that could increase exposure to these triggers (e.g., beginning to isolate from friends, which leads to red zone trigger of loneliness and being unloved; beginning to avoid schoolwork, which leads to red zone trigger of conflict with parents over grades).

> *Description Checklist:*
> __ *Cues that define this zone are specific and maladaptive cues are highlighted.*
> __ *Cues highlight risk for triggering red zone.*
> __ *Frequency/length of time typically spent in this zone is listed.*

Coping plan:
— I communicate that I am in this zone by (what words will you use?):
Explore communication with anyone in the social support network who can facilitate problem solving or help the patient avoid trigger exposure (e.g., parents, school staff, peers).

— Others can respond to me by (what can they say and do?):
Identify common triggers that link patient from yellow zone to red zone. Support patient in identifying how others can help them avoid these and support problem solving to return to green.

> *Communication Checklist:*
> __ *Language chosen is specific enough that family will understand patient's distress*
>   *and be able to distinguish this communication from communication in other zones.*
> __ *Specific supportive behaviors for parents/helpers were identified.*
> __ *Specific parent/helper behaviors that could exacerbate patient's distress in this zone*
>   *were explored and alternatives identified.*
> __ *If behaviors that parents are asked to avoid are of eventual necessity (e.g.,*
>   *discussing school progress), plan has been made to identify when/how these*
>   *conversations can occur in a more controlled setting. For example, scheduling time*
>   *limited conversations in the home and/or postponing discussions until therapy*
>   *sessions.*
> __ *Potential triggers for red zone escalation have been identified and plan made*
>   *for how patient/family can minimize exposure to these triggers.*

— I can use the following coping skills:
Provide psychoeducation on problem-focused coping, trigger avoidance, and self-care. Prompt for patient to identify coping strategies that have previously been effective. Facilitate problem-solving on how to access support for early intervention for common trigger patterns (e.g., reaching out to teachers for help when falling behind, calling IEP meeting, calling a goal-oriented family meeting).

> *Coping Checklist:*
> __ *Red zone prevention: Explored coping tools that focus on trigger avoidance,*
>   *including addressing any maladaptive coping patterns that place patient at risk (red*
>   *zone prevention).*
> __ *Green zone promotion: Explored coping tools that focus on problem-solving and*
>   *self-care.*

Figure 10–1. Stoplight Safety Plan template with prompts. (*continued*)

During this collaborative process, clinicians should remain attentive to the potential vulnerabilities and lack of supports in place to make the plan realistic and reliable. For example, adolescents may plan to communicate suicidal ideation to parents while not accounting for relationship dynamics that may impede communication in times of acute distress. Clinicians can address modifiable barriers by conducting brief interventions with the patient and family during which concrete communication and support plans are outlined. By defining specific parental behaviors that would be perceived by the patient as effectively supportive, providers can coach families to respond to crises in a manner that optimizes communication. For some teens, this may mean coaching parents to emphasize supportive validation and avoid problem-solving recommendations

Describe the GREEN ZONE:
Thoughts: Prompt for adaptive thinking about self, others, and the future.
Feelings: Prompt for emotions that represent adaptive regulation in the face of stressors.
Actions: Prompt for actions that represent adaptive daily functioning.

> *Description Checklist:*
> __ *Cues that define this zone are specific and maladaptive cues are highlighted.*
> __ *Frequency/length of time typically spent in this zone is listed.*

Coping plan:
Things I can do to stay in the green zone:
Prompt for strategies targeting any issues that made patient vulnerable to crisis and hospitalization. Emphasize self-care and stressor prevention when possible. Examples include plans for targeting school challenges, family communication, treatment adherence, etc. Most plans include goals for school reentry/504 meetings, increasing family check-ins, increasing structure and routine, and increasing regular self-care activities.

> *Coping/Self-Care Checklist:*
> __ *Explored need for sleep hygiene plan.*
> __ *Explored need for medication adherence plan.*
> __ *Explored need for commitment to change in level of care or style of therapy.*
> __ *Explored plan to address school stressors (e.g., IEP/504 or reentry meeting).*
> __ *Explored plan for patient to address social stressors (i.e., modify communication with triggering individuals or increase communication with helpful individuals).*
> __ *Explored plan for behavioral activation by increasing physical and recreational activities available.*
> __ *Explored need for substance use plan (i.e., plan for reduced access to substances and/or tox monitoring by parents or providers).*
> __ *Explored need for further consultations/supports from other providers (e.g., if patient needs additional support for eating disorder, gender dysphoria, ASD supports, among others).*
> __ *Established patient commitment to frequency and type of communication that will happen daily with family regarding level of distress until this plan is further modified by outpatient team (e.g., twice daily check-ins? Verbal/written? Number scale/zone/emotion labels?).*

Things others can help me do to stay in the green zone:
Prompt for concrete ways in which family/helpers can support patient in enacting self-care and coping plan described above. When reviewing plan with family, provide any psychoeducation handouts to facilitate their support (e.g., resources on validation strategies, collaborative problem solving, or educational support).

> *Support Checklist:*
> __ *Explored ways in which parents can facilitate any of the items that patient is committing to in the green zone (e.g., facilitate enrollment in activities, provide transportation, plan supervision for patient to spend time with friends).*
> __ *Explored commitment that family is willing to make to daily family routine to reduce triggers/stressors (e.g., family screen time curfew, family meals, work/life balance).*
> __ *Explored parental commitment to frequency and type of patient daily communication about distress.*
> __ *Explored parent role in reducing school-related stressors by working with school to establish accommodations.*

National Suicide Prevention Lifeline 1-800-273-8255
Text: CONNECT to 741741
[Clinicians to put other (local) resources, warm lines here]

Figure 10–2. Stoplight Safety Plan template with prompts. (*continued*)

until distress is reduced. For others, it may involve reducing all verbal communication and relying on visual supervision of the teen to ensure safety, while the patient agrees to use distress tolerance skills independently. A parent's contract with this plan is equally important to a patient's safety plan because it may impact an adolescent's willingness to follow through on safety communication.

At times, patients may be admitted after challenges in enacting previously created safety plans. In these circumstances, the specific barriers to safety plan adherence should be explored because they can inform

10	**Describe the RED ZONE:** (typical duration: 1–2 days monthly) **Thoughts:** I hate life, everything is my fault, it'd be better if I wasn't here anymore **Feelings:** Sad, low, anxious, more sensitive to parent's negative feedback **Actions:** Self-isolation (in room-hard share my thoughts and feelings clearly), crying, bottling up emotions, cutting (9) making plans to kill myself, or trying to kill myself (10) *Coping plan:* — I communicate that I am in this zone by (what words will you use?): I can tell/text my parents "I'm really low right now" and give number (preferably mom). If only dad is available, I can say or text code word: "red." If at 9 and unable to reach others, will call suicide hotline.
9	— Others can respond to me by (what can they say and do?): — Ask "how are you feeling right now?" — If I don't want to talk, respect that and give me physical and verbal space until I'm lower on the scale. — If I do want to talk, listen and avoid problem solving. Tell me that you hear me. Wait until I'm in yellow zone to pick a time to problem solve. — Offer me my Hope box If I don't already have it. — Let me facetime my girlfriend (I will use the call as distraction and not talk about suicidal thoughts). — During a meal, bring it up to me so I don't have to go get it. — Put my pet in my room.

8	**Safe Space Plan:**
	    — If 10, parents will be with me physically
	    — If 9, parents/sister can watch me from their room or in common area downstairs
	    — If 7–8, visual check ins every 60 minutes
	    — I will provide texts with my number and short description every 30 minutes
	    — Bedroom door to stay open when in red zone, leaving the house must be with supervision
	
	    Triggers to be avoided:
	    — Yelling/fighting with me
	    — When someone tells me I have to tell them exactly what is going on (hard for me to think clearly)
	    — Trying to solve my problems
	    — Blind affirmations
	    — Constantly checking social media, or posting about my feelings and waiting for responses

7	— I can use the following coping skills: — Use the sensory tools in my HOPE box and try an ice pack on the back of my neck. — Scroll through my photo albums. — Share my feelings with my girlfriend, sister, or one of the "trusted friends" my family and I agreed on. — Writing thoughts down through lyrics and poetry. — Listening to music while drawing. — Try my "thought stop" trick and watching TV for distraction. — Skateboarding (in front of house where parents can keep track of my location). **It is important to go to the hospital or call 911 when:** I want to kill myself (10), when I show I'm not able to follow the safe space plan in this zone, if parents notice I'm looking for or hiding means to hurt myself, if I'm taking any actions that show I'm trying to kill myself.
6	**Describe the YELLOW ZONE:** (typical duration: about 2 weeks or more every couple months) **Thoughts:** life sucks right now, I'm stuck, questioning if I'm stupid, questioning whether my friends actually care **Feelings:** switching between apathy and sadness, anxiety, constant self-doubt **Actions:** pushing friends away, procrastinating on work, skipping skating days to avoid friends, snapping at my parents and sister, less effort to do things I like, skipping meals
5	*Coping plan:* — I communicate that I am in this zone by (what words will you use?): — I can tell my mom my zone color and number during evening check in (usually right after dinner). — Tell my school counselor my yellow zone number during weekly check in (if going up, get a sooner appt).
4	— Others can respond to me by (what can they say and do?): — Ask me if I want to talk about it. If I say no, we can pick a time to talk about it later within 48 hours. Keep these check-ins shorter than 30 minutes when they do happen. — Avoid asking me about schoolwork immediately after school. Ask me during family check in twice a week. — Help me plan to see my girlfriend or friends more so I can avoid isolating (isolating is a red zone trigger). — Send my teachers/school counselor a note to check-in with me so I can make a work plan or get support to avoid falling behind (piled up work is a red zone trigger). — Work with me to avoid arguments when I'm irritable, If I snap at you, remind me "I know things are hard for you right now, and we need to keep an effort to be kind to each other." — Use validation statements when we do talk about feelings. — Make a coping recommendation or hand me the coping menu and ask me to pick one for the day. — I can use the following coping skills: — Red zone prevention: spend less than 30 minutes max in one sitting scrolling social media. Stick to my hang out commitments. Use my coping journal to track that I'm practicing my DBT skills. Get one assignment done to feel productive. Sit with my planner to map out my week. Make a list of things I'm looking forward to. When parents make a recommendation for coping, I will accept at least 1 out of every 3 suggestions. — Green zone promotion: playing guitar, watching a movie, going skating, going for ice cream with the family, baking something new, working on my comic book.

Figure 10-2. Specific example of a Safety Stoplight Plan.

(continued on page 191)

3	**Describe the GREEN ZONE:** **Thoughts:** Life is going better, I'm doing better, I've handled hard times before, take things one step at a time, not taking things personally **Feelings**: Keeping hope that things will improve, staying motivated despite obstacles, keeping a sense of humor about things when they don't go the way I planned
2	**Actions:** Doing more activities, hanging out with friends, talking more to my parents, keeping on top of my work *Coping plan:* **Things I can do to stay in the green zone:** — Keep activities in my life (hanging with friends/girlfriend, skating, music, kickboxing, walking dog, spending time with mom). Schedule at least one per day.
1	— Attend my IEP meetings so I can help decide the best way to get support from my teachers and counselor. — Avoid all substances. — Use my sleep hygiene tips (avoid screen time before bed, family phones all plugged in downstairs by 10 pm). — Eat 2.5–3 meals per day plus snacks. — Take my medication daily. **Things others can help me do to stay in the green zone:** — Create a family activity menu for fun things we can do as a family (learning to cook, museums, skiing, movies). Schedule one per week. — Work on validation skills. — Work on understanding that time with friends and girlfriend are important to my mental health and not just taking time away from studies. Drive me to activities when possible. — Reserve homework check in times for designated check in times (twice a week). If something school-related comes up and needs to be addressed sooner, ask me to pick a time to talk about it rather than springing it on me. — Keep up with my IEP meetings.

National Suicide Prevention Lifeline 1-800-273-8255
Text: CONNECT to 741741
[Clinicians to put other (local) resources, warm lines here]

Figure 10-2. Specific example of a Safety Stoplight Plan. *(continued)*

both pharmacological and nonpharmacological interventions needed to increase adherence in the future. For example, certain safety plans may have been effective when crises occurred in the home but may not have been able to be implemented in the school context. In these situations, collaboration with school staff is essential in ensuring that the patient has adequate outlets for support in different environments. In other situations, lack of adherence to safety planning may bring to light the potential need for fast-acting as-needed medication that should be made accessible to patients who are still struggling to apply distress tolerance skills rapidly enough to remain safe.

Given the broad scope of these issues, interventions are ideally delivered by an interdisciplinary team, including the integration of psychologists, psychiatrists, nurses, recreational therapists, occupational therapists, and social workers. This allows for the formulation of a more robust treatment plan that can address several goals in a more time-limited manner (Gathright et al. 2016; Lelonek et al. 2018). The collaborative roles of the interdisciplinary team can also facilitate varied opportunities for family involvement in the patient's care, which has repeatedly been shown to promote better outcomes for the mental health treatment of youth (Foster et al. 2016; Gross and Goldin 2008). Milieu staff, such as nursing and behavioral health aides, are particularly important in redirecting patients toward adaptive coping strategies and for reinforcing safety communication. Appropriate training in nonpharmacological behavioral interventions and collaborative problem solving for crisis management is essential to reducing risk of overmedication by reducing the need for as-needed medication as well as unnecessary restraints and seclusion (Allen et al. 2009; Dean et al. 2007; Martin et al. 2008).

As patients progress through inpatient treatment, the use of assessment tools such as scales that track symptom improvement can help gauge treatment gains, including response to medication for certain conditions. These tools can also demonstrate treatment efficacy to patients and families in a manner that builds hopefulness, thus increasing motivation and feelings of self-efficacy. As previously described, adherence to treatment recommendations can be fostered by maintaining a strong therapeutic alliance with patients and their families, in part through nonconfrontational and nonjudgmental approaches, including MI.

RECOGNIZING AREAS FOR FUTURE RESEARCH

Optimizing the effectiveness of time-limited inpatient hospitalizations is of great interest to clinicians, patients, families, and health care systems, but there are barriers to studying this vulnerable population. Given the nature of an inpatient psychiatric hospitalization, designing a study guided by appropriate ethical considerations, including avoidance of real or perceived coercion, is crucial. Another barrier to research is the heterogeneity in the patient population, because these patients have varied presenting complaints and come from diverse backgrounds, posing challenges in both recruitment and randomization. Among areas of future research to be considered are the efficacy of the therapeutic concepts used in an inpatient setting such as cognitive-behavioral therapy, acceptance and commitment therapy, and dialectical behavior therapy. Additionally, it is important to develop more robust metrics and valid scales to track improvement while in the hospital and beyond because those currently available are limited in application. Although we have very experienced psychiatrists and teams in the community who are able to monitor and assess patients, having available objective metrics and measures will allow for more robust and detailed treatment planning while also ensuring for continued positive outcomes upon discharge. Mobile applications and other technologies for symptom tracking, patient reporting, and provider check-ins may offer additional support and continuity for patients and families during often-fraught transitions between an inpatient hospitalization and establishment of outpatient care (Gipson et al. 2017).

Conclusion

In the current era of medical care in the United States and elsewhere, there are ever-escalating pressures to shorten expensive inpatient admissions while adhering to a rigorous standard of care. The core task of the inpatient psychiatric provider is a multifaceted, complex one: leverage the strengths of the inpatient psychiatric unit quickly and with a clear vision, to effectively stabilize the patient and best prepare the patient and their family for discharge home, where often much of the work of healing still remains to occur. It is, doubtless, a potentially daunting and burdensome task to providers. Compassion fatigue and burnout, including among psychiatrists, are increasing at a pace commensurate with the rising expectations of productivity, expedience, and precision so emblematic of modern medical practice. Approaching the assessment, formulation, treatment planning, and engagement in treatment in a dynamic but structured way, with the support of a team approach, will best position the inpatient psychiatric provider, patient, and family to develop a solid therapeutic alliance on the road to successful outcomes when time is limited and stakes are high.

References

Allen DE, de Nesnera A, Souther JW: Executive-level reviews of seclusion and restraint promote interdisciplinary collaboration and innovation. J Am Psychiatr Nurses Assoc 15(4):260–264, 2009 21665812

Blanz B, Schmidt MH: Preconditions and outcome of inpatient treatment in child and adolescent psychiatry. J Child Psychol Psychiatry 41(6):703–712, 2000 11039683

Bolton Oetzel K, Scherer DG: Therapeutic engagement with adolescents in psychotherapy. Psychotherapy: Theory, Research, Practice, Training 40(3):215–225, 2003

Colby SM, Nargiso J, Tevyaw TOL, et al: Enhanced motivational interviewing versus brief advice for adolescent smoking cessation: results from a randomized clinical trial. Addict Behav 37(7):817–823, 2012 22472523

Day JC, Bentall RP, Roberts C, et al: Attitudes toward antipsychotic medication: the impact of clinical variables and relationships with health professionals. Arch Gen Psychiatry 62(7):717–724, 2005 15997012

Dean AJ, Duke SG, George M, Scott J: Behavioral management leads to reduction in aggression in a child and adolescent psychiatric inpatient unit. J Am Acad Child Adolesc Psychiatry 46(6):711–720, 2007 17513983

DiLallo JJ, Weiss G: Motivational interviewing and adolescent psychopharma-cology. J Am Acad Child Adolesc Psychiatry 48(2):108–113, 2009 20040823

Foster K, Maybery D, Reupert A, Gladstone BA: Family focused practice in mental health care: an integrative review. Child Youth Serv 37(2):129–155, 2016

Gathright MM, Holmes KJ, Morris EM, Gatlin A: An innovative, interdisciplin-ary model of care for inpatient child psychiatry: an overview. J Behav Health Serv Res 43(4):648–660, 2016 26659088

Gipson SYT, Torous J, Maneta E: Mobile technologies in child and adolescent psychiatry: pushing for further awareness and research. Harv Rev Psychi-atry 25(4):191–193, 2017 28537949

Gross V, Goldin J: Dynamics and dilemmas in working with families in inpa-tient CAMH services. Clin Child Psychol Psychiatry 13(3):449–461, 2008 18783126

Ingoldsby EM: Review of interventions to improve family engagement and re-tention in parent and child mental health programs. J Child Fam Stud 19(5):629–645, 2010 20823946

Joshi SV: Teamwork: the therapeutic alliance in pediatric pharmacotherapy. Child Adolesc Psychiatr Clin N Am 15(1):239–262, 2006 16321733

Katz LY, Cox BJ: Dialectical behavior therapy for suicidal adolescent inpatients. Clin Case Stud 1(1):81–92, 2002

Lave JR, Frank RG: Factors affecting Medicaid patients' length of stay in psychi-atric units. Health Care Financ Rev 10(2):57–66, 1988, 10313087

Lelonek G, Crook D, Tully M, et al: Multidisciplinary approach to enhancing safety and care for pediatric behavioral health patients in acute medical set-tings. Child Adolesc Psychiatr Clin N Am 27(3):491–500, 2018 29933797

Martin A, Krieg H, Esposito F, et al: Reduction of restraint and seclusion through collaborative problem solving: a five-year prospective inpatient study. Psychiatr Serv 59(12):1406–1412, 2008

Stanley B, Brown GK: The Safety Plan Treatment Manual to Reduce Suicide Risk: Veteran Version. Washington, DC, U.S. Department of Veterans Af-fairs, 2008

Stanley B, Brown GK: Safety Planning Intervention: a brief intervention to mit-igate suicide risk. Cogn Behav Pract 19(2):256–264, 2012

Teich JL, Mutter R, Gibbons B, et al: Use of inpatient behavioral health services by children and adolescents with private insurance coverage. Psychiatr Serv 69(9):1036–1039, 2018

Totura CMW, Fields SA, Karver MS: The role of the therapeutic relationship in psychopharmacological treatment outcomes: a meta-analytic review. Psy-chiatr Serv 69(1):41–47, 2018 28945182

Twenge JM, Cooper AB, Joiner TE, et al: Age, period, and cohort trends in mood disorder indicators and suicide-related outcomes in a nationally represen-tative dataset, 2005–2017. J Abnorm Psychol 128(3):185–199, 2019 30869927

Valenkamp M, Delaney K, Verheij F: Reducing seclusion and restraint during child and adolescent inpatient treatment: still an underdeveloped area of research. J Child Adolesc Psychiatr Nurs 27(4):169–174, 2014 25100241

Winters NC, Hanson G, Stoyanova V: The case formulation in child and adoles-cent psychiatry. Child Adolesc Psychiatr Clin N Am 16(1):111–132, 2007 17141121

CHAPTER | 11

TELEPSYCHIATRY GOES VIRAL

Psychotherapeutic Aspects of Prescribing Via Telemedicine Amid (and After) COVID-19

Jeff Q. Bostic, M.D., Ed.D.
Sean Pustilnik, M.D.
David Kaye, M.D.

By early 2020, the World Health Organization announced that the novel coronavirus (COVID-19) was a pandemic, signaling a seminal event that would rapidly change society as a whole, including systems delivering health care (Shore et al. 2020). The need for social distancing and isolation strategies to flatten the curve of virus transmission and mitigate mortality forced clinicians to adopt remote communication strategies such as videoconferencing—in all social interactions across all venues, from telepsychiatry to team meetings, to even leisure activities. What previously took large organizations months to years was accomplished in days to weeks through adaptability and technical innovation; for example, a Northern California clinic changed over more than 800 mental health patients to telepsychiatry in 3 days (Yellowlees et al. 2020). The ability to rapidly transform clinics into virtual psychiatry practices became almost a matter of survival, in a literal sense for practitioners and their families in limiting exposure to infection but also in a figurative sense of being able to continue to work and sustain practices. At the same time, other colleagues in medicine and pediatrics were furloughed because of decreased patient volumes or inability to perform nonurgent or elective surgeries, while mental health evaluation and treatment remained in high demand. Everything changed, including psychopharmacology, with some aspects actually improving, some being more difficult, and some just requiring adaptations or novel approaches, as depicted in Table 11–1.

A Uniquely Shared Experience

The psychotherapeutic aspects of psychopharmacology treatment were fundamentally altered because each patient, family, and provider had unique reactions to COVID-19. Although the experience of going together through a disaster or shared trauma might unify some patients and providers, other youth experienced the COVID-19 pandemic differently based on individual circumstances (Wagner 2020). Some children dealt with infected family members and even losses, but others lived in regions largely untouched, and life events (from birthday parties to graduations, weddings, and vacations) were limited or even canceled, changing the stress load of every patient. Children of frontline medical providers and those whose parents lost jobs may have been particularly affected. Similarly, providers faced unique stresses and fears depending on institutional preparedness, geographic location, and specific work setting (inpatient, consult, outpatient balance). Child and adolescent psychiatrists who were able to maintain social distancing and continue to work at full volume, compared with colleagues facing intensive frontline exposure, were vulnerable to "survivor guilt."

Child and adolescent psychiatrists' acknowledgment of their own stress and difficulty coping may lead to a joining process with youth. Limitations in usual strategies such as physical activity, social engagement, and enjoyable activities for both youth and providers could lead to exploration of new strategies. Patients may be more willing to explore psychotherapeutic content, or parents may be more willing to consider medication options they were previously reticent toward because of a perceived limitation of other options. Child and adolescent psychiatrists must also balance the tension of wanting to help and perhaps ex-

Table 11–1. Impacts of COVID-19 on medical care

Easier aspects	More challenging aspects	Different or new impacts
Loosening of regulatory burdens, licensing, and oversight	24/7 interaction with each other and no or few other supports available	May not be able to monitor optimally (vital signs, electrocardiograms, laboratory tests)
Improved insurance reimbursement	Loss of in-person contact with other healthy influences	May have to resort to medications earlier, given limitations of other services
Decreased no-show rates (fewer scheduling demands, transition and transportation not barrier)	General stress level of children, parents, and providers	Opportunity to see into patients' and families' homes
With no school, families see pathology and progress themselves	Technology at home may not be optimized as in office	No family travel time; family may be involved differently in virtual compared with in-office visit
	Parents' knowledge/comfort with technology may be limited	Confidentiality can be challenging
	Physical aspects of provider's home, including boundary issues	
	Different demands on children and families	

peditiously prescribe, with the added uncertainties that symptoms may be more adjustment reactions than indicated diagnoses.

Telepsychiatry became a necessity for providers during the COVID pandemic but also illuminated how this tool worked well for many and perhaps not so much for others. Hearing patients poorly and seeing "parts" of them while they attended to a world beyond one's screen were among a few of the many technical obstacles. Areas unfamiliar to providers have forced us to think differently about the therapeutic components of our patient interactions on video compared with sharing space in a room together. Occurrences that would previously have been thought of as intrusive to the telepsychiatry process on both ends of the screen (e.g., other family members or pets) have become more accepted by providers, at least because of the shared lack of a sense of control. This has led to reconsideration of usual therapeutic boundaries while also creating opportunities for new avenues of rapport with selected patients. Perhaps most important, telepsychiatry will likely become a normal part of every provider's treatment armamentarium, so deciding how to best use and adapt this tool, consonant with one's personal practices, may best position providers to integrate important therapeutic components into their unique use of telepsychiatry.

The Emergence of Telepsychiatry

Telepsychiatry refers to a relationship in which the patient and provider are not in the same room physically but instead in a "virtual" room, albeit usually far away, in which the clinician is unable to see beyond what the patient allows to appear in the frame, and in which the clinician is limited to seeing and hearing the patient. The nature of this relationship is thus different, although initial evidence suggests that both patients and providers like it well enough, particularly when balancing its use against the time, cost, and logistic hurdles of trying to meet at the clinician's site (American Academy of Child and Adolescent Psychiatry 2017). *Telepsychiatry* refers to the use of secure, Health Insurance Portability and Accountability Act (HIPAA)–compliant videoconferencing to connect the psychiatric provider at the destination site with youth or their families at the origination site (Roth et al. 2019). Fundamentally, a clinician and patient (and sometimes other providers or parents) "see" each other on a screen (from computer screens to "pads" to even cell phones) in a secure space where others cannot see or overhear the encounter.

Telepsychiatry has attained prominence for multiple reasons. First, psychiatric disorders remain major contributors to the global health burden, with only some 10% of persons with mental disorders in low- and middle-income countries receiving even basic psychiatric care (Manjunatha et al. 2018). In the United States, only one-third of children with mental disorders ever receive treatment, often because of lack of available providers or feasible access. Telepsychiatry has been particularly useful to expand access to care (e.g., rural areas, or areas with few providers) and to provide greater anonymity for patients (e.g., not seeing their providers in local stores, not being seen in a provider's parking lot) (Kocsis and Yellowlees 2018). Similarly, parental efforts to get the patient to an on-site provider impede children's receiving care. At the same time, more than 70% of American youth regularly use social media and video technology, such that they are familiar and comfortable with this modality for interactions, so telepsychiatry appears particularly useful for youth with mental health needs (Roth et al. 2019).

Telepsychiatry has accelerated access to care for youth (Greenberg et al. 2006). It appears to be similar to conventional on-site treatment for youth in terms of both diagnostic accuracy and treatment effectiveness, including for those with bipolar disorder, depression, anxiety, ADHD, and adjustment disorders, and for parent training (Xie et al. 2013). Moreover, telepsychiatry appears to be cost-effective, with expenditures approximately 10% less than those for conventional on-site treatment (Stiens 2019). Finally, patient satisfaction appears high with telepsychiatry, comparable to on-site treatment (Hubley et al. 2016), including when delivered at patients' schools (improving time options for both youth and clinicians) (Cunningham et al. 2013).

The Psychotherapeutic Relationship When Prescribing in Telepsychiatry

IMPLEMENTING TELEPSYCHIATRY

In addition to clinical considerations, using telepsychiatry requires ongoing attention to evolving federal regulations, widely varying state practices, and administrative and technological parameters. For psychopharmacology, typically the clinician must be licensed in the state where practicing and usually where the patient is located as well. (Some states allow patients to receive telepsychiatry by clinicians in neighboring states, but this varies and changes frequently.) Age at consent for treatment, confidentiality parameters, and civil commitment procedures vary by state. In addition, many states require that the clinician see the patient in person face-to-face initially, before medications, particularly controlled substances, can be prescribed. Emergency procedures, such as at proximate hospitals and contact information for others (e.g., caregivers), should be established before telepsychiatry encounters (Kramer and Luxton 2016). The Center for Connected Health Policy maintains an updated website that has detailed information about telehealth regulations for each state (www.cchpca.org). Administratively, child and adolescent psychiatrists need to address HIPAA issues, including use of video or other platforms that are HIPAA compliant. Technology needs for telepsychiatry have become inexpensive, and platforms are now easily available, are HIPAA compliant, include business associate agreements, and may be compatible with electronic medical record systems. Bandwidth should be a minimum of 5 Mbps up- and download speed, and data should be sufficiently encrypted (American Psychiatric Association 2020a, 2020b).

Implementing telepsychiatry effectively appears to be based on four core components: 1) *providers* who are receptive and interested in the telepsychiatry modality to deliver care; 2) *stakeholders* (e.g., caregivers, school staff) committed to collaborating with providers through telepsychiatry; 3) *coordinators* positioned to identify space, devices, and electronic connections to bring providers, patients, and stakeholders together; and 4) *system supporters* (e.g., school, clinic, hospital administrators) willing to support both the telepsychiatry encounters and the infrastructure (space, devices, costs) to sustain telepsychiatry (Myers et al. 2010). Systemic therapy skills are often needed to align all these participants:

1. Clarifying both the interest level and apprehensions of each participant alone and addressing these with factual information and collaborative solutions diminishes resistance.
2. Managing identified resistance by empathic responses to not only the stated obstacle but also potential underlying fears (e.g., "I don't know how to use this software and could be embarrassed in front of patients or others") may be required (e.g., "Let's practice these encounters first, and then let's pilot this first with familiar, collaborative patients").
3. Anticipating resistance that may not be stated or acknowledged but instead acted out (e.g., complaints that the service was too slow or the patient's devices were too old to continue a telepsychiatry encounter)

requires thoughtful interventions to support participants who just cannot seem to "do" telepsychiatry.

4. Coalescing the participants is a high priority because one participant can derail telepsychiatry interventions; obtaining feedback from all participants often illuminates patterns or themes (e.g., "Our telepsychiatry room is too often needed for emergency or crisis events"), which then can be directly problem-solved by participants or may require intervention with specific participants who do not fulfill their telepsychiatry functions.

   a. Clarifying roles and whom to contact about specific components decreases frustration (which, if not addressed, can lead to fragmentation of services or scapegoating of participants).

   b. When problem-solving with particular participants is ineffective, backing up to the participant's perceptions about telepsychiatry (e.g., "It's just a way of connecting all of us so service can be centralized with providers at one site") may be helpful.

   c. Rarely, patterns of dysfunction may persist with particular participants such that either the process needs to be simplified (e.g., "Sounds like you [the clinician] may need to enter the identified room 30 minutes early, set up, do phone calls, so that the room remains available and ready for telepsychiatry sessions"), or sometimes, clinicians may not really be invested in using telepsychiatry options, signaling the need to address their resistances.

5. Reviewing the telepsychiatry process with these participants can help sustain momentum and coalesce this team, particularly by identifying patient successes (both clinically and logistically; e.g., "This is the only way this specific patient or family would ever get seen by us"), so that ongoing efforts and improvements in this process occur.

PSYCHOTHERAPEUTIC ASPECTS OF PRESCRIBING VIA TELEPSYCHIATRY

Using Electronic Devices to Enhance the Therapeutic Alliance in Medication Treatment

Telepsychiatry conditions the patient to connect virtually. This allows the patient more control than is possible in the conventional practice of going to a clinician's office. Kocsis and Yellowlees (2018) have reported that even in intensive psychotherapy settings (including psychoanalysis), increased eye contact in telepsychiatry appears to be moderated by the physical distance afforded by telepsychiatry; patients appear more comfortable discussing intimate or distressing subjects (sexual activity, substance use) because of the "protection of the virtual space." Patients are able to control what the clinician sees (from their faces to their home environments). This affords several advantages in ongoing medication treatment:

1. Patients can provide "virtual tours" of their homes to clarify where medications are stored, to more accurately "count" remaining pills, and to provide additional understanding about the patient's environment. Even "meeting the family" in their natural environment through telepsychiatry may help the provider recognize considerations for storing medicines, where to place reminders, and even variables to monitor (e.g., the patient's adherence to a daily schedule, managing their bedroom, destruction of property).
2. Patients may record and provide visual depictions of possible side effects of medication so that the clinician may "see" what patients are reporting.
3. Patients may use cell phone apps to remind themselves to take medication, to record changes in symptoms, and to recognize side effects so that encounters include more "data" than recollections only during the encounter (Stiens 2019, p. 13; see also Kim et al. 2016).
4. Patients may use their many electronic devices to enhance mental health by including positive images (e.g., pictures that always bring a smile to counter daily "down times") or music playlists throughout the day to help improve their clinical functioning.

For optimizing clinical encounters, configuring the electronics effectively can lead to a significant positive impact. Preferred practices for creating connectedness with patients and to develop good "webside manner" are described in Table 11–2 (Roth et al. 2019).

The Therapeutic Telepsychopharmacology Interview

Configuring telepsychiatry with each patient. The patient's familiarity and comfort level with technology impact telepsychiatry visits, so youth already engaged with electronic media adapt more easily to telepsychiatry visits (Wang and Alexander 2014). Telerapport appears favored by the following (Myers et al. 2008):

1. A more casual style by the clinician

Table 11–2. Preferred practices for telepsychiatry configuration

Telepsychiatry condition	Preferred practices
Camera placement	Place atop the computer screen so that the patient and clinician are looking at eyes versus the image on the screen below; if using a mobile device, place so that it does not move around during the encounter.
Room: background	Use warm color background (close or draw curtain over windows); minimize "busy-ness" (i.e., distractions or items hard to see or make sense of behind the clinician).
Lighting	Ensure that face and expressions are clearly visible; avoid using lights behind you and halos (from backlighting); use indirect lighting by lamps in front of the clinician and equipment.
Sound	Make it easy to hear what patient says; consider a headset; have minimal ambient noise; add pillows, curtains, tapestries, and so on to walls to absorb sound.
Size	Adjust size to allow patient, parent, or child to play on the floor and be seen at his or her location.
Eye contact	Maintain eye contact (vs. looking down and typing); eyes should be about one-third down from the top of the image patients see.
Facial expression	Keep face aimed toward the screen (not sideways) and smile often.
Body position	Maintain upright and open posture, but situate yourself about 2–3 feet from camera so that head, torso, and arms can be seen; young patients may need to sit in parent's lap with parent in middle of screen.
Gestures	Remember that nodding and smaller gestures can enhance communication (e.g., thumbs-up, point at ear if cannot hear), but they should be slowed so as not to appear blurry on-screen.
Speaking	Speak at normal rate and volume, but increase pause time to avoid talking over each other.
Screen empathy and "webside manner"	Nod (and smile) instead of saying "Yes," "Tell me more," and so on; move in to show interest; move back when patient may feel trapped, defensive, paranoid, or uncomfortable.
Movement	Avoid drifting off the screen; minimize charting and instead favor maintaining eye contact with patient.

Table 11–3. Interview questions to prepare patients for televisits

---

1. What is your **experience** with videocalls, FaceTime, or Skype? (Note whether the patient may associate such calls with negative events, such as breakups or bad news from others.)

2. Is there anything you particularly **like** about videocalls? Is there anything you don't like about these videocalls?

3. How do you think you would **feel** while doing our visits by video (on a computer, laptop, pad, or cell phone)?

4. What would help make you **comfortable** during these telesessions? (Sometimes patients may want to have fidgets next to them, beverages, and so on.) Where would you feel most comfortable and safe doing a telesession? (Particular rooms or spaces can be discussed to ensure acceptable viewing or lighting, confidentiality, and so on.)

5. Would you like to **show me** your room, home, other family members during the session?

6. What might be some good **cues** for us to use if we're having trouble hearing or seeing each other or if you're feeling uncomfortable during the telepsychiatry session?

---

2. Demystifying the experience by direct, open answers about where the clinician is during the session
3. Showing audiovisual controls (e.g., zooming in, muting) to the patient and allowing the patient to try using them and making adjustments based on individual preferences
4. Having adults present (for child patients) to provide appropriate structure, including assisting the child in remaining, when needed, within the frame

In addition, younger patients and those with behavioral issues report feeling less stigma when visits are by telehealth, and anxious patients report that telepsychiatry tends to be less anxiety provoking than face-to-face visits in a clinician's office (Mucic and Hilty 2020). Patients describe a greater sense of safety and control when dealing with an unfamiliar adult (e.g., mental health clinician) and a greater sense of personal space (Roth et al. 2019). However, patients with histories of trauma sometimes report feeling more detached or disconnected during televisits (Wang and Alexander 2014). The framework provided in Table 11–3 may be helpful for clinicians to assess a patient's receptivity to televisits.

Patient responses to these items help position the clinician to configure telepsychiatry sessions around the unique needs and preferences of each patient, fostering a collaborative therapeutic relationship. In addition, this approach allows problem solving to be practiced with the patient about which devices to use and how they will ensure confidentiality; assessment for any fantasies the patient may have about these sessions being recorded and later viewable by others; or assessment of other potential barriers that may impede enthusiasm for telepsychiatry visits.

In addition, positive psychology approaches may be integrated into telepsychopharmacology sessions, as shown in Table 11–4.

Psychotherapeutic aspects within telepsychopharmacology sessions. Individualizing telepsychiatry sessions through a collaborative approach also sets the stage for the collaborative therapeutic relationship. Greetings for meetings may include gestures (e.g., fist pumps or unique tele-handshakes on the screen) to move beyond the often-sterile doorbell sounds signifying entrance to many video platforms. Cues used to signal that audio and video quality are good (e.g., thumbs up) also help increase connection for the session to begin.

Clinicians should anticipate unexpected lapses (e.g., frozen frames) in the audio and video quality during sessions. Not only does this disrupt the patient's narrative flow, but it may also artificially cause the patient to pause about comments made, to reconsider them, and even to imagine such audiovisual malfunctions (Freudian blips) are not coincidental but instead a signal from the tele-universe to reconsider sharing such information.

Patient diagnoses may also influence how telesessions are provided. Even patients with psychosis tolerate the virtual distance afforded by telepsychiatry and report decreased anxiety via telesessions, in which turning away or speaking without eye contact may be needed (Sharp et al. 2011). Patients with anxiety who may be unable to leave home or to come into an office consistently may benefit from a "hybridized" model of telesessions when unable to get to the office but with goals of being able to get out and navigate to the office. Patients with autism spectrum disorder may engage with computer or electronic devices more eagerly than in an office, and screen sharing to put other items or games onto the screen for parts of the session may increase patient cooperation. Patients with past trauma report decreased anxiety and more openness discussing sensitive material in telesessions. Boundary concerns may require attention to personality disorder concerns, such as patients engaging in other activities or multitasking during telesessions (Kocsis and Yellowlees 2018), although this may also occur in patients who are young or who have ADHD. Teleclinicians who engage in other tasks or multitask during telesessions may similarly need to recognize potential im-

Table 11–4.	The pharmacotherapy evaluation using a positive psychology approach (adolescent version)

Initial pharmacotherapy evaluation

1. What **positive symptoms or emotions** do you wish to regain or feel?

    a. How have you been feeling serenity, hope, awe, love, joy, inspiration, and gratitude recently?

    b. Have you been feeling fear, regret, envy, shame, hate, guilt, anger, or sadness recently?

    c. What would you wish treatment could alter about your current emotions?

2. How are you **engaging** with things that matter to you?

    a. Do you lose yourself in desirable activities?

    b. What are you noticing instead of losing yourself in preferred thoughts or activities?

3. How are your **relationships**? How are you connecting to others?

    a. How will others who matter to you think about your diagnosis?

    b. How will they react to you taking medication?

4. What has **meaning** to you?

    a. What does it mean to you to have a psychiatric diagnosis?

    b. What does it mean to you to take a medication?

5. What are you **accomplishing** these days?

    a. Despite your current distress, what are you continuing to do well?

    b. What is interfering with your accomplishing tasks?

"Homework" exercises between sessions

1. Log your emotions frequently (daily if possible).

    a. Which are most prominent?

    b. How intensely are you feeling positive emotions?

    c. What survival emotions have been most prominent?

2. How are you engaging in those things that really matter to you?

3. Who are you reaching out to? How are you stepping up your interactions with others?

4. What are you doing to create meaning during this chapter or time in your life?

Table 11–4. The pharmacotherapy evaluation using a positive psychology approach (adolescent version) *(continued)*

"Homework" exercises between sessions *(continued)*

5. Add to your weekly accomplishment log.

   a. What accomplishments each week are you noticing?

   b. How's your exercise going?

   c. How's your nutrition going?

   d. How's your sleep routine going?

   e. How's your spiritual side doing?

Follow-up pharmacotherapy evaluations

1. How have your positive or survival emotions changed on your current medication regimen?

2. How are you now engaging or being involved with those things that really matter to you?

3. How are your relationships now going with others (family, school staff, and friends)?

4. What has it meant to you to be taking medication? How do you feel about taking it?

5. What things have you accomplished (that you wanted to) since our last meeting?

---

pacts of their boundary breaches on their therapeutic relationships with patients.

Clinicians should also examine how telesessions feel for them. It may be difficult to take notes or to chart during telesessions while trying to remain empathic and attuned to patients. Clinicians may also feel "on-stage" rather than "in the room" with the patient, which requires patience to alter. Countertransference reactions may also arise because patients may have more technical expertise about audio-video technology, such that the clinician feels embarrassed or inadequate with such patients or triggered by telepsychiatry technology to feel uncomfortable and distracted or preoccupied. However, clinicians may also feel more relaxed and open to discuss topics via this protective space, particularly with patients having a history of volatility or violence (Kocsis and Yellowlees 2018).

Prescribing within telepsychiatry has remained a bit more complicated because the clinician does not hand the patient a prescription as in conventional practice. Several models have emerged, from the clinician sending prescriptions or contacting the pharmacy to the clinician interacting with the patient's primary care provider, who will then write prescriptions for the patient (Myers et al. 2008).

Side effects should always be investigated during psychopharmacology visits, and possible side effects may be shown or demonstrated to the clinician via telepsychiatry. Similarly, the clinician may demonstrate side effects (e.g., tics) to better ensure accurate detection of side effects.

Treatment planning can be enhanced by easier participation of others engaged with the patient. Time with the patient alone is usually preferred so that delicate information or concerns by the patient may be more easily shared. Collateral input and treatment planning often benefit by participation of others, including on-screen. Shared screen video platforms allow multiple people to simultaneously be on the screen (e.g., parents, significant others, teachers) or for rating scales, school reports, or events to be reviewed by all to improve alignment and problem solving around treatment goals.

Future Directions

Telemedicine expands opportunities for clinical care both through different clinical options and through the integration of emerging technology:

1. Virtual reality (VR) affords options for increasing therapeutic density of treatment options. For example, VR exposure therapy has been found effective in the treatment of patients with anxiety disorders, phobias, social anxiety disorder, PTSD, panic disorder, addiction disorders, eating disorders, autism spectrum disorder, and schizophrenia. User satisfaction has been high, and refusal rates significantly lower than in traditional therapies. VR programs can be constructed with a variety of circumstances and elements to best meet the individual needs of each patient (Maples-Keller et al. 2017).
2. Similarly, "virtual" providers may further enhance the options and palatability of psychiatric care to expand treatment options as well as the "match" between patients and providers (Mucic and Hilty 2020, p. 4).
3. Among the most powerful psychotherapeutic opportunities available through telepsychiatry will be the ultimate "capturing" of patient symptoms and patterns, which can then be more objectively examined by the patient and treater. Although recording patient encounters may be initially concerning to patients and providers, ultimately, recording patient encounters (or segments of them) will enhance clinical care. Through recording patient encounters, patients' (and

providers') awareness of changes in symptoms may be "seen" more easily, as well as side effects or residual symptoms. Resistances may be addressed objectively and quickly as the patient and treater review what symptoms were on the screen, and the treatment alliance can be strengthened by "seeing" the actual symptoms or side effects being targeted. In addition, when treatment is initiated and the patient can provide appropriate informed consent, subsequent sessions in which the patient exhibits psychotic, manic, or profound anxiety symptoms, often unrecallable by the patient after an acute exacerbation, can be viewed to improve the patient's awareness of differences when taking or not taking different medications.

4. Emerging technologies to monitor mood or anxiety responses (now even with "rings" or watches) may allow the patient and provider to wire up together during sessions to more objectively monitor mood responses and physical reactions during these sessions.

COVID-19: Not Treatment as Usual

So often in medicine, and especially telemedicine, an intervention is compared to the concept of "treatment as usual" to determine efficacy, even when usual treatment may not be available.

Before the COVID-19 pandemic, telepsychiatry was used to help expand access to mental health treatment for children to areas where it was unlikely to be available or for those who had significant barriers to coming to a clinic (e.g., distance to clinic, limited financial means to travel/transport to clinic, severe developmental disabilities). With child psychiatry clinics and other services unable to operate as usual, the previous provider resistances (noted earlier in this chapter) were dwarfed compared with the need to continue to provide care to patients, and telepsychiatry adoption surged. This may partly be attributable to the easing of regulatory and licensing burdens and payment barriers that previously seemed overwhelming for providers to figure out. However, providers may experience additional unease if not able to perform certain monitoring tasks such as vital signs, laboratory studies, or electrocardiograms if indicated. The lack of familiarity with telepsychiatry may also compound provider vulnerability without the "prop" of being in their office and the confidence conveyed to families with diplomas, volumes of books, and awards (Carlson and Wilens 2020).

Because of circumstances of isolating together, family dynamics (both adaptive and unhelpful) were sometimes amplified. Without reliance on school and other social supports and activities, parents become more intimately aware of what is going on with their child throughout the day (when not teleworking themselves) and develop a more robust understanding of the child's functioning. Parents who may have been uninterested or logistically unavailable to engage in the child's mental health treatment may be within earshot or have the opportunity to join in. More than ever, an assessment of all family members' coping during the shared stressor can shed light on the index child's struggles.

Telepsychiatry makes it easier for families to engage in and sustain regular treatment. For some families, this is a preferable, more comfortable mode of interaction and is logistically easier for ongoing treatment. Yet telepsychiatry also requires a more distant mode of relating, including both patient and provider difficulties in recognizing nuances particularly of nonverbal communication not fully visible on the screen. Concerns of social media impacts on a child's ability to communicate verbally and form meaningful relationships may creep into telepsychiatry as well. Providers report telepsychiatry is an acceptable way to interact, but many do not describe it as rewarding or impactful as meeting in person. So, likely the future will be a hybrid model of in person face-to-face meetings alongside telepsychiatry, VR, and telephonic communication, and coalescing of current and emerging technologies to balance forging optimal patient-provider relationships with accessibility and sustainable treatment.

It is likely that someday, telepsychiatry, and possibly all of medicine, will look back at how things were before the COVID-19 pandemic and then during or afterward. The genie may have been let out of the bottle on aspects such as licensing and regulatory requirements enough for patients, families, and providers to realize some of the real advantages of telepsychiatry within child psychiatry practice. It is unclear how much things will return to the "previous normal," but hopefully as providers increase their comfort and sophistication with telepsychiatry practice, we will be able to provide more high-quality mental health treatment for youth in need.

References

American Academy of Child and Adolescent Psychiatry, Committee on Telepsychiatry and AACAP Committee on Quality Issues: Clinical update: telepsychiatry with children and adolescents. J Am Acad Child Adolesc Psychiatry 56(10):875–893, 2017 28942810

American Psychiatric Association: Telepsychiatry Practice Guidelines (video). Available at: https://www.psychiatry.org/psychiatrists/practice/telepsychiatry/toolkit/practice-guidelines. Accessed May 18, 2020a.

American Psychiatric Association: Telepsychiatry Toolkit. Available at: https://www.psychiatry.org/psychiatrists/practice/telepsychiatry/toolkit. Accessed May 18, 2020b.

Carlson G, Wilens T: AACAP screenside chats—episode 3: managing medication remotely. Podcast/video. 2020. Available at: https://www.aacap.org/ScreensideChats

Cunningham DL, Connors EH, Lever N, Stephan SH: Providers' perspectives: utilizing telepsychiatry in schools. Telemed J E Health 19(10):794–799, 2013 23980938

Greenberg N, Boydell KM, Volpe T: Pediatric telepsychiatry in Ontario: caregiver and service provider perspectives. J Behav Health Serv Res 33(1):105–111, 2006 16636911

Hubley S, Lynch SB, Schneck C, et al: Review of key telepsychiatry outcomes. World J Psychiatry 6(2):269–282, 2016 27354970

Kim J, Lim S, Min YH, et al: Depression screening using daily mental-health ratings from a smartphone application for breast cancer patients. J Med Internet Res 18(8):e216, 2016 27492880

Kocsis BJ, Yellowlees P: Telepsychotherapy and the therapeutic relationship: principles, advantages, and case examples. Telemed J E Health 24(5):329–334, 2018 28836902

Kramer GM, Luxton DD: Telemental health for children and adolescents: an overview of legal, regulatory, and risk management issues. J Child Adolesc Psychopharmacol 26(3):198–203, 2016 26259027

Manjunatha N, Kumar CN, Math SB, Thirthalli J: Designing and implementing an innovative digitally driven primary care psychiatry program in India. Indian J Psychiatry 60(2):236–244, 2018 30166682

Maples-Keller JL, Bunnell BE, Kim SJ, Rothbaum BO: The use of virtual reality technology in the treatment of anxiety and other psychiatric disorders. Harv Rev Psychiatry 25(3):103–113, 2017 28475502

Mucic D, Hilty DM: Psychotherapy using electronic media, in Intercultural Psychotherapy. Edited by Schouler-Ocak M, Kastrup MC. Cham, Switzerland, Springer Nature, 2020, pp 205–229

Myers K, Cain S; Work Group on Quality Issues, American Academy of Child and Adolescent Psychiatry Staff: Practice parameter for telepsychiatry with children and adolescents. J Am Acad Child Adolesc Psychiatry 47(12):1468–1483, 2008 19034191

Myers KM, Vander Stoep A, McCarty CA, et al: Child and adolescent telepsychiatry: variations in utilization, referral patterns and practice trends. J Telemed Telecare 16(3):128–133, 2010 20197356

Roth DE, Ramtekkar U, Zekovic-Roth S: Telepsychiatry: a new treatment venue for pediatric depression. Child Adolesc Psychiatr Clin N Am 28(3):377–395, 2019 31076115

Sharp IR, Kobak KA, Osman DA: The use of videoconferencing with patients with psychosis: a review of the literature. Ann Gen Psychiatry 10(1):14, 2011 21501496

Shore JH, Schneck CD, Mishkind MC: Telepsychiatry and the coronavirus disease 2019 pandemic—current and future outcomes of the rapid virtualization of psychiatric care. JAMA Psychiatry 2020 [Epub ahead of print] 32391861

Stiens L: Uses, benefits, and future directions of telepsychiatry. Creative Components 251, 2019. Available at: https://lib.dr.iastate.edu/creativecomponents/251. Accessed March 31, 2021.

Wagner KD: Addressing the experience of children and adolescents during the COVID-19 pandemic (editorial). J Clin Psychiatry 81(3):20ed13394, 2020

Wang L, Alexander C: Telepsychiatry: technology progress, challenges, and language and transcultural issues. Journal of Translational Medicine and Developmental Disorders 1:1–11, 2014

Xie Y, Dixon JF, Yee OM, et al: A study on the effectiveness of videoconferencing on teaching parent training skills to parents of children with ADHD. Telemed J E Health 19(3):192–199, 2013 23405952

Yellowlees P, Nakagawa K, Pakyurek M, et al: Rapid conversion of an outpatient psychiatric clinic to a 100% virtual telepsychiatry clinic in response to COVID-19. Psychiatr Serv 71(7):749–752, 2020 32460683

PART IV

POPULATIONS

CHAPTER 12

ALLIANCE ISSUES TO CONSIDER IN PHARMACOTHERAPY WITH TRANSITION-AGE YOUTH

Jennifer Derenne, M.D.
Farrah Fang, M.D.
Anthony L. Rostain, M.D., M.A.

The term *transition-age youth* refers to a developmental stage between adolescence and adulthood (16–26 years) (Fuchs and Martel 2017). The term came to prominence as various systems of care (e.g., health care, child welfare) struggled with helping young people who were "aging out" of pediatric services and transitioning to adult care. These systems recognized that mental disorders arising in childhood and adolescence rarely remit spontaneously on achieving the age of majority. Given that child and adolescent psychiatrists are trained to work with adults as well as with children and adolescents, they are in a unique position to help transition-age youth populations and their families prepare for the move to adult mental health services (Chan et al. 2014; Derenne and Martel 2013b; Derenne and Usher 2019). In this chapter we review the challenges and opportunities facing this clinical group and offer specific guidance to practitioners in their efforts to help vulnerable youth and their families prepare for the transition to adulthood.

Vulnerabilities and Barriers

Transition-age youth populations with mental health issues are especially vulnerable for several reasons. They have high rates of risky behaviors, including experimenting with substance use (Substance Abuse and Mental Health Services Administration 2019) and multiple sexual partners, and low rates of participation in health maintenance behaviors and preventive medical visits. This may be secondary to the fact that they are often otherwise healthy and maintain that they are "invincible" or that nothing bad will happen to them. They are less likely to be covered by insurance, especially if they are employed part time and are no longer students (Narendorf et al. 2017). They are also prone to risk taking at this developmental stage because they are in the process of separating and individuating from their family of origin (Leebens and Williamson 2017). From a neurobiological perspective, their frontal lobes are still in the process of pruning and myelination, which means the circuits undergirding executive functioning are relatively immature. This developmental lag can lead to poor judgment and decision making, impulsivity, excessive risk taking, and difficulties with emotional regulation (Chung and Hudziak 2017).

Young adults can present for mental health treatment in many different settings. Although college has become the expected next step for many after finishing high school, not all transition-age youth want to or have the skills necessary to attend university (Pao 2017). Some choose to enter the workforce directly. Others sign up for military service. Still others defer postsecondary education and take a gap year to travel, work, or volunteer. Community college and technical school programs offer additional options for those who are not interested in a traditional 4-year university program of study (Derenne 2018). Of those who do enter college, many struggle with suboptimal transitions that result in medical leaves of absence or dropping out altogether. Students with a history of mental health treatment sometimes benefit from choosing schools that are closer to home or those that have bridge programs to provide additional structure and support. Some find it helpful to take a few classes at a community college and live at home with their parents to practice implementing independent living skills before moving out on their own. More severely impaired transition-age youth may not be able to work or go to school and are cared for in community mental health centers or specialized facilities (Derenne 2018).

In spite of the challenges and barriers presented above, there are many opportunities for TAY populations who are college-bound to connect and thrive. Developing a sense of belonging with a group of peers or with specific ethnocultural communities can be key, especially for students who are the first in their families to attend college, students from low-income households, and those from BIPOC (Black, Indigenous and Persons of Color) communities. An example follows from a previous review on this topic (Wang and Joshi 2018, p. 392):

> DB attended an elite university as a first-generation student whose parents were Central American immigrants. During her first year, she had good academic results and made numerous social connections through the on-campus Latino community center. However, she struggled to maintain these connections during her sophomore year, after some of her friends dropped out of school. She began to expand her social connections to include many students from the dominant (white, non-first-generation) student culture and at times felt estranged from her culture of origin. She felt a loss of belongingness and also began to experience a growing acculturation stress, as she tried to live her life as a bicultural young adult. DB insightfully comments on her own experience: "What really helped me the most was being able to share my story with people who got me. This included not only resident fellows and counselors but also my friends (both Latino and 'other') and my former counselor from high school. Also, there were classes I took that helped me focus on my own wellness, and that honored my story."

Significant barriers may impact the successful transition from pediatric to adult mental health care. When a patient reaches the age of majority, he or she now has the legal right to refuse treatment or to restrict contact between parents and clinicians (Chan 2018). Often, patients express the hope that moving into a new phase of life will mean no longer needing mental health services. They may believe that increased autonomy and independence will lead to decreased stress and diminished symptoms. It is common for young adults to stop taking medications or to experiment with decreasing the frequency of psychotherapy appointments when they turn 18. The myth of invulnerability, fear of being chronically ill (and the stigma it implies), and worries about the long-term effects of medication all work to reduce the young person's motivation to remain in treatment. Unfortunately, such thinking is often misguided because decreased structure, support, and parental oversight combined with increased expectations and autonomy are more commonly associated with an exacerbation of symptoms.

Those who go to college may procrastinate or defer connecting to the counseling center or disability office out of shame, embarrassment, or concerns about stigma. Others may be misinformed about the services available to them. For example, many campuses have limits on the number of sessions available through the counseling center. Others refer students with long-standing mental health issues to community providers for ongoing care. Some college campuses are too rural or remote to have subspecialty mental health services available. Transportation issues may also impact access to care. Financial concerns are also very widespread in the young adult population and may limit treatment options. Those who are still students may remain on their parents' insurance plan until age 26 years through the Affordable Care Act (Chan 2018). However, those who are working jobs without health benefits or those who are unable to work or attend school may be uninsured or underinsured.

Differences in philosophy and approach may also make it easy for diverse transition-age youth populations to slip through the cracks when making the transition from pediatric to adult clinics. Pediatric providers tend to involve families and other stakeholders (e.g., teachers, coaches, and guidance counselors) in care and offer a lot of structure and support for making and keeping follow-up appointments. They are likely to call when an appointment is missed and reach out to teachers and parents as needed. Adult clinics tend to value autonomy and assume that patients will schedule appointments when they are ready to access care and are less likely to reach out or offer support when appointments are missed. They are also less likely to recommend that individuals sign releases of information to allow clinicians to have contact with parents and other important individuals involved in their care.

Functional Domains in Transition Planning

Members of the American Academy of Child and Adolescent Psychiatry Transition-Age Youth and College Student Mental Health Committee have described six domains of functioning that are important for helping older youth seamlessly transition to adulthood (Derenne and Martel 2013a, 2015) (Table 12–1). Although initially developed to assist with making the transition to college, these domains can also be used in the

Table 12–1. Essential functional domains in transition planning

Health condition knowledge and skills

Self-advocacy knowledge and skills

Independent life skills

Psychosocial development

Academic skills and executive function

Anticipatory guidance

Source. Leebens 2018.

non-college-bound transition-age youth population. The hope is that if youth are given opportunities to practice independence while still living with their parents, they will have the scaffolding, support, and safety net of parental oversight to nurture and protect them before they leave home. Clinicians who work with teens and young adults can help anticipate and assess specific needs and guide parents and families through the process. The remainder of this chapter reviews each of these functional domains in greater detail.

HEALTH CONDITION KNOWLEDGE AND SKILLS

Young people need to gain an accurate understanding of their symptoms, diagnoses, and treatment options. They should know what their conditions are called, the names and doses of their medications, and what the medications are used to treat, and they need to know the important signs and symptoms of their illnesses. It is also important that they understand the effects of nutrition, sleep, stress, and exercise on their underlying disorders. When they are experiencing symptom exacerbation, they need to know how to access additional help and support. It is important that youth get experience making and keeping medical, psychiatric, and psychotherapy appointments before being on their own. They also need to practice filling and refilling prescriptions before they run out of medication and to get into the routine of independently taking medications as directed.

SELF-ADVOCACY KNOWLEDGE AND SKILLS

Young adults in transition should be helped to understand the importance of understanding and advocating for one's needs. They should understand mental health law, their right to privacy, and their right to determine their own treatment course. They should also understand their rights to accommodations at school or in the workplace and should know how to advocate for themselves with employers or campus administration. College students need to be aware of the services that the disability office provides, including contacting professors about any accommodations that have been granted. Students may need to reinforce this information with their teachers. This is a marked difference from high school, where the onus is on the educational system to identify students with learning challenges and provide them with the appropriate support.

INDEPENDENT LIFE SKILLS

Many of these young adults are dependent on their parents, teachers, and coaches guiding them through their daily activities. They may not have a lot of experience managing their own schedules, especially when these may change from day to day. It is imperative that they learn to implement a daily routine of adequate sleep, regular wake-up times (setting an alarm and getting up when it goes off), moderate exercise, balanced diet, and consistent attendance at classes, jobs, practices, and appointments. They also need to be able to manage a budget, do laundry, and keep their living space clean and orderly. This can be challenging for those who are not used to having virtually unlimited and unmonitored access to video games, parties, and other fun activities. It is even more difficult for individuals experiencing mood, anxiety, or inattention symptoms that adversely affect energy, motivation, and concentration.

PSYCHOSOCIAL DEVELOPMENT

In addition to navigating newfound independence around scheduling and activities, adolescents and young adults are neurodevelopmentally programmed to experiment with new roles and behaviors as they search for and form their identities. They may be deepening friendships, establishing romantic relationships, and learning to navigate conflicts with roommates or coworkers. Meeting people from different backgrounds and cultures may enable them to challenge their personal values and beliefs. This may be especially novel for young adults in the first-generation and low-income categories. Changing attitudes and behaviors may cause tensions with family or friends, especially if they are distancing from close relationships. This can be destabilizing in some situations, particularly if others are threatened by these changes. It is important to remember that psychosocial development is not linear and that there are inevitable ups and downs in the journey toward achieving a stable sense of self.

ACADEMIC SKILLS AND EXECUTIVE FUNCTION

Teens transitioning to adulthood, especially those who are college bound, may have a lot of experience with progressively increasing academic workloads, but they may not have as much experience organizing themselves with the competing demands of sleep, relationships, and managing independent living skills. Those who have previously used tutors, coaches, instructional accommodations, and other strategies to support their executive functioning skills often struggle with the loss of these supports as they move on to the next phase of life. Practicing these skills and increasing independence and autonomy throughout high school can help smooth this transition. Equally important is the process of finding sources of support and guidance in the college environment or in the workplace.

ANTICIPATORY GUIDANCE

It is important for patients and families to consider and openly discuss potential challenges and pitfalls while considering the opportunities that lie ahead. For example, moving to a new part of the country for college might allow for new experiences that shape identity in positive and meaningful ways. At the same time, increased freedom offers the temptation to experiment with risky behaviors that might have negative effects on academics, social relationships, and health. For instance, experimenting with illicit substances can result in medical complications, injury, arrest, addiction, or relapse of psychiatric symptoms. Clinicians should foresee potential pitfalls and encourage young people to consider how they might face them in the future. This may require a motivational interviewing approach, whereby the patient is asked to consider the pros and cons of experimenting with substances and other risky behaviors.

Treatment Implications for Psychiatric Pharmacotherapy

The Institute of Medicine's 2014 report "Investing in the Health and Well-Being of Young Adults" (Institute of Medicine and National Research Council 2014) somberly notes that up to two-thirds of the burden of disability in transition-age youth is associated with either mental health or substance use disorders, and only one-fourth of these youth are receiving treatment. Moreover, the report notes a conspicuous absence of research evidence demonstrating the effectiveness of medical and psychosocial interventions with transition-age youth populations (Stroud et al. 2015). As Skehan and Davis (2017) point out: "There is no research to date that assesses the pharmacologic effectiveness of FDA-approved treatments specifically in transition age youth." This presents major challenges to clinicians working with this population. Not only is the choice of medication difficult to determine in the absence of good evidence, but there are no long-term studies examining the impact of psychotropic medications on disease outcome, functional status, or long-term health. Safety concerns are especially important when considering the use of agents that are associated with weight gain, metabolic syndrome, or cardiovascular risks and subject to misuse and abuse.

The issue of medication adherence, a challenge throughout all of clinical medicine, is especially difficult with transition-age youth populations. A combination of factors, such as systems barriers (e.g., insurance, access to care), cultural biases, developmental variables (e.g., limited insight and judgment), and individual differences (e.g., cognitive abilities, attitudes, habits), contributes to poor adherence to treatment. In general, a shared-decision-making model is favored in working with older teens and young adults insofar as this emphasizes patient autonomy regarding treatment options as well as individual responsibility for maintaining or modifying the treatment regimen (Skehan and Davis 2017).

Using a shared-decision-making framework, clinicians can improve treatment adherence by providing thorough information about the patient's diagnosis, education about the medication regimen being proposed (including the most common side effects), ongoing discussions about target symptoms that the medication is aimed at addressing, and close communication during the initial phases of treatment. It is also important to address predictable barriers to treatment adherence in a matter-of-fact way, pointing out how forgetfulness, ambivalence, side effects, and suboptimal clinical response can all reduce one's motivation to continue taking a medication. Open dialogue about the pros and cons of medication using a motivational interviewing approach can also enhance the chances that patients will make a commitment to carrying out behaviors that promote treatment adherence. It is also important to listen carefully to expressions of doubt, anxiety, or fearfulness and to give the young adult an opportunity to explore their feelings about taking medication. Reports of side effects, no matter how minor, should be taken seriously, and when possible, practical tips on how to reduce these should be offered. Adopting a nonjudgmental, compassionate, and hopeful stance toward the value of continuing medication treatment can help a reluctant patient to put up with the daily hassle of taking pills and with dealing with bothersome side effects.

Beyond engaging the youth or young adult in decisions about medication management, it is generally advisable to include the family in similar discussions, especially with respect to treatment goals, medication choices, predictable side effects, and likely barriers to successful adherence. When they can be successfully enlisted to support the patient's decision to pursue treatment, there is a greater likelihood of good adherence. By contrast, if family members object to the introduction of psychiatric medications or if they signal their displeasure about pharmacotherapy in less open ways, adherence is much harder to achieve. The critical role of the family in the lives of young adults is more fully explored in the next sections.

Importance of Family Relationships in Development

The transition to adulthood is highly dependent on and influenced by family relationships. By providing adequate scaffolding and support, the family can alter the trajectory of development in positive directions (Wood et al. 2018).

The definition of family has evolved over recent years to expand beyond the traditional nuclear family. Members might include parents, siblings, caregivers, grandparents, and friends. During this period, peers have an integral role in identity formation, normalizing changes, and identifying beliefs. The role of supportive peers is especially important in groups in which biological family might not be accepting of one's identity, such as the LGBTQ community. It is important to ask older teens and young adults whom they identify as their chosen family (Livesey and Rostain 2017). For the purpose of this chapter, the term *family* will refer to parents and caregivers of diverse transition-age youth populations.

Challenges in the Transition of Care and Changes in the Role of Family

Taking responsibility for managing one's own health care can be a struggle for young adults. Many are learning for the first time how to navigate medical insurance (identifying in-network providers and understanding expenses such as copays and deductibles), schedule appointments and understand policies around cancellations and no-shows, and remember to take medication and obtain timely refills. They must acquire these new skills while navigating normal developmental tasks, which include, for those in college, learning how to balance increased academic demands with multiple distractions. This shift in locus of control to the young adult can cause friction within the family system and can give rise to situations that have the potential to disrupt treatment. The clinician has an important role in facilitating this transition. Goals of this transition include helping transition-age youth populations understand, seek, and manage services for their conditions; involving families in treatment in a way that promotes mutual understanding, growth in autonomy, and safety; and highlighting that these tasks are opportunities for independence (Martel 2018).

Before age 18 years, the clinician should prepare young adults and their families for the adult approach to care. This process requires several visits to review legal changes around decision making, privacy, consent, and access to information; planning for optimal timing of transfer; identifying and transitioning care to an adult provider; and providing resources about insurance and community and campus supports (Got Transition 2020). The clinician should use these meetings to obtain consent from the young person for relevant releases of information (family, new provider, college, and so on). If the youth agrees to sign a release of information for family involvement, it is helpful to consider the level of involvement of family members, preferences around communication, and decision-making autonomy regarding treatment options. Will the provider reach out to the family only as needed, such as to clarify treatment history? Or does the young person want the family to be involved in all decisions about treatment? How often and in what ways will the provider communicate with the family? Will the young person be the primary point of contact to relay information, or does the family expect to be able to reach out to the provider directly? Are there circumstances in which the provider will initiate contact with the family, such as concerns about safety, worrisome declines in functioning, or missed appointments?

The conversations surrounding transition of care are also opportunities to highlight hallmarks of normal development that can threaten to disrupt treatment. The energy and excitement of this time of great change may result in transient improvement of symptoms. Many transition-age youth decide reactively during this transition that they no longer need treatment even if actual remission of the underlying symptoms has not truly occurred. College-bound youth may wish to start fresh in their new environment, without the need for ongoing treatment relationships (Derenne 2019). Concerns about confidentiality and fears about the negative impact on academic transcripts, social relationships, or future job prospects are also barriers to seeking treatment. Young adults may be reluctant to start over and see new providers, or they may not even agree with the diagnosis or need for treatment. Although denial of illness, limited insight, a sense of invulnerability, and the desire for independence may be developmentally normal, they can lead to poor decision making and adverse health outcomes (Martel 2018). In their desire to stay in step with their peers, young adults may think that it is safe to skip medications, to drink, or to self-medicate with substances as an alternative to prescribed medications (Leebens 2018). Often, they may need to experience discomfort from medication discontinuation or a relapse of symptoms to grasp the benefits of treatment. This cycle may need to recur several times before acceptance of treatment benefit sinks in. The provider should prepare them and their families about these challenges to support young persons' strivings for independence in managing their health and so as to minimize possible disruptions to treatment stemming from family dynamics and power struggles.

Managing Conflict With Different Parenting Styles

The process of achieving independence for older teens and young adults requires a balance between autonomy, boundary setting, and support from family in challenging situations. The dual reality of the need for support and the need for independence can result in tensions in the family system. Proactively addressing conflicts that might arise with family involvement can help to optimize support and minimize disruptions in treatment. Providers can expect to be dragged into these complex and problematic dynamics. Both overly engaged and disengaged parenting styles can impact a young person's developmental progression toward self-reliance and independence (Livesey and Rostain 2017).

Helicopter parenting is characterized by overly intrusive, controlling, and hovering family involvement. This style includes behavioral and psychological control and reinforced dependence (Luebbe et al. 2018). Helicopter parenting can limit the development of autonomy, diminish self-perception of competence, and increase the risk of depression and anxiety (Schiffrin et al. 2014). These families have trouble with the concept of letting go and transitioning ownership of treatment to the transition-age youth. Helicopter parents often try to schedule and attend appointments even after the young person is no longer living with them. They may contact the provider directly, bypassing the patient, to question treatment decisions or to report concerns about the patient's behavior. Often, these concerns may simply reflect the youth's normal striving for autonomy rather than pathology. The family may go so far as to track the young adult's whereabouts using GPS locating services on his or her phone. For those who attend college, the family may inappropriately reach out to the dean of students or to professors in an effort to "rescue" their child from potential academic difficulties. In treatment, the provider should promote autonomy by establishing clear boundaries with the family while at the same time acknowledging the family's good intentions and empathizing about their anxiety about letting go. The provider should explain how overinvolvement can be counterproductive because it interferes with the treatment alliance and undermines the young person's confidence and ability to manage their own treatment and to make appropriate decisions that promote self-management. It is important for overinvolved parents to learn to accept the notion that their child may indeed make mistakes at times, and that learning from mistakes is part of growing up.

In other cases, providers may feel that more parental support would be beneficial, but the transition-age student may disagree. Families who are distant or who adopt a "hands off" approach may be overwhelmed with their own stressors, such as caring for other family members, psychiatric illness, or financial strain. The relationship may be estranged because of differences in cultural or religious beliefs (a factor often cited by LGBTQ youth), abuse or trauma, or lack of support for mental health diagnoses and treatment. In situations other than abuse or trauma, the provider should encourage consent for family involvement and reach out directly to obtain additional perspectives on developmental issues, past psychiatric history, and family relationships. The provider may find that the family was not aware of the extent of a young person's struggles. After being informed, they may respond with increased support and guidance. The provider should use every opportunity to convey concern for the transition-age student's well-being and offer concrete suggestions on how the family can provide support (e.g., financial resources, affection, and encouragement to remain in treatment). If the family remains disengaged, the provider should work with the transition-age student to find alternative sources of support, such as extended family or friends. The clinician should always explore the quality of sibling relationships, especially if there is friction within the family system (Livesey and Rostain 2017), because continued strong attachment is positively correlated with socioemotional well-being and perceived support and negatively correlated with depression and school failure. Campus resources such as counseling and health services, victim advocates, or other student life support staff can be very helpful, depending on specific circumstances.

Boundary and Transference Issues

The clinician should be aware of boundary and transference issues, based in parent-child dynamics, that often arise during the course of treatment. For instance, young adults may react negatively to recommendations from providers if they feel like they have heard similar advice from their parents, especially regarding self-care ("Make sure you get enough sleep, go to your classes, don't drink or use drugs"). Psychoeducation based on best practices and published evidence can help the young person to accept treatment recommendations and distinguish them from parental "nagging." Conversely, the provider may develop a sense of parental responsibility toward the young adult and may wonder, "What if this were my child?" The family may reinforce this obligation by assuming that the provider will act in loco parentis. Sometimes the family explicitly states this expectation. At other times, this negative dynamic emerges during periods of stress, such as when treatment goals do not align with parents' career or academic goals for the transition-age student; when the provider does not side with parents during inevitable family disagreements; or when the parents start to regularly contact the provider directly, bypassing the transition-age student, even in the absence of urgent treatment concerns. The provider needs to be careful to distinguish a positive relationship with parents from an alliance that marginalizes the young adult from his or her own treatment.

These pitfalls can best be addressed by establishing a schedule of regular family meetings during which parents and patient can review treatment goals and progress and can also raise concerns about these in a safe and respectful environment. Issues of confidentiality and respect for boundaries can be raised at the time the young person signs a release of information to involve his or her family. It can be helpful for the provider to reassure the family that the release will be used to notify them about safety concerns but that otherwise, one of the most important goals of treatment is for the young person to learn how to self-advocate and navigate treatment.

Conclusion

The transition from adolescence to adulthood is a time of significant change and development, with an end goal of achieving independence. The family has an essential role in this process: an appropriate level of support can provide scaffolding to achieve this goal, but overly intrusive engagement or lack of involvement can hinder development. Child and adolescent psychiatrists and other clinicians can help young adults and their families navigate this journey using best practices as guidance, but they need to be aware of the dynamics and pitfalls that might negatively affect treatment, including their own transference-based reactions to the unfolding process of separation and individuation.

Resources

American Academy of Child and Adolescent Psychiatry (AACAP) Youth in Transition Resource Center. Available at: www.aacap.org/ AACAP/AACAP/Families_and_Youth/Resource_Centers/ Youth_In_Transition_Resource_Center/Youth_In_Transition_Re-source_Center_Home.aspx.
The Jed Foundation: Set-to-Go. Available at: www.settogo.org. This eas-ily navigated website provides tools and resources focused on the emotional and mental health aspects of the high school–young adult transition.

References

Chan V: Understanding campus mental health services and the campus system of care, in Promoting Safe and Effective Transitions to College for Youth With Mental Health Conditions. Edited by Martel A, Derenne J, Leebens P. New York, Springer, 2018, pp 37–42

Chan V, Derenne J, Martel A, Leebens P: Launching our patients to college. AACAP News 45(5):193–194, 2014

Chung WW, Hudziak JJ: The transitional age brain: "the best of times and the worst of times." Child Adolesc Psychiatr Clin N Am 26(2):157–175, 2017 28314448

Derenne J: The range of postsecondary options and thinking about the differ-ences between high school and college, in Promoting Safe and Effective Transitions to College for Youth With Mental Health Conditions. Edited by Martel A, Derenne J, Leebens P. New York, Springer, 2018, pp 29–36

Derenne J: Eating disorders in transitional age youth. Child Adolesc Psychiatr Clin N Am 28(4):567–572, 2019 31443875

Derenne J, Martel A: Successfully transitioning youth to college: a hands-on approach. The Scientific Proceedings of the 2013 Annual Meeting of the American Academy of Child and Adolescent Psychiatry, Vol XL. 2013a

Derenne J, Martel A: Training in college student mental health: a compelling argument. AACAP News 44(3):138–140, 2013b

Derenne J, Martel A: A model CSMH curriculum for child and adolescent psychiatry training programs. Acad Psychiatry 39(5):512–516, 2015 25895628

Derenne J, Usher C: CAPs and college. J Am Acad Child Adolesc Psychiatry 58(9):921–922, 2019 31445622

Fuchs DC, Martel A: Successful transition to young adulthood with mental illness: common themes and future directions. Child Adolesc Psychiatr Clin N Am 26(2):395–396, 2017 28314463

Got Transition: The six core elements of health care transition 3.0. Washington, DC, National Alliance to Advance Adolescent Health, 2020. Available at: www.gottransition.org/resourceGet.cfm?id=206. Accessed May 25, 2020.

Institute of Medicine and National Research Council: Investing in the Health and Well-Being of Young Adults. Washington, DC, National Academies Press, 2014

Leebens P: Essential domains in transition planning and the roles of various constituents, in Promoting Safe and Effective Transitions to College for Youth With Mental Health Conditions. Edited by Martel A, Derenne J, Leebens P. New York, Springer, 2018, pp 11–27

Leebens PK, Williamson ED: Developmental psychopathology: risk and resilience in the transition to young adulthood. Child Adolesc Psychiatr Clin N Am 26(2):143–156, 2017 28314447

Livesey CM, Rostain AL: Involving parents/family in treatment during the transition from late adolescence to young adulthood: rationale, strategies, ethics, and legal issues. Child Adolesc Psychiatr Clin N Am 26(2):199–216, 2017 28314451

Luebbe AM, Mancini KJ, Kiel EJ, et al: Dimensionality of helicopter parenting and relations to emotional, decision-making, and academic functioning in emerging adults. Assessment 25(7):841–857, 2018 27561986

Martel A: Adaptation of pediatric health care transition guidelines for use with youth heading to college with mental illness: building a toolkit, in Promoting Safe and Effective Transitions to College for Youth With Mental Health Conditions. Edited by Martel A, Derenne J, Leebens P. New York, Springer, 2018, pp 43–82

Narendorf SC, Wagner R, Fedoravicius N, Washburn M: Prior experiences of behavioral health treatment among uninsured young adults served in a psychiatric crisis setting. Community Ment Health J 53(7):782–792, 2017 28676940

Pao M: Conceptualization of success in young adulthood. Child Adolesc Psychiatr Clin N Am 26(2):191–198, 2017 28314450

Schiffrin HH, Miriam L, Miles-McLean H, et al: Helping or hovering? The effects of helicopter parenting on college students' well-being. J Child Fam Stud 23:548–557, 2014

Skehan B, Davis M: Aligning mental health treatments with the developmental stage and needs of late adolescents and young adults. Child Adolesc Psychiatr Clin N Am 26(2):177–190, 2017 28314449

Stroud C, Walker LR, Davis M, Irwin CE Jr: Investing in the health and well-being of young adults. J Adolesc Health 56(2):127–129, 2015 25620297

Substance Abuse and Mental Health Services Administration: Key substance use and mental health indicators in the United States: results from the 2018 National Survey on Drug Use and Health (HHS Publ No. PEP195068, NSDUH Series H-54). Rockville, MD, Center for Behavioral Health Statistics and Quality, Substance Abuse and Mental Health Services Administration, 2019. Available at: www.samhsa.gov/data/sites/default/files/cbhsq-reports/NSDUHNationalFindingsReport2018/NSDUHNationalFindingsReport2018.htm. Accessed March 11, 2020.

Wang R, Joshi SV: First-generation college students, in Student Mental Health: A Guide for Psychiatrists, Psychologists, and Leaders Serving in Higher Education. Edited by Roberts LW. Washington, DC, American Psychiatric Association Publishing, 2018, pp 389–398

Wood D, Crapnell T, Lau L, et al: Emerging adulthood as a critical stage in the life course, in Handbook of Life Course Health Development. Edited by Halfon N, Forres CB, Lerner RM. New York, Springer, 2018, pp 123–143

CHAPTER 13

THE PHARMACOTHERAPEUTIC ALLIANCE WHEN WORKING WITH DIVERSE YOUTH AND FAMILIES

Takesha Cooper, M.D., M.S.
Michelle Tom, M.D.
Erin Fletcher, M.D., M.P.H.

Over the years, we have increased our understanding of the psychological factors behind prescribing medication. Still, there is much to decipher surrounding the complicated dynamics behind a doctor ordering a medication for a patient. Pruett et al. (2010) opined that when considering medication, it is the patient, not the drug, that should get our primary focus. This is an important lesson, particularly when shifts in managed care and dwindling appointment times tempt providers to resort to the drug-focused, time-limited "med management visit."

Anecdotally, most prescribers appreciate that when we write a prescription for a patient, many factors can influence whether or not that patient takes the medicine as prescribed. A strict medical model training approach to psychopharmacology leads to the fallacy that the process is simple and obscures the genuine complex processes that inevitably play out during the act of prescribing and taking (or not taking) medications (Mintz 2005). *Adherence* is defined as the extent to which a person's behavior (in regard to taking medication, executing lifestyle changes, and so on) concurs with the prescriber's recommendation (Sackett 1979). Therefore, adherence to medication involves many components. Health care providers must prescribe a medication while clearly communicating its utility for the patient, and the patient or family must fill the prescription (initiation); the patient then takes the medicine as prescribed (implementation) and continues taking it as long as recommended by the prescriber (discontinuation) (Vrijens et al. 2012). Although this may seem simple, we must recognize that adherence can be further impacted by many factors, including transference (and countertransference) gone unexplored, the patient's resistance to change, a parent's validation that there indeed is a disorder in need of treating, the patient's overt attitudes about medication or about their physician and conversely the physician's attitude toward the patient, the affordability of and access to the medication, expected efficacy, and side effects.

Even less is understood about psychological factors involved as they relate to prescribing to a culturally diverse youth population. Malik and colleagues (2010) taught us that culture plays a pivotal role in how children with mental disorders function and in how children are subsequently understood and treated (Malik et al. 2010). Differences in culture between the prescriber and the patient often lead to differing perspectives and, if not explored, can interfere with the treatment alliance and subsequently with treatment adherence. In particular, racial discordance between patient and physician almost always predicts poorer communication in the domains of satisfaction, information giving, partnership building, participatory decision making, visit length, and supportiveness and respect of conversations (Shen et al. 2018). Although racial concordance is thought to be beneficial for the doctor-patient relationship, some studies report this not to be the case. Cultural concordance, being that much harder to achieve, is even less likely; therefore, perhaps the most important alternative is to teach physicians how to appreciate the cultural background unique to each patient in a way that values and honors both similarities and differences with the clinician.

One important aspect of culture is socioeconomic status (SES), and several studies have assessed medication adherence in different racial or ethnic groups and among varying SESs. In patients with lower SES and minority backgrounds, medication adherence rates tend to be lower (Salt and Frazier 2011; Simoni et al. 2012). Poorer outcomes are associated with medication nonadherence. Thus, better understanding the underlying factors, particularly the cultural factors involved, is of paramount importance.

When factors involved in prescribing to diverse youth and collaborating with families are being considered, various factors should be measured as contributors. In this chapter, we discuss several concepts, including the impact that implicit bias has in the physician-patient relationship as it relates to prescribing medication; physician attitude toward patients, particularly patients from minority backgrounds; differences in medication usage between patients of different ethnicities; and the importance that cultural humility can play in helping physicians understand the importance of maintaining a stance of curiosity, humbleness with regard to patient-family-physician power dynamics, and a lifelong commitment to self-evaluation and self-critique. These concepts are particularly suited to further understanding the complex influences involved in prescribing to a diverse pediatric patient population.

Implicit Bias

It has been widely documented that effective communication is an integral part of clinical practice and serves as the foundation of clinician-patient relationships. The quality of this relationship is often associated with outcomes of care, including patients' adherence to treatment, satisfaction with care and clinical care outcomes, improved ability to recall information, decision to continue care with a clinician, and health outcomes (Zolnierek and DiMatteo 2009). Patient-centered communication, including greater patient input into medical decisions, has been associated with better patient recall of information, treatment adherence, satisfaction with care, and health outcomes (Chapman et al. 2014).

It is no wonder that clinician bias can impact communication, alliance building, and trust in ongoing clinical relationships. Implicit biases are composed of associations, thoughts, and feelings that are often outside conscious awareness. These attitudes can unintentionally lead to negative judgments of a person on the basis of perceived characteristics such as gender, race, age, or ability status. The implicit biases that are most relevant to clinicians are those that operate to the disadvantage of those who are already vulnerable, including children, minority groups, immigrants, LGBTQ youth, women, people with disabilities, and those with low SES (Martin et al. 2014).

The attitudes and behaviors of physicians are two of the many elements that contribute to health disparities. Numerous studies have used various methods to test for correlations with clinicians' behavior, with the most common being the assumption method and implicit association testing (IAT). Illustrating measurable implicit bias among physicians does not prove that this bias affects patient-doctor interactions or alters the treatment patients receive. However, research studies underscore a link between patient care and physician bias in ways that could reinforce health care disparities. One study examined patient-doctor communication and revealed that physicians' implicit pro-white bias on the IAT corresponded with poorer communication and lower-quality care as perceived by Black patients (Blair et al. 2013). Another study demonstrated that Black patients were less satisfied with providers who had low explicit but high implicit race bias, rating them as less friendly, open, and collaborative than clinicians with equivalent measures of implicit and explicit bias (Cooper et al. 2012).

Physician Dominance

The sense of trust and open communication that physician and patient share are critical components of the overall therapeutic relationship and have been shown to influence a wide array of outcomes while helping to avoid misunderstandings that can be detrimental to clinical outcomes (Ha and Longnecker 2010). In addition, the collaborative process between clinician and patient is vital to ensuring that the patient's values and needs, along with the clinician's medical acumen, guide the decision-making process, leading to greater patient satisfaction. However, these outcomes become more difficult to achieve when clinician attitudes hamper communication (FitzGerald and Hurst 2017). One study showed physicians were more verbally dominant and less collaborative in their approach with African American patients than with white patients (Cooper et al. 2012). This could be demonstrated by the extent to which providers collaborate with patients in systematic yet unintentional ways in weighing treatment options based on patients' appearance. For example, during a follow-up appointment for new-onset hypertension, a provider may presume that a Black patient has low health literacy and decide to prescribe what they believe is best, forgoing discussion of alternatives rather than asking open-ended questions about the patient's understanding of hypertension and listening carefully for their response.

Differences in Medication Use: Race and Ethnicity

In the past 10 years, the rate at which psychotropic medications are prescribed in the pediatric population has slowed down compared with their use in decades prior (Lopez-Leon et al. 2018). Racial and ethnic differences in psychotropic medication use pose an important public health concern because they may identify groups of people who do not have access to medication or highlight overuse in a particular group. Data analysis of insurance claims can provide information about differences in psychotropic medication use in children and adolescents between different racial and ethnic groups. One study using the Medicaid's person summary database (patient demographics) and prescription drug file (claims for filled prescriptions) showed that non-Hispanic white children were greater than two times more likely to have an antipsychotic prescription filled compared with African American, Hispanic, and Asian children (Cataife and Weinberg 2015). The same study also showed that white children were more likely than nonwhite children to receive psychiatric services. Another study reinforced that African American and Hispanic youth were less likely than white youth to fill psychotropic medications (Cook et al. 2017).

In many studies, the differences between psychotropic medication use among different races and ethnicities are identified, but few address the issues that lead to such discrepancies, whether due to families of youth not being offered or not accepting medication recommendations. However, there are known disparities in access to outpatient child and adolescent mental health providers and psychotropic medication use. Such disparities can be due to family and patient preferences and greater stigma among certain racial or ethnic groups toward mental health and mental health treatment (Cook et al. 2017). Surveys show that Black and Hispanic parents are more reluctant to seek mental health care than white parents and are more skeptical of the medical system (Cooper et al. 2003). However, whether families in different racial or ethnic groups refuse to accept mental health treatment when offered has yet to be determined (Cooper et al. 2003). Studies show that underuse of mental health services among Hispanic families is largely attributable to language and cultural barriers, and Asian families tend to underuse services because of the stigma associated with mental illness (Rothe et al. 2008).

Differential use of psychotropic medication in youth based on race or ethnicity may be possibly explained by differences in access to care and treatment. Studies have shown that despite having accessed mental health services, racial or ethnic minorities are less likely to continue treatment. Underuse of mental health services, including pharmacotherapy, can be attributable to distrust of the mental health system and medication, religious practices, and social support, among other factors (Fortuna 2008). Culturally based beliefs about health practices can affect the psychiatric assessment and thus affect pharmacotherapy recommendations. For example, a psychiatrist may find it concerning that a Hispanic child reports seeing her late grandmother every night before falling asleep and may want to treat a possible psychotic symptom. However, the child's experience may be culturally acceptable to the parent and child, who may not want to address it with psychotropic medication. Many patients from different ethnic groups may present initially with somatic instead of psychological complaints. They may also hold shared cultural beliefs that may be easily misinterpreted as delusions if the clinician is unaware or unfamiliar with these beliefs or customs (Pi and Simpson 2005). Culture may impact how parents respond to their child's behavioral cues and the beliefs about how effective psychotropic medications can be for their child (Fortuna 2008).

Cultural Humility

In 1998, Melanie Tervalon, M.D., M.P.H., and Jann Murray-García, M.D., M.P.H., introduced the term *cultural humility*, which emphasizes ongoing self-reflection with regard to culture and appreciating that one can never know all there is to know about someone's identity and experiences. By definition, *humility* means "freedom from pride or arrogance, or the quality or state of being humble" (https://www.merriam-webster.com/dictionary/humility). Physicians are not immune to feelings of arrogance; therefore, it takes a shift for doctors to set aside the years of training and expertise in service of allowing patients to be the expert of their own experience. Whereas cultural competence implies an end point, as if one has learned all one could learn about a person's culture, cultural humility allows for an evolution of understanding and accounts for the fact that patients, especially children, develop and evolve in many ways over time. Disadvantaged youth in particular might resonate with a seemingly all-powerful physician who demonstrates humility in his or her interactions with them and their families. This can yield a strengthened treatment alliance and improved self-esteem for a child who feels genuinely respected by an authority figure.

In essence, cultural humility reinforces four concepts: a lifelong process of self-reflection and self-critique, reduction of power imbalances in the patient-provider dynamic, development of mutually beneficial partnerships within communities, and endorsement of institutional accountability that reflects these principles (Tervalon and Murray-García 1998). By nature of its humanistic approach, cultural humility allows for reducing the hierarchy between patient and physician, which is particularly important when working with diverse families. The concept of cultural humility was developed further in its application to youth populations as cultural sensibility in a review by Karnik and Dogra (2010).

CASE EXAMPLE: TROUBLE WITH THE LAW: AN INNOCENT QUESTION OR OVERT BIAS?

A PGY-2 resident begins his child psychiatry rotation at a busy outpatient children's mental health clinic. A 10-year-old African American boy is brought to the clinic by his mother for an assessment. The chief complaint is "inattention." The attending physician, an African American woman, typically observes new residents perform assessments to provide them feedback and now sits back to watch the assessment. The resident, a white man, refers to the parent by her first name, Mildred, and asks her to exit the room as a normal part of the history and physical examination. The resident then performs the assessment and as part of the social history asks the child if he has "ever been in trouble with the law." The child seems a bit taken aback by the question but answers, "No," and the assessment continues. After the visit is over, the attending physician is left feeling uneasy about the question asked by the resident.

Perhaps most obvious is the resident referring to the parent by her first name, which in many cultures is considered disrespectful (e.g., not calling an older adult by their surname proceed by *Mr.* or Mrs.). This case also involves the layered impact of asking an African American male child about law enforcement encounters, which could be interpreted as an underlying implicit bias about African Americans and criminal activity. Ten years old is indeed young to have had problems with the law, and for the child this might bring up issues of highly televised police misuse of force in the African American community. A physician who is seen as an authority figure asking such a question may make the child feel stigmatized and stereotyped. One wonders if the resident would have asked this question in the parent's presence or would have framed the question differently such as to show more respect for the child, or perhaps if the child were from a different background or female, whether the question would have been asked at all. Given that the parent was not in the room, if the child shares with his parent the question he was asked, consider how the parent might experience her child being asked such a question and how this might impact the therapeutic alliance process and likelihood of seeking help in the future.

CASE EXAMPLE: SIMPLY "NERVIOS"? A DOWNFALL OF PHYSICIAN DOMINANCE IN COMMUNICATING WITH PATIENTS

A mother and her 6-year-old daughter, both immigrants from Guatemala, arrive at an outpatient mental health clinic for an initial evaluation, per the recommendation of an emergency medicine physician. The mother took her daughter to the emergency room about six times in the past 3 months for complaints of "shortness of breath and sudden crying." They are seen by a PGY-1 resident, a South Asian woman, who participated in her medical school's medical Spanish course. The resident begins her interview without a Spanish interpreter and occasionally pauses to formulate sentences and questions. Very early in the evaluation, the resident believes that the child may be experiencing panic attacks and describes them to the mother as "nervios." The mother and child remain fairly quiet during the interview, and the resident continues to present possible treatment options. The resident presents the case to her attending physician, who then reevaluates the parent and child with a Spanish interpreter. The mother becomes more open and describes that the child's "nervios" would occur randomly during the day and that it once occurred in the middle of the child's sleep. It is revealed that the child was about 5 years old when her family fled Guatemala because of gang-related violence and that she had witnessed her older brother's murder that same year. It now becomes clear to the resident that the child may be experiencing symptoms of PTSD.

In this case, the resident chose not to use a Spanish interpreter, which created a language barrier between the physician, parent, and child. The mother was hesitant to speak much during the interview because she worried she would not be understood. The situation was further exacerbated by the resident's continuing the evaluation and eventually using the term "nervios" to explain the child's symptoms without gathering all the needed information to formulate a thorough differential diagnosis. The mother interpreted it as "nervousness" or "anxiety" and was left confused by what she thought was a minimization of her child's symptoms. Using a Spanish interpreter and allowing the mother to speak more freely during the interview created a more inviting environment for the mother to disclose more of the child's history. Two factors created a barrier for the parent and child: one due to language and one due to physician verbal dominance. One may argue that the resident might have been able to procure the details of the child's trauma, even without the use of a Spanish interpreter, if she had allowed for a more patient-focused exchange.

Areas for Future Research

Culture often plays a silent role between patient and physician. Incorporating our patient's and family's culture into all aspects of care, from the initial contact through the treatment formulation to ongoing follow-up, allows us to provide the most comprehensive and compassionate care. More research is needed in the area of how the implementation of cultural humility and cultural sensibility can improve outcomes and reduce health disparities. Additional studies on the impact of implicit bias and stigma's impact on pediatric mental health are also needed, particularly in patients who come from immigrant backgrounds. Also needed are further data that shed light on differences in health care utilization and adherence patterns of children from different cultural backgrounds, including those of sexual and gender minority groups.

TAKE-AWAY POINTS

- Systematically work to reduce institutional racism to allow for increased diversity of providers and increased access to care for all.

- Decrease language barriers by having certified interpreters available at all visits.

- Strive to provide education programs in multiple languages for families to improve their mental health literacy.

- Provide cultural awareness trainings for clinicians, which should include the concepts of cultural humility, cultural sensibility, and implicit association testing. These trainings should also include a review of health disparities among communities of color and sexual and gender minority populations.

References

Blair IV, Steiner JF, Fairclough DL, et al: Clinicians' implicit ethnic/racial bias and perceptions of care among Black and Latino patients. Ann Fam Med 11(1):43–52, 2013 23319505

Cataife G, Weinberg DA: Racial and ethnic differences in antipsychotic medication use among children enrolled in Medicaid. Psychiatr Serv 66(9):946–951, 2015 25975884

Chamsi-Pasha M, Albar MA, Chamsi-Pasha H: Minimizing nocebo effect: pragmatic approach. Avicenna J Med 7(4):139–143, 2017 29119079

Chapman SC, Horne R, Chater A, et al: Patients' perspectives on antiepileptic medication: relationships between beliefs about medicines and adherence among patients with epilepsy in UK primary care. Epilepsy Behav 31:312–320, 2014 24290250

Cook BL, Carson NJ, Kafali EN, et al: Examining psychotropic medication use among youth in the U.S. by race/ethnicity and psychological impairment. Gen Hosp Psychiatry 45:32–39, 2017 28274336

Cooper LA, Gonzales JJ, Gallo JJ, et al: The acceptability of treatment for depression among African-American, Hispanic, and white primary care patients. Med Care 41(4):479–489, 2003 12665712

Cooper LA, Roter DL, Carson KA, et al: The associations of clinicians' implicit attitudes about race with medical visit communication and patient ratings of interpersonal care. Am J Public Health 102(5):979–987, 2012 22420787

FitzGerald C, Hurst S: Implicit bias in healthcare professionals: a systematic review. BMC Med Ethics 18(1):19, 2017 28249596

Fortuna LR: Disparities in Child and Adolescent Psychoactive Medication Prescription Practices by Race and Ethnicity. Worcester, University of Massachusetts Medical School, 2008

Ha JF, Longnecker N: Doctor-patient communication: a review. Ochsner J 10(1):38–43, 2010 21603354

Karnik NS, Dogra N: The cultural sensibility model: a process-oriented approach for children and adolescents. Child Adolesc Psychiatr Clin N Am 19(4):719–737, 2010 21056343

Lopez-Leon S, Lopez-Gomez MI, Warner B, Ruiter-Lopez L: Psychotropic medication in children and adolescents in the United States in the year 2004 vs 2014. Daru 26(1):5–10, 2018 30159759

Malik M, Lake J, Lawson WB, Joshi SV: Culturally adapted pharmacotherapy and the integrative formulation. Child Adolesc Psychiatr Clin N Am 19(4):791–814, 2010 21056347

Martin AK, Tavaglione N, Hurst S: Resolving the conflict: clarifying 'vulnerability' in health care ethics. Kennedy Inst Ethics J 24(1):51–72, 2014 24783324

Mintz DL: Teaching the prescriber's role: the psychology of psychopharmacology. Acad Psychiatry 29(2):187–194, 2005 15937266

Pi EH, Simpson GM: Cross-cultural psychopharmacology: a current clinical perspective. Psychiatr Serv 56(1):31–33, 2005 15637188

Pruett K, Joshi S, Martin A: Thinking about prescribing: the psychology of psychopharmacology, in Pediatric Psychopharmacology: Principles and Practice. Edited by Martin A, Scahill L, Kratochvil C. Oxford, UK, Oxford University Press, 2010, pp 422–433

Rothe EM, Pumariega AJ, Rogers KM: Cultural aspects of the pharmacological treatment of depression: factors affecting minority and immigrant youth. Psychiatr Times 25(5):21–24, 2008

Sackett DL: Introduction, in Compliance With Therapeutic Regimens. Edited by Sackett DL, Haynes RB. Baltimore, MD, Johns Hopkins University Press, 1979, pp 1–6

Salt E, Frazier SK: Predictors of medication adherence in patients with rheumatoid arthritis. Drug Dev Res 72(8):756–763, 2011 22267889

Shen MJ, Peterson EB, Costas-Muñiz R, et al: The effects of race and racial concordance on patient-physician communication: a systematic review of the literature. J Racial Ethn Health Disparities 5(1):117–140, 2018 28275996

Simoni JM, Huh D, Wilson IB, et al: Racial/ethnic disparities in ART adherence in the United States: findings from the MACH14 study. J Acquir Immune Defic Syndr 60(5):466–472, 2012 22595873

Tervalon M, Murray-García J: Cultural humility versus cultural competence: a critical distinction in defining physician training outcomes in multicultural education. J Health Care Poor Underserved 9(2):117–125, 1998 10073197

Vrijens B, De Geest S, Hughes DA, et al: A new taxonomy for describing and defining adherence to medications. Br J Clin Pharmacol 73(5):691–705, 2012 22486599

Zolnierek KBH, DiMatteo MR: Physician communication and patient adherence to treatment: a meta-analysis. Med Care 47(8):826–834, 2009 19584762

CHAPTER | 14

THE PSYCHOPHARMACO-THERAPEUTIC ALLIANCE WHEN RESOURCES ARE LIMITED

Arthur Caye, M.D., Ph.D.
Brandon A. Kohrt, M.D., Ph.D.
Christian Kieling, M.D., Ph.D.

INTERVIEWER: Did you ever receive any treatment for depression?
PATIENT: My mother took me to the primary health clinic. At that time, I hadn't tried to kill myself yet; she had only seen the marks on my wrist....Then she...it took a while, it took one, two...a month I

We are thankful to Anna Viduani (UFRGS) for drafting and sharing the transcript of an interview with a participant of a qualitative study on adolescent depression. This work is part of a multisite study funded by MQ: Transforming Mental Health, Brighter Futures grant named "Identifying Depression Early in Adolescence" (MQBF/1 IDEA).

think for me to do it, because…It took a little while, because if it were another case, because my brother is still waiting today. Because my brother was taking medicine, and until today, they couldn't find a place for him; for me, it was faster. And then, I went there. They prescribed medicine for me. I didn't want to take it. My mom bought it, I took it for two days, and then I didn't want it anymore. Then, afterwards, I had to call to schedule a follow-up appointment.

INTERVIEWER: Did you schedule the follow-up?

PATIENT: No, because I was rescheduled one day and had to wait for the scheduling to open for the next month, and it hadn't opened yet. You have to keep calling to ask if it's open for scheduling or not.

INTERVIEWER: But, so, did you think about seeking help at that point?

PATIENT: I thought….

INTERVIEWER: What did you think?

PATIENT: But I didn't think about taking medication.

INTERVIEWER: No? Why not taking medication?

PATIENT: I thought, why do I have to take medication? Medication for me will be for the rest of my life….

INTERVIEWER: I understand….Are you currently taking any medication?

PATIENT: (*Shakes head no*) Because my mother told me she wasn't going to give it to me anymore. She said I have to go to the psychiatrist once again because I stopped. I took it for 2 days and stopped taking it. She said, "I'm not going to give it to you. You're going to keep going on and off…."

This vignette of a 16-year-old girl treated in the Brazilian public health system illustrates several challenges relevant in the clinical practice of psychopharmacology with youth and families in a low- to middle-income country (LMIC). In contrast to the focus of most of the medical literature on evidence-based treatment strategies, the care of the child or adolescent with a mental health condition usually begins much earlier than having to formulate a diagnosis or decide what kind of intervention to recommend. In most parts of the globe, specialized youth mental health services are simply not available to most children and adolescents. Even when services are available (Fatori et al. 2019), barriers include lack of awareness, reduced demand, stigma, economic costs, lack of time for delivery in resource-stretched health systems, and inconsistencies in the availability of medications. In this chapter, we present some of the challenges for the treatment of children and adolescents with mental illnesses with medications in low-resource settings around the world. We begin by outlining the state of mental health services in these settings and then discuss the cultural, economic, and systems-level factors that shape the delivery and experience of prescribing psychiatric medications for young people and their families.

The Math Doesn't Add Up, But Could It?

Working in low- and middle-income settings often brings up complex dilemmas concerning the gap between mental health needs and resources available to address them. Although each patient's suffering is unique, when treating diverse youth and their families, prescribing clinicians undoubtedly face patterns of inequalities in society that reflect on the specific individual who is struggling with a mental health issue (Metzl and Hansen 2014).

A worldwide perspective unveils the gap between resources needed and resources available. Almost 9 of 10 children and adolescents live in LMICs. In these countries, they account for up to 50% of the population (www.unicef.org/reports). Furthermore, the frequency of exposure to early life stressful events and other predisposing factors to mental disorders, from high blood lead levels to harsh parenting and negligence, is inversely related to a country's wealth and development (Heise and Kotsadam 2015; Viola et al. 2016; Walker et al. 2007). However, indicators of mental health resources specific to this population reveal alarming shortages and disparities: In 2017, there were fewer than 0.09 child psychiatrists for every 100,000 people in LMICs compared with 1.19 for every 100,000 in high-income countries (World Health Organization 2018). Not only human resources but also mental health facilities and strategies aimed at mental health promotion are grossly imbalanced and out of proportion with necessities worldwide. Research and science efforts, possible pathways to narrow resource gaps (Kieling and Martin 2013), follow the same pattern: 90% of the research on treatment for child and adolescent mental disorders is conducted in high-income countries (Kieling and Rohde 2012). The math simply does not add up.

An optimistic perspective, however, holds that the most significant challenges can also be the greatest opportunities for change. There is now consistent evidence to support that most mental disorders begin early in life, and many risk factors for psychiatric conditions have been identified (Kim-Cohen et al. 2003). Young people are usually physically healthy but prone to experience behavioral and emotional problems with lifelong consequences—for instance, increasing their likelihood of having age-related diseases many years later (Scott et al. 2016). Mitigating risk factors and preventing the onset of mental disorders, as well as identifying and treating psychiatric conditions, can simultaneously help child and adolescent populations and alleviate the burden of disease across the entire life span (Moffitt and Caspi 2019). Concentrating efforts and resources on identifying and treating children and adolescents with mental disorders and preventing these disorders is not only an ethical imperative but also clever public policy because it has the potential to increase productivity and decrease the economic burden to society in the long run (Caspi et al. 2016). A paradigm shift with this perspective might multiply limited resources in LMICs and promote human and economic development.

Influence of Culture on Perceptions About Psychiatric Care and Medication

When we think about "low-resource" settings, we think not simply about financial poverty (McDaid et al. 2008) but also about *knowledge* as a limited resource (Acharya et al. 2016). LMIC mental health care is often framed as health workers lacking the knowledge to provide treatment and parents and teachers lacking the knowledge to recognize signs and symptoms of mental illness that would trigger help seeking for their children and students. The term *culture* is often invoked as a proxy for ignorance. In this section, we take a more holistic perspective of culture to understand influences of why—or why not—and how psychiatric medications play a role in LMICs.

Culture, rather than a fixed characteristic of a group, is better understood as something that emerges as an interaction of context (resources and constraints), history, and the human processes of learning and development (Hruschka 2009; Kohrt 2014). Therefore, the culture of medical care is strongly impacted by the resources of time, materials, medication, and so on, which we discuss later. In this section, we review other aspects of culture that influence mental health care encounters.

The first issue relates to autonomy and decision making when it comes to young people's mental health. Although young people in LMICs may take on adult responsibilities of employment, marriage, and child-rearing at earlier ages than young people in high-income countries, cultural models of how families operate may emphasize decision making relegated to older—and typically male—members of the household. The United Nations Convention on the Rights of Persons with Disabilities (https://www.un.org/development/desa/disabilities/convention-on-the-rights-of-persons-with-disabilities.html) emphasizes recovery models in which persons with mental illness are able to live independently. However, in some cultural groups, family interdependency is seen as positive, and autonomy and isolation may be considered risk factors (Cratsley and Mackey 2018). Because of this, parents or guardians are frequently present throughout health consultations and are responsible for help-seeking decisions and providing consent for treatment choices. Involving families is the rule rather than the exception in most settings. In the World Health Organization Mental Health Gap Action Programme Humanitarian Intervention Guidelines, health workers are trained to begin consultations with the patient alone and then engage the family. However, a cultural adaptation and contextualization process in Nepal revealed that this would not be acceptable and that the consultation needs to begin with the entire family (Richards 2016).

Family members also have a range of different explanatory models for signs and symptoms of mental illness. An explanatory model refers to the ways that they understand an illness, the symptoms that they emphasize, their understanding of the cause, and their expectations of what type of help seeking is needed (Kleinmann 1980). In some public health research, explanatory models are presented as if static and singular. However, individuals typically have multiple, and at times contradictory, explanatory models (Groleau et al. 2006). An ethnographic study in LMICs demonstrated that children and their parents could all have multiple explanations for psychiatric symptoms, ranging from attributing the symptoms to a gastrointestinal illness, to a spiritual affliction, to a terrifying experience (Kohrt and Harper 2008). Health workers—especially when non–mental health specialists are trained to deliver care—may also hold multiple explanatory models. Tools exist to help health care providers and their supervisors elicit explanatory models to inform the treatment planning process: the Cultural Formulation Interview includes both patient and family member versions that have been piloted around the world, including in LMICs (Lewis-Fernández et al. 2017).

With regard to cultural aspects of psychiatric medication use, a number of factors need to be considered. One aspect of this is the biocultural interaction: Because prescribing standards are dominated by high-income, typically English-speaking cultural contexts, the recommendations may not take into account the diversity of young people around the world. Studies of ethnopharmacology in adults have shown that patients in some settings may be more sensitive to certain types of side effects because of the cultural meaning of these side effects (Ninnemann 2012). For example, dizziness among Cambodian refugees is highly distressing, and psychiatric medications that are associated with side effects of dizziness may be considered to be worsening the problem rather than treating it (Hinton et al. 2010). In other cultural contexts, headaches are a warning sign, and this may lead to discontinuing medication before it impacts psychological states (Darghouth et al. 2006). Gastrointestinal symptoms in settings of high parasitic infections, cholera, and other forms of dysentery may be highly alarming in settings where childhood diarrheal diseases are a leading cause of death. Another factor to consider is that metabolism may differ because of population differences in cytochrome P450 and micro- and macronutritional content (Taylor and Werneke 2018).

The cultural interpretation of medication may also play a role. In many LMICs, public health efforts have predominantly focused on infectious diseases, and chronic disease treatment has only received attention in recent years (Gong et al. 2019). Consequently, the majority of encounters with the health system have focused on short-term medication treatments (e.g., short courses of antimalarial drugs and antibiotics). This leads to an understanding that medications are taken for a brief period of time. The idea, as with many psychiatric medications, that medication will need to be taken for many years—or a lifetime—can be deeply distressing. With few adults having access to chronic medication treatment for conditions such as hypertension, hyperlipidemia, or diabetes, it may come as a shock to be told that a child will need to take a medication on a long-term basis (Gong et al. 2019). There are also financial concerns about this, which may lead to discounting the recommendations for ongoing medication use. In the next section, we discuss more about the financial resources and other aspects that play an even greater role in influencing care.

It's Not All About the Money

When we think about resources in health care, it is very common to oversimplify the question by narrowing it down to financial aspects. The scarcity of financial resources is certainly a central aspect of the challenge. However, focusing exclusively on this perspective is rather counterproductive on our primary aim to help children and adolescents in resource-limited settings. First, it ignores the fact that money is not an ultimate resource in itself but only a means to allocate the actual resources in health care, such as specialized human resources and dedicated settings that promote mental health. Second, as assisting clinicians, we can usually do very little about how many financial resources our patients are assigned to receive but a great deal on how to best allocate those toward more useful purposes in the service of better outcomes.

TIME IS PROBABLY THE MOST VALUABLE RESOURCE

Modern society is experiencing an increasingly faster pace of living. In every area, we feel like less and less time is available for our work to be done, our homes to be taken care of, and our children to be raised. We are expected to multitask more and to avoid idleness beyond all costs. Health care is no different. For half of the world's population, a primary care doctor visit, one that should cover a wide range of medical complaints and history, lasts less than 5 minutes (Irving et al. 2017). For some countries, that number goes down to 48 seconds.

In low-resource settings, access to specialists is much less frequent, and prescribing clinicians usually have less time to interact with young patients and their families. Psychiatry is arguably the most time-intensive medical specialty (Hing et al. 2006; Hutton and Gunn 2007). The patient's presenting problem needs to be translated from a subjective narrative of distress to a hierarchized web of symptoms that can be understood as one or more psychiatric syndromes. Feedback and psychoeducation are essential for engagement into treatment (Becker et al. 2015; Martinez et al. 2017). Close monitoring of symptoms over time increases treatment success (Hiemke et al. 2018). Good practice also involves reasonable questioning, listening, and empathic human interaction. On the other hand, shorter appointment lengths lead to less rapport, trust, and patient satisfaction. Building a therapeutic alliance invariably requires time.

Practicing in resource-limited settings undoubtedly forces us to encounter inevitable dilemmas. Even the best-intentioned clinician might need to rush through hasty psychiatric interviews after walking into a crowded waiting room, and he or she will do so to collectively protect the best interest of all the patients that wait for him or her. In such cases, rational allocation of time is paramount. Screening for general common symptoms and monitoring of treatment response might be conducted with self-rated instruments before and after the appointment. Standardized patient-friendly educational material could be provided to assist in psychoeducation, saving time for patients to raise specific doubts that arise during reading. As we will discuss further later in this chapter, efficient task sharing in multiprofessional teams allows each professional to make the most out of the time that is available to him or her. But most important of all, we should avoid falling into the ambush of saving time to produce more. In psychiatry's measure of time, more is more. Patients who receive more precise and carefully assigned diagnoses get more effective treatment, and those with higher adherence tend to get better more often and more quickly. This all leads to lessening their need for care in the future; in other words, they tend not to overcrowd offices (or emergency departments) months afterward. In resource-limited settings, at many times we will need to play a defender role, helping our goalkeeper patients deflect balls hurled their way. But if we want to maximize our scarce resources, we should save time to serve as trainers, planning ahead and preventing balls getting near the goal in the first place. The good news is that we do not need to play the game alone. Team play is as essential to health care as it is to soccer.

TWO HEADS THINK (AND PROBABLY PRESCRIBE) BETTER THAN ONE

From clinical guidelines and randomized clinical trials to the books and movies that portray the cliché of the mysterious therapist in a dimly lit room full of overstuffed couches, the standard representation of mental health care generally consists of a series of time-intensive encounters with a very specialized and experienced psychiatrist (Gabbard 2017; Garcia 2008). This imagination shapes the expectations of patients, families, and therapists themselves. From our own perspective, most of our training and even the body of evidence that supports the treatments that we offer rely on assumptions of access that simply do not hold for most youth around the world who need our help today, right now. Most children and adolescents live in countries where the ratio of child psychiatrists to the population goes down to 1 per 4 million (Malhotra and Padhy 2015), but we estimate the proportion of youth who have any mental disorder to be around 1 in 7 (Polanczyk et al. 2015). How do we narrow this millionfold gap in our practice? We should probably change our mindset on how to provide care.

Collaborative care models have been studied as a promising strategy to tackle the shortage of medical specialists in specific areas, such as cardiology (Ledwidge et al. 2013), psychiatry (Katon et al. 2010), and child and adolescent psychiatry (Asarnow et al. 2015). This is a patient-centered approach in which different levels of care are managed by one clinician (usually, the primary care provider) throughout time. It assumes that most psychiatric problems in youth can be effectively managed in the primary care setting, provided that proper training and supervision are available. Accordingly, there is evidence that collaborative care is superior to usual primary care for a wide scope of behavioral health problems in children and adolescents (Kolko 2015).

As child and adolescent psychiatrists in settings with minimal resources, we can dedicate part of our time to providing training and clinical consulting for our colleagues in primary care, and even general (adult) psychiatrists, in prevalent disorders that most of the time do not need our in-person direct care (e.g., ADHD in school-age children, social anxiety in adolescents). This model requires that we define, in our setting, what the patient will be prescribed and by whom. Not only factors related to the patient (i.e., severity of the disorder) affect referral. Availability of resources certainly modulates the threshold at which primary care doctors refer patients. In Brazil, there is a government-funded hierarchically structured system in which all primary care doctors in the country can call at any time to speak to a specialist in several fields, including psychiatry and child and adolescent psychiatry, to discuss clinical cases on a real-time basis. The initiative, called Telessaúde (Telehealth), also created guidelines with very objective criteria on why, when, and where (to what level of care) to refer patients (Ministério da Saúde 2020). This program has been helping to reduce waiting lists to child and adolescent psychiatry services by several months.

In practice, our role as local specialists could be to identify, select, and adapt established protocols and to organize an accessible training platform with the health care system and stakeholders. Of course, complex and refractory cases might still need to be further referred to specialized services.

The Psychopharmacotherapeutic Alliance, Contextualized

> There is no power for change greater than
> a community discovering what it cares about.
>
> Margaret J. Wheatley

As prescribing clinicians, we are inclined to focus on our own roles and responsibilities toward our patients and their families, easily forgetting that every youth belongs to an extended network of relationships in their school, church, sports team, neighborhood, and town. Indeed, organized communities can have meaningful impacts on promoting mental health and yet are among the most overlooked resources worldwide.

A pivotal role of mental health specialists is to promote awareness and reduce stigma in local communities. This could be achieved through periodic campaigns of psychoeducation focused on laypeople with accessible vocabulary. Lower stigma means that youth with psychiatric conditions might waver less to seek help or to accept medication (Radez et al. 2020; Tully et al. 2019; Wright et al. 2006). A community with increased levels of awareness and familiarity with the anguishes of mental disorders can probably experience an enhanced ability to behave empathically toward children and adolescents with psychiatric disorders (Furnham and Sjokvist 2017; Heyes 2018; Jorm 2012; Wolff et al. 1996). Empathy is crucial toward building solidarity.

However, eliciting solidarity within communities without further guidance does not in itself allocate resources to their utmost potential. As child and adolescent psychiatrists who are connected at the same time with the limitations of our particular community and with the evidence on risk and protective factors and mental health promotion worldwide, it is our role to channel voluntary efforts toward effective actions. We can merge intelligence with creativity. Giving just one example, we can stimulate the creation of sports teams and competitions of children and adolescents, offering voluntary outposts for retired older adults to train the teams, organize the games, and promote their own well-being by being in contact with the youth. We would at once promote mental health through physical exercise for young people and increase social contact for older adults.

Access to Treatment and How It Shapes Clinical Practice

After we assess a patient and generate a case formulation, several factors need to be weighed to select the adequate treatment for the individual patient. If we recommend psychotherapy, we ought to reflect on how the strengths and weaknesses of each modality could impact our individual patient and the probability of response to the intervention. When the balance favors medication, we should consider expected efficacy, side effects profile, and posology of each possible drug. For instance, an adolescent who develops psychotic symptoms and is also obese could probably have their condition managed with antipsychotics with a lower likelihood of weight gain and dyslipidemia. Sharing our deliberations and even our doubts with the youth and the family and sharing the responsibility for each choice are essential steps for a strong therapeutic alliance and increase the chance that the treatment will be followed (Cheng et al. 2017; Pieterse et al. 2019). Although this is true for every therapeutic interaction, in resource-limited settings, we also face important restrictions on what treatments are actually available for the children and adolescents who seek our services. This further complicates our treatment decision algorithm and extends the distance from the up-to-date, state-of-the-art practice we read about in the latest scientific articles to the practice that we can actually offer to our patients.

LMICs are affected by a cycle of supply and demand failures. Because access to mental health services is so meager in these countries, the actual demand is underestimated, and priority becomes low. This results in an erratic supply chain with frequent shortages and excessive prices in relation to the international market (Barbui et al. 2017). For some countries, medication availability has an episodic nature, depending on a specific nongovernmental organization that eventually moves away or on politicians who change health priorities after an election. A number of actions have been proposed by the World Health Organization and other researchers to improve access to psychiatric medications in LMICs (World Health Organization 2017). At the international level, they encourage rational selection of psychotropic medication based on evidence-based guidelines and the provision of adequate exemptions of intellectual property and patent rights. Among the actions at the national level are the implementation of reliable supply and control systems and the training of local health staff. Going down to the community level, effective advocacy from service use organizations may have a role in improving access to medicines for patients with mental disorders.

Similarly, specialist-delivered psychotherapies are also unavailable in many places, not to mention their cost in financial and time aspects. Furthermore, there seems to be a tendency not to equate psychotherapy with medication in the conception of essential health care. For instance, in Brazil, it is common for patients to engage (and win) in judicial processes against the government for the right to receive medication that is expensive and unavailable in the public system. It is very rare to see similar judicial demands for psychotherapies. This is probably influenced by a more traditional perspective on what constitutes "medical" care, in a shared vision of the patient and the clinician.

As a result, a clinician working in resource-limited systems has to deal with the availability and costs of the therapies being considered for the patients. Because psychiatric conditions tend to have a chronic course, it might be wise to prefer the drugs with more predictable and stable supplies (i.e., nationally produced drugs and feedstocks versus drugs or raw materials that are imported) to ensure the possibility of long-term continuous treatment. Moreover, cost-effectiveness needs to be discussed with the family: Many new psychiatric drugs enter the market with substantial marketing investment and high prices but no proven superiority over traditional medication that is widely available at a fraction of the cost (Cipriani et al. 2016). Sometimes we need to thoroughly explain to family members why we think it is worth spending a little bit more on a specific medication—for instance, to guarantee a lower like-lihood of side effects to which a patient is particularly susceptible. We might hear that the difference in cost will mean that the patient's brother will have to stop taking guitar lessons, and the pros and cons will have to be weighed within a shared-decision framework. At other times, a family will demand the latest medication available that they saw in the newspaper, but we know that it has no clinical advantage for the indi-vidual youth. Unfortunately, people can be prone to associate price with quality and effectiveness, and this can even moderate the placebo effects of psychiatric medication (Andrade 2015). This kind of conver-sation has to be handled gently and considerately, lest the child or ado-lescent believe that he or she does not deserve the "best medication" or the family feel that we are not telling the whole true story. It is our role to clarify these kinds of questions and misunderstandings, ensuring that the patient and their family are empowered with information based on evidence.

Finally, as prescribing clinicians, we can and should work to influence public policies that guarantee access to treatments that we consider es-sential to provide adequate care for our patients. The World Health Or-ganization provides a Model List of Essential Medicines that inspired many countries around the world (World Health Organization 2019). However, we do not need to be constrained by their suggestions because they include only three antidepressants and two atypical antipsychot-ics. We are in a favored position to inform local authorities about the im-portance of including other options in the list of essential medicines made available for our community, as well as the specific situations in which each medication is recommended.

Conclusion

Prescribing in resource-limited settings is as challenging as it sounds. On top of the dilemmas that are inherent to the care of youth with men-tal distress, as clinicians, we also have to deal with several adversities that are beyond our control, including restricted access to medication, stigma within communities, lack of minimal state welfare support, and overburdened clinics in need of our scarce time. We might end up feel-ing lost and hopeless amid so many hardships and obstacles to provid-ing good psychiatric care to our patients.

In this chapter, we aimed to light a candle of hope to enlighten those who embraced their duty and lingered beyond all the difficulties. We can use local culture in our favor to engage people into treatment and communities to stigmatize less and cooperate more. Working collaboratively and closely with our colleagues in primary care, we can maximize resources to make sure each patient is treated at the right place by the right person, saving resources for those who are in greater need of specialized care. Finally, we encourage professionals involved in child and adolescent psychiatry to become agents of change beyond the individual care by influencing local advocacy and politics. At least, we should spread the information that leads us to think that the mental health of our youth is a priority—and the best investment we can make.

References

Acharya B, Hirachan S, Mandel JS, van Dyke C: The mental health education gap among primary care providers in rural Nepal. Acad Psychiatry 40(4):667–671, 2016 27259491

Andrade C: Cost of treatment as a placebo effect in psychopharmacology: importance in the context of generic drugs. J Clin Psychiatry 76(4):e534–e536, 2015 25919852

Asarnow JR, Rozenman M, Wiblin J, Zeltzer L: Integrated medical-behavioral care compared with usual primary care for child and adolescent behavioral health: a meta-analysis. JAMA Pediatr 169(10):929–937, 2015 26259143

Barbui C, Dua T, Kolappa K, et al: Mapping actions to improve access to medicines for mental disorders in low and middle income countries. Epidemiol Psychiatr Sci 26(5):481–490, 2017 28067194

Becker KD, Lee BR, Daleiden EL, et al: The common elements of engagement in children's mental health services: which elements for which outcomes? J Clin Child Adolesc Psychol 44(1):30–43, 2015 23879436

Caspi A, Houts RM, Belsky DW, et al: Childhood forecasting of a small segment of the population with large economic burden. Nat Hum Behav 1:0005, 2016 28706997

Cheng H, Hayes D, Edbrooke-Childs J, et al: What approaches for promoting shared decision-making are used in child mental health? A scoping review. Clin Psychol Psychother 24(6):O1495–O1511, 2017 28752631

Cipriani A, Zhou X, Del Giovane C, et al: Comparative efficacy and tolerability of antidepressants for major depressive disorder in children and adolescents: a network meta-analysis. Lancet 388(10047):881–890, 2016 27289172

Cratsley K, Mackey TK: Health policy brief: global mental health and the United Nations' sustainable development goals. Fam Syst Health 36(2):225–229, 2018 29369647

Darghouth S, Pedersen D, Bibeau G, Rousseau C: Painful languages of the body: experiences of headache among women in two Peruvian communities. Cult Med Psychiatry 30(3):271–297, 2006 17031551

Fatori D, Salum GA, Rohde LA, et al: Use of mental health services by children with mental disorders in two major cities in Brazil. Psychiatr Serv 70(4):337–341, 2019 30651056

Furnham A, Sjokvist P: Empathy and mental health literacy. Health Lit Res Pract 1(2):e31–e40, 2017 31294250

Gabbard GO: Long-Term Psychodynamic Psychotherapy: A Basic Text. Washington, DC, American Psychiatric Publishing, 2017

Garcia R (producer): In Treatment (American TV series), 2008

Gong E, Lu H, Shao S, et al: Feasibility assessment of invigorating grassroots primary healthcare for prevention and management of cardiometabolic diseases in resource-limited settings in China, Kenya, Nepal, Vietnam (the FAITH study): rationale and design. Glob Health Res Policy 4:33, 2019 31742234

Groleau D, Young A, Kirmayer LJ: The McGill Illness Narrative Interview (MINI): an interview schedule to elicit meanings and modes of reasoning related to illness experience. Transcult Psychiatry 43(4):671–691, 2006 17166953

Heise LL, Kotsadam A: Cross-national and multilevel correlates of partner violence: an analysis of data from population-based surveys. Lancet Glob Health 3(6):e332–e340, 2015 26001577

Heyes C: Empathy is not in our genes. Neurosci Biobehav Rev 95:499–507, 2018 30399356

Hiemke C, Bergemann N, Clement HW, et al: Consensus guidelines for therapeutic drug monitoring in neuropsychopharmacology: update 2017. Pharmacopsychiatry 51(01/02):9–62, 2018

Hing E, Cherry DK, Woodwell DA: National Ambulatory Medical Care Survey: 2004 summary. Adv Data 23(374):1–33, 2006 16841616

Hinton DE, Pich V, Marques L, et al: Khyâl attacks: a key idiom of distress among traumatized Cambodia refugees. Cult Med Psychiatry 34(2):244–278, 2010 20407813

Hruschka DJ: Culture as an explanation in population health. Ann Hum Biol 36(3):235–247, 2009 19381984

Hutton C, Gunn J: Do longer consultations improve the management of psychological problems in general practice? A systematic literature review. BMC Health Serv Res 7:71, 2007 17506904

Irving G, Neves AL, Dambha-Miller H, et al: International variations in primary care physician consultation time: a systematic review of 67 countries. BMJ Open 7(10):e017902, 2017 29118053

Jorm AF: Mental health literacy: empowering the community to take action for better mental health. Am Psychol 67(3):231–243, 2012 22040221

Katon WJ, Lin EH, Von Korff M, et al: Collaborative care for patients with depression and chronic illnesses. N Engl J Med 363(27):2611–2620, 2010 21190455

Kieling C, Martin A: Catalyzing the publication of international research in child and adolescent mental health. Child Adolesc Psychiatry Ment Health 7(1):23, 2013 23899334

Kieling C, Rohde LA: Child and adolescent mental health research across the globe. J Am Acad Child Adolesc Psychiatry 51(9):945–947, 2012 22917207

Kim-Cohen J, Caspi A, Moffitt TE, et al: Prior juvenile diagnoses in adults with mental disorder: developmental follow-back of a prospective-longitudinal cohort. Arch Gen Psychiatry 60(7):709–717, 2003 12860775

Kleinmann A: Patients and Healers in the Context of Culture: An Exploration of the Borderland Between Anthropology, Medicine, and Psychiatry. Berkeley, University of California Press, 1980

Kohrt BA: Child maltreatment and global health: biocultural perspectives, in Handbook of Child Maltreatment. Edited by Krugman RD, Korbin JE. Dordrecht, The Netherlands, Springer, 2014, pp 553–577

Kohrt BA, Harper I: Navigating diagnoses: understanding mind-body relations, mental health, and stigma in Nepal. Cult Med Psychiatry 32(4):462–491, 2008 18784989

Kolko DJ: The effectiveness of integrated care on pediatric behavioral health: outcomes and opportunities. JAMA Pediatr 169(10):894–896, 2015 26259063

Ledwidge M, Gallagher J, Conlon C, et al: Natriuretic peptide-based screening and collaborative care for heart failure: the STOP-HF randomized trial. JAMA 310(1):66–74, 2013 23821090

Lewis-Fernández R, Aggarwal NK, Lam PC, et al: Feasibility, acceptability and clinical utility of the Cultural Formulation Interview: mixed-methods results from the DSM-5 international field trial. Br J Psychiatry 210(4):290–297, 2017 28104738

Malhotra S, Padhy SK: Challenges in providing child and adolescent psychiatric services in low resource countries. Child Adolesc Psychiatr Clin N Am 24(4):777–797, 2015 26346389

Martinez JI, Lau AS, Chorpita BF, et al: Psychoeducation as a mediator of treatment approach on parent engagement in child psychotherapy for disruptive behavior. J Clin Child Adolesc Psychol 46(4):573–587, 2017 26043317

McDaid D, Knapp M, Raja S: Barriers in the mind: promoting an economic case for mental health in low- and middle-income countries. World Psychiatry 7(2):79–86, 2008 18560485

Metzl JM, Hansen H: Structural competency: theorizing a new medical engagement with stigma and inequality. Soc Sci Med 103:126–133, 2014 24507917

Ministério da Saúde: TelessaúdeRS. Brasilia, Brazil, Ministerio de Saude, 2020. Available at: www.ufrgs.br/telessauders. Accessed May 10, 2020.

Moffitt TE, Caspi A: Psychiatry's opportunity to prevent the rising burden of age-related disease. JAMA Psychiatry 76(5):461–462, 2019 30916735

Ninnemann KM: Variability in the efficacy of psychopharmaceuticals: contributions from pharmacogenomics, ethnopsychopharmacology, and psychological and psychiatric anthropologies. Cult Med Psychiatry 36(1):10–25, 2012 22286864

Pieterse AH, Stiggelbout AM, Montori VM: Shared decision making and the importance of time. JAMA 322(1):25–26, 2019 31002337

Polanczyk GV, Salum GA, Sugaya LS, et al: Annual research review: a meta-analysis of the worldwide prevalence of mental disorders in children and adolescents. J Child Psychol Psychiatry 56(3):345–365, 2015 25649325

Radez J, Reardon T, Creswell C, et al: Why do children and adolescents (not) seek and access professional help for their mental health problems? A systematic review of quantitative and qualitative studies. Eur Child Adolesc Psychiatry 2020 31965309 [Epub ahead of print]

Richards HJ: Documenting the contextualization and implementation of mhGAP-HIG in postearthquake Nepal. Unpublished master's thesis, Duke University, Durham, NC, 2016. Available at: http://dukespace.lib.duke.edu/dspace/bitstream/handle/10161/12297/Richards_duke_0066N_11486.pdf?sequence=1. Accessed May 10, 2020.

Scott KM, Lim C, Al-Hamzawi A, et al: Association of mental disorders with subsequent chronic physical conditions: world mental health surveys from 17 countries. JAMA Psychiatry 73(2):150–158, 2016 26719969

Taylor DM, Werneke U: Ethnopharmacology. Nord J Psychiatry 72 (suppl 1): S30–S32, 2018

Tully LA, Hawes DJ, Doyle FL, et al: A national child mental health literacy initiative is needed to reduce childhood mental health disorders. Aust N Z J Psychiatry 53(4):286–290, 2019 30654614

Viola TW, Salum GA, Kluwe-Schiavon B, et al: The influence of geographical and economic factors in estimates of childhood abuse and neglect using the Childhood Trauma Questionnaire: a worldwide meta-regression analysis. Child Abuse Negl 51:1–11, 2016 26704298

Walker SP, Wachs TD, Gardner JM, et al: Child development: risk factors for adverse outcomes in developing countries. Lancet 369(9556):145–157, 2007 17223478

Wolff G, Pathare S, Craig T, Leff J: Community knowledge of mental illness and reaction to mentally ill people. Br J Psychiatry 168(2):191–198, 1996 8837909

World Health Organization: Improving Access to and Appropriate Use of Medicines for Mental Disorders. Geneva, World Health Organization, 2017

World Health Organization: Mental Health Atlas 2017. Geneva, World Health Organization, 2018. Available at: https://www.who.int/mental_health/evidence/atlas/mental_health_atlas_2017/en. Accessed May 10, 2020.

World Health Organization: WHO Model List of Essential Medicines, 7th List. Geneva, World Health Organization, 2019. Available at: https://www.who.int/publications/i/item/WHOMVPEMPIAU201907. Accessed February 28, 2021.

Wright A, McGorry PD, Harris MG, et al: Development and evaluation of a youth mental health community awareness campaign—The Compass Strategy. BMC Public Health 6:215, 2006 16923195

PART V

RESEARCH

CHAPTER 15

BUILDING A THERAPEUTIC ALLIANCE IN PSYCHOPHARMACOLOGY DURING CLINICAL TRIALS

Ethical and Practical Considerations

Manpreet K. Singh, M.D., M.S.
Janice Cho, M.D.

Youth presenting with psychiatric disorders have a limited range of therapeutic options. What happens when these options have been exhausted? As is true for many areas of medicine, we do not currently have something good for everything that is bad, such as challenging symptoms that are resistant to available interventions. As a result, we must look with hope into the future to improve on currently available interventions and create a rational road map for discovering them. A healthy research portfolio including clinical trials in child and adolescent psychiatry may be our best hope for better treatments on the horizon (Stringaris 2014). However, to expediently bring these treatments to our patients, key participants in the conduct of research and mission-engaged stakeholders must work collaboratively (Greenhill et al. 2003) and within the bounds of contemporary ethical standards to ensure that risks, benefits, and alternatives for treatment are weighed thoughtfully in discussions with prospective participants and without coercion. Here, we consider some ethical and practical issues that arise while prescribing medications or conducting interventional psychiatric treatments (repetitive transcranial magnetic stimulation [TMS], electroconvulsive therapy, dialectical behavior therapy) in the discovery space.

Because of the lack of adequate pediatric clinical trials, evidence for medications and interventional psychiatry in children is largely based on studies performed in adults. This is problematic because of the fundamental differences in physiology, development, psychology, and pharmacology in children compared with adults (Shirkey 1968). Although the number of randomized controlled trials (RCTs) for adults published in high-impact general medical journals has doubled over the past 20 years, the number of clinical trials for children has remained stagnant (Cohen et al. 2007). In addition, pharmaceutical companies have allocated greater funding to investigate novel therapies in adults (65%) compared with those in youth. Advocacy for more research in youth includes an evidence-informed research agenda and policies that address deficiencies in the quantity and quality of clinical trials, given that current off-label and untested standards of care frequently result in the use of questionably effective medications with unknown or potentially harmful side effects.

Although psychotherapeutic interventions were the initial first-line treatments in child and adolescent psychiatry, the advent of clinical trials validated the integration of pharmacological modalities into the armamentarium of interventions for youth with psychiatric disorders. The efficacy of evidence-based drug trials involving large effect sizes enabled exciting advances in pediatric psychopharmacology for the treatment of patients with psychotherapy-resistant ADHD, enuresis, depression, anxiety disorders, obsessive-compulsive disorder (OCD), and psychosis. However, current challenges to the further advancement of pediatric psychopharmacology stem from a number of factors, including concerns about adverse effects of medication, overmedication, and inadequacy of long-term drug surveillance (Rapoport 2013). Approximately half (40%–50%) of pediatric patients demonstrate incomplete response or intolerance to medications, underscoring the need for new directions in treatment. Moreover, very few interventions have a lasting effect (Fonagy 2015), suggesting a need to shift away from the focus on elusive cures toward a mechanistic understanding of brain-behavior-environment interactions that lend themselves to prevention, adaptive outcomes, and sustained health for youth (Fearon 2017).

In the field of child and adolescent psychiatry, the therapeutic alliance between the patient, caregiver, and the provider is of utmost importance to ensure positive clinical outcomes (Joshi 2006; Krupnick et al. 1996; Weiss et al. 1997). Of equal value to the intervention itself are the interpersonal skills of the provider (Pruett et al. 2010) and a trusting relationship that facilitates a judicious evaluation of the relative risks, benefits, and alternatives of a proposed intervention. Indeed, the power of the therapeutic alliance alone has been well documented in our field. For example, among 225 cases of depressed patients who received interpersonal psychotherapy, cognitive-behavioral therapy, imipramine with clinical management, or placebo with clinical management, the positive impact of the therapeutic alliance on both psychotherapies and pharmacotherapies was clearly apparent (Krupnick et al. 1996). This therapeutic alliance permeates not only the doctor-patient relationship but also the relationship between the clinician and caregiver(s) (Joshi 2006). Just as in clinical settings, clinical researchers in youth mental health work to protect a participant's self-esteem, emote an understanding and acceptance of the relevant symptoms, and engage in realistic discussions about implications of participation in clinical research (Joshi 2006). Indeed, by integrating the therapeutic alliance into the historical precedence that established research in child psychiatry and contemporary ethical standards, researchers in child psychiatry can build a foundational framework for successful research in our field. In this chapter, we describe the historical, ethical, and practical ingredients for any successful research endeavor, including clinical trials being conducted in the field of child and adolescent psychopharmacology today.

Historical Context for Contemporary Treatment Approaches

The first description of the role of psychotropic drugs in pediatric patients occurred serendipitously after the illustration of positive effects by the stimulant agent Benzedrine on school behavior (Bradley 1937) and tricyclic antidepressants (TCAs) on enuresis (Griffiths 1979). Demonstrated by numerous double-blind, placebo-controlled studies, the efficacy of psychostimulants on task behavior and motor activity reduction in children with ADHD propagated the initial incorporation of medication to treat pediatric psychiatric disorders (Rapoport et al. 1978, 1980). Interestingly, studies showed a difference in the participant response as well as a difference in *caregiver* response to participants who received stimulants versus placebo (Barkley 1989; Wells et al. 2006). This observation suggested that pharmacological interventions could have effects beyond the physiological systems on which they were working to modulate a change in behavior. Changes in a child's behavior had an observable impact on the parent as well, with different behaviors noted in the active versus placebo conditions, foreshadowing the importance of understanding the effects of both the active and placebo conditions in the design of clinical trials in youth. However, the impact of discovery was dampened by difficulties reproducing initial trials with TCAs, as well as concerns about the risk of suicidality (Hammad et al. 2006; Keller et al. 2001). Other challenges in the conduct of clinical trials in children persisted, including the inadequacy of funding needed to address the important issues raised by clinical trial design in youth, ethical concerns about studying this vulnerable population, and emerging challenges in diagnostic accuracy.

Although antidepressants were initially used to treat enuresis in children, their use was subsequently extended for the treatment of pediatric depression and anxiety through serendipitous discovery (Mikkelsen and Rapoport 1980; Puig-Antich et al. 1987). However, challenges in the diagnosis of depressive symptoms in children were frequently reported (Cytryn and McKnew 1986; Kashani et al. 1981). Perhaps in response to the skeptics, researchers developed semi-structured clinical interviews that systematically assessed for disorders and symptoms in the context of clinical trials. These semi-structured interviews, which integrate multi-informant reports from parents and youth, have become the gold standard approach to psychiatric diagnostic assessment in clinical trials; efforts are being made to practically implement the rigor of these interviews in clinical settings (Young et al. 2016). Antidepressant use was extended to treat children with anxiety disorders (Ballenger 2004; de Beurs et al. 1999; Klein et al. 1992; Pine et al. 2009). Although anxiety disorders are commonly comorbid with depression, prescribing antidepressants for anxiety could cause confusion in patients simply on the basis of nomenclature alone (Sultan et al. 2018). Nevertheless, comorbidity is the rule rather than the exception in child psychiatry (Avenevoli et al. 2015). Further, the field has long recognized the importance of combining proven psychotherapeutic interventions with pharmacological treatments to target complexity in phenotypes. In fact, these multimodal treatment approaches demonstrated superiority in treating depression and anxiety (Domino et al. 2008), including OCD (Flament et al. 1985; Swedo et al. 1992), compared with monotherapeutic alternatives. Multimodality became a feature of clinical trial design rather than an exclusion criterion (Reeves and Anthony 2009).

With the passage of time and with a better understanding of phenomenology and the neuroscience underlying prevalent symptoms, interventions have become increasingly sophisticated, particularly for complex psychiatric presentations, and multi-use indications have typically prevailed (Findling et al. 2011). Although safety concerns are persistently cited as a barrier to pursuing more advancements in treatment for youth, off-label treatments without U.S. Food and Drug Administration (FDA) approval abound in clinical practice. Polypharmacy, in the absence of evidence-supported guidelines, is also worthy of consideration. As clinical trials in the field of child and adolescent psychiatry have increased, prescriptions for psychotropic medications and rates of polypharmacy have risen, especially in the United States (Barnett et al. 2019; Findling et al. 2000; Zito et al. 2008). Pediatric patients remain on stimulant medications for longer and have them prescribed at earlier ages than before, and individuals in institutional or foster care frequently receive high doses and multiple medications. Among child psychiatrists, polypharmacy and off-label prescribing have exceeded the number of child diagnoses (Kearns and Hawley 2014), reflecting the prevalence of increasingly complex phenomenology and comorbidity.

These complexities necessitate a therapeutic alliance not just with patients and families but also with key operational personnel (e.g., research coordinators, study monitors) and regulatory bodies (e.g., institutional review boards, the FDA) to build an understanding of the considerations unique to the field of child and adolescent psychiatry. By proactively striving to promote understanding and mitigation of common misconceptions in child psychiatry research, we may extend the therapeutic alliance to these key participants in research implementation. Thus, researchers can ensure that the pursuit of discovery is harmonious with contemporary ethical standards established by the historical precedent that has brought us here today. Simultaneously, in the context of a limited evidence base, the practice of child and adolescent psychiatry merits critical and continuous evaluation of recommendations proffered to patients and prospective participants. In this effort, it is useful to highlight some ethical considerations.

The Immorality of Not Knowing: The Imperative to Conduct Research in Pediatric Psychiatry and Other Ethical Principles

A central question to ponder in the field of child psychiatry, then, is, in the absence of a strong evidence base for most interventions in childhood-onset psychopathology, what are the ethics of not conducting research to measure treatment effects or to understand treatment mechanisms? If the promise of discovery and precision medicine conveys hope to families, does research become a moral imperative (Hattab 1996)? The dilemma of pediatric clinical trials involves finding an equilibrium between the imperative to conduct trials (pursuit of knowledge in research) and the potential harms associated with making off-label recommendations about untested or yet to be tested treatments (needing to provide clinical care without empirical knowledge to support the approach).

TRANSFERENCE, COUNTERTRANSFERENCE, AND WORKING WITH PARENTS

All doctor-patient relationships, even in a research setting, involve some degree of transference (unconscious projection of emotions by the patient onto the provider) and countertransference (unconscious projection of emotions by the provider onto the patient) (Hochhauser 2005). According to Jay Katz's *The Silent World of Doctor and Patient* (Katz 2002), "paternalistic and authoritarian" physicians may fail to discuss certain topics during their encounters with "childlike" patients whom they believe to have a limited understanding of medicine. Countertransference and transference may complicate the recruitment process for clinical trials. Although certain measures from Federal Regulations (45 CFR 46: Federal Policy for the Protection of Human Subjects ["Common Rule"]; Office for Human Research Protections, n.d.), the Declaration of Helsinki (World Medical Association 2013), and the Belmont Report (National Commission for the Protection of Human Subjects of Biomedical and Behavioral Research 1978) have attempted to address ethical considerations in selecting patients for clinical trials, transference and countertransference in clinical research have not been adequately addressed in the literature (Hochhauser 2005).

Both positive and negative transference may complicate the clinical research process. Positive transference, in which a patient decides to participate in research based on emotions such as love and trust regardless of informed consent discussions, may be likely when a patient's physician is also the researcher. In addition, patients with serious illnesses may be motivated to participate because of a lack of treatment options, which places unrealistic expectations on the outcome of the clinical trial. To decrease the likelihood for emotionally charged decisions regarding participation in a clinical trial, some physicians aim to give patients and their families time and space to accept the diagnosis and treatment recommendations or dissociate the role of clinician and researcher entirely to mitigate role confusion. Negative transference, in which a patient is deterred from participating in clinical trials, can occur when patients mistrust doctors and the health care system because of prior unpleasant experiences. At the center of many unpleasant experiences is distrust built by a sad history of maltreatment and exploitation of marginalized minorities (Washington 2006), as well as ongoing contemporary tensions between academic institutions and the communities where they reside. What recent history has taught us, however, is that we must not confuse reluctance with refusal, and ensure equity in access to research studies as we would to clinical care.

Countertransference may be more harmful than transference, especially because doctors hold positions of power over vulnerable patients. A physician may "overpromise" the positive effects of an experimental drug to garner participation, or patients deemed as "problem patients" may fall victim to doctors' frustrations and inadvertently be denied participation in clinical trials. Acknowledging the vulnerability of patients during the recruitment process can guard against such potential behaviors. Patients who place complete trust in doctors and decide to participate in research without full consideration of the risks could invalidate the principles of informed consent. Alternatively, physicians may unconsciously overstate the benefits of clinical trials. Thus, awareness of and vigilance for transference and countertransference are necessary for any physician who is also conducting clinical research (Carrier et al. 2017).

Pediatric clinical trials may be fundamentally challenged by obtaining informed consent from parents or guardians for research participation while trying to manage caregiver expectations. Parents feel an immense sense of responsibility to make the best decisions to protect their sick children. Therefore, through positive interactions during recruitment in addition to the flexibility to tailor discussions to the needs and circumstances of each child, parental concerns may be adequately addressed (Shilling and Young 2009). With regard to clinical trials, whereas some parents may be influenced by the fear of negative outcomes, others may view these trials as hopeful options. When the researcher ensures that parents have a complete understanding of the research process and a sense that they have exercised their responsibility to protect their child, the process of enrollment in a clinical trial can go more smoothly than if the researcher does not ensure this understanding. Further research into the best practices of obtaining parental or caregiver consent may help improve the clinical trial recruitment process for all individuals involved (Shilling and Young 2009). Importantly, if a child refuses to participate, their wishes should be respected.

CLINICAL EQUIPOISE

The term *equipoise*, coined in 1974 by Charles Fried, means that the physician-investigator must be indifferent to the therapeutic effect of the experimental versus the control arm when conducting an RCT (Miller and Brody 2003). Fried proposed that the ethics of therapeutic medicine, especially the idea of informed consent, be also applied in a clinical research context (Miller and Brody 2003).

Clinical equipoise is the genuine uncertainty in the therapeutic outcome of a trial's arms by its investigator (Freedman 1987). In any clinical research protocol involving randomization of treatment conditions, an investigator must demonstrate impartiality (Freedman 1987), which may obstruct the therapeutic alliance. This is because if one treatment modality demonstrates superiority during the clinical trial, the investigator is ethically beholden to offer the superior treatment to all subjects (Freedman 1987). Consequently, according to clinical equipoise, placebo-controlled trials would be unethical whenever there is a proven effective treatment for a disorder under investigation (Freedman 1990). However, in child and adolescent psychiatry, there remains genuine uncertainty within the "expert community" that goes beyond the uncertainty of the individual investigator (Freedman 1987). Thus, an RCT is ethical as long as the greater professional community has not reached a consensus on a superior treatment modality. Physician-investigators can defer their "therapeutic obligation" to patients if treatments satisfy this definition of clinical equipoise (Miller and Brody 2003). In child and adolescent psychiatry, expert community consensus is challenged by many levels of disagreement, including differences between clinical and research diagnoses (Jensen-Doss et al. 2014) and an absence of comparative effectiveness trials that could demonstrate superiority of one treatment over another. Diagnostic agreement between a research-based semistructured interview and a clinical diagnostic interview can predict positive treatment outcomes (Jensen-Doss and Weisz 2008), and empirical evidence for recommended treatments is central to the research agenda in child psychiatry.

THE DISTINCTION BETWEEN RESEARCH AND THERAPY

Although clinical trials are scientific experiments distinct from standard medical care, there is a therapeutic misconception that clinical trials may serve dual roles as both research and medical treatment, referred to as "therapeutic research" (Miller and Brody 2003). According to the Belmont Report (National Commission for the Protection of Human Subjects of Biomedical and Behavioral Research 1978), clinical research is fundamentally different from the practice of clinical medicine. Although clinical medicine is ethically bound by principles of therapeutic beneficence and nonmaleficence with the aim of finding the optimal treatment for the patient, it does not aim to develop scientific knowledge to benefit the greater population (Miller and Brody 2003). In contrast, clinical research attempts to answer a scientific question with the goal of producing "generalizable knowledge" rather than providing therapeutic benefit for individual patients (Miller and Brody 2003).

Distinguishing medical care from clinical research reduces the potential to exploit research participants (Emanuel et al. 2000). In clinical medicine, the interests of the physician and the patient converge as the physician attempts to provide the patient with the means to regain or maintain health (Miller and Brody 2003). In contrast, the motivations of the physician and the patient in clinical research may diverge due to the inherent differences between the interests of the investigator and those of the research participant (Miller and Brody 2003). Thus, considerations that may help differentiate clinical research from medical care include an understanding of 1) scientific versus social value, 2) the pursuit of scientific validity, 3) fair subject selection, 4) favorable risk-benefit ratio, 5) independent review, 6) informed consent, and 7) respect for enrolled research participants (Emanuel et al. 2000).

Research subjects cannot give informed consent if they do not understand that clinical trials are aimed at discoveries to help future patients rather than their own benefit. Investigators must draw clear boundaries between medical care and clinical research. For example, the patient can trust the physician to decide the best course of action with regard to treatment. However, the same cannot be said for the participant-investigator relationship because the investigator must prioritize the interests of future patients over those of the individual participant. Participants must understand the incompatibility of certain principles of clinical treatment with the scientific method (Appelbaum et al. 1987). In contrast, the physician is ethically obligated to provide an individual patient with all available measures to maximize the chances of a successful outcome. Randomization, an important element in many clinical trials, inherently compromises the obligation of the physician to provide the best treatment to the patient if one treatment arm is known to be better than the other. Furthermore, features of research design that promote scientific robustness, such as certain interventions used to measure trial outcomes (e.g., blood draws, lumbar punctures, radiation-based imaging), may carry risk to participants without offering a therapeutic benefit (Miller and Brody 2003).

Voluntary consent of seriously ill populations, for whom clinical research may represent a last hope of rescue, can pose its own unique challenges (Bosk 2002). Research subjects who have previously tried and failed a variety of different interventions for problem behaviors are especially vulnerable and are subsequently highly susceptible to exploitation. Such patients are asked to make significant life decisions and are presented with information in moments when they are least able to process it and are heavily dependent on their clinicians to assist them with medical decision making. In a meta-analysis of 812 articles on the ethics of clinical trials in which 14 methods for obtaining informed consent were compared, the manner and timing in which information was presented made a difference to a participant's decision to enroll in research (Bosk 2002). The patient's prior relationship with a physician and the understanding that the clinical trial was "the last best hope" for treatment were the most important factors in enrollment. In addition, vulnerable populations are likely to defer decision-making to a trusted expert, as opposed to healthy populations who may be more equipped to make in-the-moment autonomous decisions. Further, seriously ill patients do not always rationally weigh the evidence before deciding on treatment and may choose to enroll in a clinical trial based on their trust in providers and their willingness to persevere regardless of the informed consent. These scenarios illustrate how the model of the neutral, rational decision-making process critical for informed consent could be compromised. Importantly, for informed consent to be morally valid, four criteria are required: disclosure, understanding, voluntariness, and competence.

Another key ethical dilemma of placebo-controlled trials is the possibility of exposing children to unnecessary risk versus meeting the need for adequate information to guide clinical care. In other words, how do you establish a therapeutic alliance in the context of a balanced risk-benefit discussion when participants must understand the possibility that they may improve, have no change, or even get worse? There have been several lessons learned from clinical trials in child psychiatry in this context (Joseph et al. 2015). Unlike in clinical trials in adults, drug formulations are important to consider in pediatric clinical trials, because dose and delivery methods may affect adherence to treatment in children. Indeed, difficulties swallowing tablets and receiving injections may affect bioavailability of the drugs and subsequently adversely affect the outcome of a clinical trial (Abdel-Rahman et al. 2007). Moreover, significant developmental changes that occur throughout childhood introduce difficulties when comparing subjects of different ages and stages (Sinha et al. 2008). Because the goals of clinical research and medical care are different, some argue that they should be dictated by distinct ethical standards because it is a misnomer to label research as either "therapeutic" or "nontherapeutic" (Brody and Miller 2003; Miller and Brody 2003). All of these issues must be carefully considered in the ethical implementation of research in child psychiatry.

Practical Applications and Strategies

UNDERSTANDING, MITIGATING, AND LEVERAGING THE PLACEBO EFFECT IN CHILD PSYCHIATRY

Clinical trials for pediatric depression have yielded significant placebo effects (Bridge et al. 2009; Emslie 2009; Rutherford et al. 2011). In a meta-analysis of 12 clinical trials testing the efficacy of second-generation antidepressants in 2,862 children and adolescents with major depressive disorder, the mean responses to placebo versus active medication were 48% and 59%, respectively. On the basis of these findings, the authors concluded that lower baseline illness severity and younger age (except in a single trial of fluoxetine in both children and adolescents) were associated with higher placebo response. Further, the strongest predictor of placebo response was the number of study sites. Because of these findings, the authors suggest that placebo response can be better controlled by careful recruitment of children and adolescents with moderate to severe depression and from fewer sites. The changes observed in these studies were attributable more to differences in response to placebo than to differences in efficacy of antidepressants.

Clinicians should not ignore placebo-controlled study results that fail to separate treatment effects between active and placebo conditions, because they can provide information about drug safety and facilitate an understanding of the placebo effect in youth. The high rate of response to placebo in multisite clinical trials does not signify that childhood depression is not clinically valid but rather highlights that trial design should be modified to decrease the likelihood of confounding effects from placebo response. According to an alternative framework, the placebo effect may be an integral component of the overall treatment effect and represents a neurobiological effect that is triggered by specific processes secondary to social and environmental factors (Zion and Crum 2018). In fact, the placebo effect may be leveraged in medicine without the use of inert placebo pills or sham conditions. This framework considers the possibility of using placebo-controlled trials to *understand the psychological meaning associated with receiving a pharmacological treatment beyond expectation formation and implicit learning.* If depressed adolescents are particularly predisposed to a high placebo effect, this finding may open opportunities to test the placebo response as a variable of interest rather than as a control condition. Strawn and colleagues have devoted an entire chapter in this book to the subject of placebos (see Chapter 16, "The Power of Placebo").

THE PROMISE OF PRECISION MEDICINE AND THE HOPE OF DRUG DISCOVERY

In child and adolescent psychiatry, as in other fields, precision medicine involves tailoring treatments for each patient rather than for a specific disease process (Posner 2018). In contrast to oncology, however, current psychiatric standards of care administer treatment irrespective of the cause of symptoms. For instance, children with anxiety or depression are prescribed selective serotonin reuptake inhibitors (SSRIs) irrespective of the eliciting cause (e.g., recent trauma, genetic predisposition). Rather than the patient's history, genetics, or environmental status, trial and error primarily dictate the course of treatment because of the scarcity of causation studies published for psychiatric disorders.

By applying concepts of precision medicine from oncology to psychiatry, providers may one day be able to select treatments based on the underlying disease mechanism and pathology rather than the diagnosis or related symptoms alone. However, there are inevitably several challenges in the application of precision medicine to child psychiatry, including the lack of homogeneity in psychiatric disorders and multidomain contributions from the environment, genetics, and brain cognition. For example, despite several recent advancements in applying pharmacogenetic research to evaluate the safety of psychotropic drug options, the clinical application of these pharmacogenetic techniques remains challenging because of a lack of prospective studies to evaluate response to psychotropic drugs based on an individual's genotype, multiple divergent pathways between medication and medication dose along with considerations about clinical response and side effects, as well as the wide therapeutic range of SSRIs in the pediatric population (Wehry et al. 2018). Clearly, more research and patient education are needed before pharmacogenetic testing is ready for prime time.

Until precision medicine can be readily applied to the field of child and adolescent psychiatry, advancing complementary treatments has been proposed by many as a reasonable next step in translational medicine. These strategies include repurposing, collaborative research participation, and trials that study or integrate mechanisms of change during psychotherapy. Repurposing is the use of medications beyond their initial purpose. There are other, more recently implemented treatments that illustrate this concept beyond the example presented earlier for multipurpose use of antidepressants in patients with enuresis, depression, and anxiety. For example, although atomoxetine was ineffective for the treatment of patients with depression, the FDA approved its use in those with ADHD because of its mechanistic similarities to desipramine (Spencer et al. 2001; Witcher et al. 2003). An increase in collaborative research participation may identify new treatment modalities for psychiatric illnesses. However, stigma and other noted challenges reviewed in this chapter continue to remain significant barriers to participant recruitment. Finally, although not inherently developed with the idea of precision medicine, psychotherapeutic approaches aim to tailor interventions to patients and may be viable to advance understanding of the science of behavior change. By uncovering the biological mechanisms underlying psychiatric disorders, treatments incorporating precision medicine will likely be welcomed by child psychiatry practitioners despite the heterogeneity and complexity of the determinants of mental illnesses. Researchers are privileged to interpret these complex processes and translate them into clinical relevance.

Strategies for Mitigating Therapeutic Misconception

Because many participants claim the hope of benefit as a primary reason for enrolling in clinical trials, they may be inherently misguided because of the different goals of research and medical care. This may result in an inherent conflict between the interests of the medical provider and that of the investigator, especially in early phase trials in which researchers are still delineating the toxicity and side effects of experimental drugs or procedures.

Take, for instance, the following illustrative scenario: A teen presents to a child and adolescent psychiatry clinic with treatment-refractory depression that has not responded to multiple trials of various psychotherapies, antidepressants, and combinations offered as part of usual clinical care. Frustrated by these treatment failures, her parents see an advertisement on their social media account about a new investigation attempting to understand the safety and efficacy of TMS for adolescent depression. They express an interest to their child psychiatrist in enrolling their daughter in this TMS study, asking for an opinion about the potential value of this novel intervention for their daughter. The parents have read reports that TMS may be effective in "curing" treatment-refractory depression. How do the clinician and then the physician-scientist address the caregivers' desire for an effective treatment versus the possibility that the child may not experience benefit from participation in the trial? Would the risk of receiving a sham comparison condition lead the parents to exercise caution in signing up for trial participation?

This vignette illustrates the importance of presenting medical care and clinical research as distinct entities. Therapeutic misconception is the ethical problem of study participants who believe they are receiving treatment (Appelbaum et al. 1982); it is incompatible with adequate informed consent and undermines the trustworthiness of the research enterprise. Consequences of misplaced trust by the subject on the investigator include damaging effects on self-trust, unfair burdens on researchers, disruption of trust relationships with medical professionals, and loss of social legitimacy of clinical research. Clinicians who refer patients, researchers, the scientific community, and oversight agencies can all play a role in helping to reduce or eliminate therapeutic misconception.

Let us consider some safeguards that can be implemented to minimize and prevent therapeutic misconception in child and adolescent psychiatry (Charuvastra and Marder 2008; de Melo-Martín and Ho 2008). The voluntary nature of research participation should be emphasized, with no promise of benefit leading up to and including the informed consent procedure. To minimize confusion, discussions about research should occur independently of medical care discussions, with education provided about their distinct roles and goals. In addition, informed consent for clinical trials in vulnerable populations may be improved if research personnel not associated with the medical care discuss the logistics of the clinical trial and allow patients time to contemplate their options before enrollment (de Melo-Martín and Ho 2008).

Another strategy to facilitate a clear understanding in the frequently clinically underresourced setting of child and adolescent psychiatry is that patients could be presented with the option of participating in a "research program," entry into which could also include general orientation to the program with an informed consent discussion that includes the key elements of disclosure, understanding, voluntariness, and competence. This can allow patients and families to make an informed decision about electing to participate in a research study that may offer diagnostic assessments or treatment recommendations in the context of a research study. Although benefit cannot be ensured when one is volunteering for research, research programs common to academic settings are reputably of high quality, evidence informed, and measurement based. Disadvantages of research program participation may include inherent risks associated with a yet-to-be-tested intervention, such as time insensitivity leading to potentially delayed treatments or blinded randomization of treatments. Collaborative care, community participatory trial designs, and implementation science models that leverage the inherent complementarity of research and clinical missions commonly espoused in academic settings have been proposed as a possible future direction for improved mental health care in a variety of academic and nonacademic settings (Lake and Turner 2017). In this context, research is not done in a silo but is directly informed by the clinical challenges faced by the most complex patients. Proper execution and success of clinical research practices entail trust among investigators, participants, research institutions, and oversight agencies to ensure alignment of ethical principles to mitigate therapeutic misconceptions that lead to under- or overestimation of risk, benefit, or both. Finally, ensuring a warm handoff between research participation and medical care into a standard clinical psychiatric practice once research participation is complete preserves therapeutic alliance and ensures continuity of care beyond a research-based intervention.

Principles derived from the past two decades of cardiovascular clinical research provide yet another perspective on how clinical research discussions are weighed in a medical setting (Califf and DeMets 2002). First, most treatments produce a combination of helpful and harmful effects, so clinicians should assist patients in evaluating the risks and benefits of therapeutic modalities in clinical trials. Second, most beneficial treatments do not immediately save money, but they may be incrementally cost-effective in the long run. Because the development of new, potentially effective treatments is costly, an effective assessment of such treatments should also evaluate prospective cost of development and the degree of benefit in the long term (i.e., incremental cost-effectiveness). Thus, efforts should be made toward promoting the use of proven, cheaper, and alternative treatments while avoiding unproven ones. Third, there is benefit derived from applying the results of clinical trials, which provide evidence-based studies to guide treatment. Well-conducted randomized trials integrated into systematic overviews and clinical guidelines determined by professional societies and disease-oriented organizations enable evidence-based clinical practice. For example, the American Heart Association and the American College of Cardiology have devised a system involving level of evidence (grade) and type of recommendation (class) for therapeutic interventions based on clinical trials. Fourth, it should be recognized that some areas of medicine are underserved. Fifth, participation is imperative; the willingness of both clinicians and patients to participate in clinical trials will help generate findings to implement evidence-based treatment.

Unsurprisingly, there are some unique barriers to implementing these principles in the field of child and adolescent psychiatry, including a different disease burden compared with cardiovascular medicine, uncertainty about risks and unknown effects, and stigma. Nevertheless, measurement-based care and digital therapeutics that apply the rigorous standards for novel drug discovery that have been facilitated through clinical trial networks may be within reach to revitalize in child and adolescent psychiatry. With the growing impact of untreated psychopathology on global health burden, perhaps these principles could hold traction in our field sooner than later.

RESEARCH DESIGN AND IMPLEMENTATION CHALLENGES AND STRATEGIES

Limited new investigational drugs are tested in pediatric trials. Of drug trials registered in the ClinicalTrials.gov database between 2006 and 2011, only 10% of pediatric trials centered on drugs developed for neuropsychiatric conditions (Murthy et al. 2013). Ideally, clinical trials should be publicly registered, and results should be promptly published to prevent duplicate studies as well as publication and reporting bias (Hoppu 2009; Viergever et al. 2014). Pharmaceutical companies have been reducing funding for neuroscience research, which has had the effect of potentially inhibiting prospects for psychopharmacological drug advancements. These challenges may directly affect pediatric psychiatric drug development in all phases of clinical translation and in both academic research and industry settings (Grabb and Gobburu 2017).

There are four phases of treatment development. Phase I tests the efficacy of a new drug, Phase II studies the safety and efficacy of the intervention, and Phase IV postmarketing trials are relatively uncommon in children (Aleksa and Koren 2002). Phase III trials, in which RCTs compare an investigational intervention with standard therapy, are the most common in youth. The field of child and adolescent psychiatry is relatively young but is receiving increased attention for better recognized, highly prevalent, and increasingly debilitating but potentially preventable health conditions. Developmental preclinical models that take into account critical sensitive windows in development and consider the important role of sex differences in phenomenology and treatment response are key for the achievement of personalized treatments. Pharmacokinetic studies in pediatric populations are also lacking because of the challenges of performing accurate tests to measure the volume and timing of sampling and the absence of sensitive techniques to determine the drug concentration of very small volume specimens (Laughon et al. 2011). To address these challenges, pharmacokinetic studies in youth could extrapolate from adult data if the disease progression is similar between children and adults, use single-dose pediatric studies in different age groups if the drugs are known to have linear pharmacokinetics in adults, and conduct opportunistic trials through the collection of pharmacokinetic samples from children and teens already receiving treatment through routine clinical care (European Medicines Agency 2007; Johnson 2005; Laughon et al. 2011). By nurturing science along all phases of the translational continuum, the field holds significant promise to meet the unmet clinical needs of a growing patient population. Indeed, meeting clinical unmet needs is fundamental to building a therapeutic alliance (Arnold et al. 2017) and could significantly influence psychiatric outcome (Reininghaus et al. 2013).

Some of the difficulty in recruiting pediatric patients for clinical trials may stem from a different set of challenges associated with disease burden in children with serious behavioral problems. Clinical trials across many areas in pediatric medicine suffer from small sample sizes that lead to problems of inadequate statistical power (Caldwell et al. 2004; Krekels et al. 2007; Lim and Cranswick 2003; Morales-Olivas and Morales-Carpi 2006). Collaborative clinical trial networks for pediatric drug development (Turner et al. 2017) enable resource sharing between trials, informative learning, and standardized processes for trial conduct, and provide an avenue for producing larger sample studies with potentially more generalizable results. Networks across a wide geographic area are often developed to facilitate translation of research into the clinic and may centralize research infrastructures for participants. Indeed, clinical trial networks have been implemented with some success in child and adolescent psychiatry (Lebowitz et al. 2003; March et al. 2004; Shapiro et al. 2009) but need to be revived with stable funding and contextualized by lessons learned from prior efforts.

Clinical trials in child and adolescent psychiatry must also be designed to systematically assess for safety. Therapeutic drug monitoring is a valid tool to optimize pharmacology and allows clinicians to adjust the dosage of drugs according to the characteristics of an individual patient (Mehler-Wex et al. 2009). Multicenter therapeutic drug monitoring studies allow researchers to identify the age- and development-dependent therapeutic ranges of blood concentrations and facilitate a standardized approach to child and adolescent psychiatric treatment. Although some parents and clinicians are hesitant to enroll children in clinical trials because of the risk of potentially introducing the harms of uncertain treatment effects, it is important to remember that other caregivers with a positive experience of clinical trials view study participation as an exciting opportunity to be part of advancing science in this relatively nascent field.

Discussion and Future Directions

Although significant progress has been made in understanding the biological mechanisms of psychiatric disorders, application toward new therapeutic agents has been slow, leaving patients with limited treatment options, which can lead to conversations of futility rather than hope in clinical settings, perhaps for good reasons. Preclinical predictors of success and failure for CNS drug discovery have been evaluated for drugs developed for schizophrenia, depression, and anxiety. Discoveries of the earliest psychotropic drugs, including the antipsychotic actions of chlorpromazine (Delay et al. 1952) and the antimanic effects of lithium (Cade 1949), were serendipitous. Further, preclinical trials have not always accurately predicted therapeutic response, as exemplified by the initial rejection of clozapine as a viable antipsychotic because of its inefficacy in rodents. There is also a need to understand the specific actions of psychotropic medications on developing brain systems. Not much is known about underlying mechanisms of psychiatric illnesses of childhood onset, which makes advancements in drug discovery challenging.

Hope for new breakthroughs in treatment can promote treatment engagement and facilitate the therapeutic alliance. There are several ways we can enhance progress in pediatric psychopharmacology (Grabb and Gobburu 2017). First, we can advance our understanding of the biological basis of mental illness, which may yield new molecular targets for drug discovery. We can also encourage random small molecular-based screening and chemical optimization in academic settings and research into basic mechanisms of drug toxicities and side effect liabilities. If we focus on target validation at every step in the drug discovery process, we may be able to accelerate the transition from biological target to a lead compound that becomes an intervention. We may also develop designs for safe, early proof-of-concept studies in humans, such that humans are the animal model of choice (Insel 2011). Finally, we may encourage a portfolio of science that identifies and validates novel targets that aim to meet clinical unmet needs and accelerate translation from preclinical to clinical, and vice versa, by integrating discovery and applied science, which has traditionally been denoted unidirectionally as translation from bench to bedside.

Pediatric psychopharmacological drug development depends on a variety of synchronous factors fueled principally to meet clinical unmet needs in child and adolescent psychiatry. These factors depend fundamentally on the desire for patients and caregivers to seek treatment. Consequently, a series of collaborative efforts on multiple fronts can ensue; these include 1) regulatory guidance and potential acceleration of regulatory processes; 2) National Institute of Mental Health, foundation, and other funding sources for drug research; 3) availability of investigational drugs provided by industry; 4) pediatric trial experts and staff skilled in conducting clinical trials; 5) enhancement of preclinical models; 6) technological improvements to enable noninvasive CNS biomarker measurement and treatment in children; 7) development of the field of pediatric CNS biomarker research; and 8) development of platforms that can provide additional patient data for clinical trials. Together, these efforts can constitute a rational approach to ensure a hopeful horizon for patients and their families, ultimately forging stronger and more trusting relations between patients and the health care system.

Thus, there are a limited number of clinical trials in the field of child and adolescent psychiatry, and application toward new therapeutic agents has been slow, leaving patients with few available treatment options. Building a therapeutic alliance focused on collaborative efforts among patients, families, and clinical research teams in academic, industry, federal, and private settings is essential to make progress in pursuit of better treatments in child and adolescent psychiatry.

TAKE-AWAY POINTS

- Currently, clinical evidence for pharmacological treatment in youth primarily stems from adapting findings from studies conducted in adults because of limited clinical trials in pediatric populations. However, differences in physiology, development, psychology, and pharmacology in children compared with adults do not obviate the need for more research studies in children and adolescents.

- Conducting clinical research in youth involves added layers of complexity because of the requirement of informed consent by a proxy (e.g., parent or caregiver) and the potential risks that may uniquely be associated with exposure to novel or yet-to-be-tested treatments in developmental populations.

- The ethical dilemma of pediatric clinical trials involves finding an equilibrium between the obligation to conduct trials and the potential harms associated with untested treatments.

- Clear distinctions can be made between medical care and clinical research. Medical care aims to find the optimal treatment for an individual patient. Clinical research is aimed at discoveries to develop scientific knowledge to benefit the greater population rather than an individual. When a clinical trial ends and further care is clinically indicated, the clinical researcher should facilitate a warm handoff to a clinician in order to facilitate a therapeutic alliance with psychiatric care.

- Research that aims to understand and leverage the placebo effect, that develops strategies for personalizing treatment based on objective biomarkers, and that utilizes existing knowledge to innovate through iteration may be among our most accessible pathways toward developing new treatments that can help patients sooner rather than later. These strategies that integrate applied science into discovery can pave an accelerated path toward novel treatments.

References

Abdel-Rahman SM, Reed MD, Wells TG, Kearns GL: Considerations in the rational design and conduct of phase I/II pediatric clinical trials: avoiding the problems and pitfalls. Clin Pharmacol Ther 81(4):483–494, 2007 17329988

Aleksa K, Koren G: Ethical issues in including pediatric cancer patients in drug development trials. Paediatr Drugs 4(4):257–265, 2002 11960514

Appelbaum PS, Roth LH, Lidz C: The therapeutic misconception: informed consent in psychiatric research. Int J Law Psychiatry 5(3–4):319–329, 1982 6135666

Appelbaum PS, Roth LH, Lidz CW, et al: False hopes and best data: consent to research and the therapeutic misconception. Hastings Cent Rep 17(2):20–24, 1987 3294743

Arnold K, Loos S, Mayer B; CEDAR Study Group: Helping alliance and unmet needs in routine care of people with severe mental illness across Europe: a prospective longitudinal multicenter study. J Nerv Ment Dis 205(4):329–333, 2017 28350783

Avenevoli S, Swendsen J, He J-P, et al: Major depression in the National Comorbidity Survey—Adolescent Supplement: prevalence, correlates, and treatment. J Am Acad Child Adolesc Psychiatry 54(1):37–44, 2015 25524788

Ballenger JC: Remission rates in patients with anxiety disorders treated with paroxetine. J Clin Psychiatry 65(12):1696–1707, 2004 15641876

Barkley RA: Hyperactive girls and boys: stimulant drug effects on mother-child interactions. J Child Psychol Psychiatry 30(3):379–390, 1989 2663900

Barnett ER, Trepman AZ, Fuson HA, et al: Deprescribing psychotropic medications in children: results of a national qualitative study. BMJ Qual Saf 29:655–663, 2019

Bosk CL: Obtaining voluntary consent for research in desperately ill patients. Med Care 40(9, suppl):V64–V68, 2002 12226587

Bradley C: The behavior of children receiving Benzedrine. Am J Psychiatry 94:577–585, 1937

Bridge JA, Birmaher B, Iyengar S, et al: Placebo response in randomized controlled trials of antidepressants for pediatric major depressive disorder. Am J Psychiatry 166(1):42–49, 2009 19047322

Brody H, Miller FG: The clinician-investigator: unavoidable but manageable tension. Kennedy Inst Ethics J 13(4):329–346, 2003 15049297

Cade JFJ: Lithium salts in the treatment of psychotic excitement. Med J Aust 2(10):349–352, 1949 18142718

Caldwell PHY, Murphy SB, Butow PN, Craig JC: Clinical trials in children. Lancet 364(9436):803–811, 2004 15337409

Califf RM, DeMets DL: Principles from clinical trials relevant to clinical practice: part II. Circulation 106(9):1172–1175, 2002 12196347

Carrier F, Banayan D, Boley R, Karnik N: Ethical challenges in developing drugs for psychiatric disorders. Prog Neurobiol 152:58–69, 2017 28268181

Charuvastra A, Marder SR: Unconscious emotional reasoning and the therapeutic misconception. J Med Ethics 34(3):193–197, 2008 18316462

Cohen E, Uleryk E, Jasuja M, Parkin PC: An absence of pediatric randomized controlled trials in general medical journals, 1985–2004. J Clin Epidemiol 60(2):118–123, 2007 17208117

Cytryn L, McKnew DH: Treatment issues in childhood depression. Pediatr Ann 15(12):856–858, 1986 3808766

de Beurs E, van Balkom AJ, Van Dyck R, Lange A: Long-term outcome of pharmacological and psychological treatment for panic disorder with agoraphobia: a 2-year naturalistic follow-up. Acta Psychiatr Scand 99(1):59–67, 1999 10066008

Delay J, Deniker P, Harl JM: Therapeutic method derived from hiberno-therapy in excitation and agitation states. Ann Med Psychol 110(22):267–273, 1952

de Melo-Martín I, Ho A: Beyond informed consent: the therapeutic misconception and trust. J Med Ethics 34(3):202–205, 2008 18316464

Domino ME, Burns BJ, Silva SG, et al: Cost-effectiveness of treatments for adolescent depression: results from TADS. Am J Psychiatry 165(5):588–596, 2008 18413703

Emanuel EJ, Wendler D, Grady C: What makes clinical research ethical? JAMA 283(20):2701–2711, 2000 10819955

Emslie GJ: Understanding placebo response in pediatric depression trials. Am J Psychiatry 166(1):1–3, 2009 19122009

European Medicines Agency: Guideline on reporting the results of population pharmacokinetic analyses. June 21, 2007; legal effective date: January 1, 2008

Fearon RMP: Making clinical trials smarter (and more interesting) (editorial). J Child Psychol Psychiatry 58(2):113–115, 2017 28102619

Findling RL, McNamara NK, Gracious BL: Paediatric uses of atypical antipsychotics. Expert Opin Pharmacother 1(5):935–945, 2000 11249501

Findling RL, Horwitz SM, Birmaher B, et al: Clinical characteristics of children receiving antipsychotic medication. J Child Adolesc Psychopharmacol 21(4):311–319, 2011 21851189

Flament MF, Rapoport JL, Berg CJ, et al: Clomipramine treatment of childhood obsessive-compulsive disorder: a double-blind controlled study. Arch Gen Psychiatry 42(10):977–983, 1985 3899048

Fonagy P: What Works for Whom? A Critical Review of Treatments for Children and Adolescents, 2nd Edition. New York, Guilford, 2015

Freedman B: Equipoise and the ethics of clinical research. N Engl J Med 317(3):141–145, 1987 3600702

Freedman B: Placebo-controlled trials and the logic of clinical purpose. IRB 12(6):1–6, 1990 11651265

Grabb MC, Gobburu JVS: Challenges in developing drugs for pediatric CNS disorders: a focus on psychopharmacology. Prog Neurobiol 152:38–57, 2017 27216638

Greenhill LL, Vitiello B, Abikoff H, et al: Developing methodologies for monitoring long-term safety of psychotropic medications in children: report on the NIMH conference, September 25, 2000. J Am Acad Child Adolesc Psychiatry 42(6):651–655, 2003 12921472

Griffiths AO: Enuresis and tricyclic antidepressants (letter). Br Med J 1(6172):1213, 1979 445010

Hammad TA, Laughren T, Racoosin J: Suicidality in pediatric patients treated with antidepressant drugs. Arch Gen Psychiatry 63(3):332–339, 2006 16520440

Hattab JY: Ethics and Child Mental Health. Jerusalem, Gefen, 1996

Hochhauser M: Psychodynamic influences on human subject recruiting practices. SOCRA Source 2:20–23, 2005

Hoppu K: Can we get the necessary clinical trials in children and avoid the unnecessary ones? Eur J Clin Pharmacol 65(8):747–748, 2009 19521694

Insel TR: A bridge to somewhere. Transl Psychiatry 1:e2, 2011 22832390

Jensen-Doss A, Weisz JR: Diagnostic agreement predicts treatment process and outcomes in youth mental health clinics. J Consult Clin Psychol 76(5):711–722, 2008 18837589

Jensen-Doss A, Youngstrom EA, Youngstrom JK, et al: Predictors and moderators of agreement between clinical and research diagnoses for children and adolescents. J Consult Clin Psychol 82(6):1151–1162, 2014 24773574

Johnson TN: Modelling approaches to dose estimation in children. Br J Clin Pharmacol 59(6):663–669, 2005 15948929

Joseph PD, Craig JC, Caldwell PHY: Clinical trials in children. Br J Clin Pharmacol 79(3):357–369, 2015 24325152

Joshi SV: Teamwork: the therapeutic alliance in pediatric pharmacotherapy. Child Adolesc Psychiatr Clin N Am 15(1):239–262, 2006 16321733

Kashani JH, Husain A, Shekim WO, et al: Current perspectives on childhood depression: an overview. Am J Psychiatry 138(2):143–153, 1981 6109452

Katz J: The Silent World of Doctor and Patient. Baltimore, MD, Johns Hopkins University Press, 2002

Kearns MA, Hawley KM: Predictors of polypharmacy and off-label prescribing of psychotropic medications: a national survey of child and adolescent psychiatrists. J Psychiatr Pract 20(6):438–447, 2014 25406048

Keller MB, Ryan ND, Strober M, et al: Efficacy of paroxetine in the treatment of adolescent major depression: a randomized, controlled trial. J Am Acad Child Adolesc Psychiatry 40(7):762–772, 2001 11437014

Klein RG, Koplewicz HS, Kanner A: Imipramine treatment of children with separation anxiety disorder. J Am Acad Child Adolesc Psychiatry 31(1):21–28, 1992 1347039

Krekels EHJ, van den Anker JN, Baiardi P, et al: Pharmacogenetics and paediatric drug development: issues and consequences to labelling and dosing recommendations. Expert Opin Pharmacother 8(12):1787–1799, 2007 17696784

Krupnick JL, Sotsky SM, Simmens S, et al: The role of the therapeutic alliance in psychotherapy and pharmacotherapy outcome: findings in the National Institute of Mental Health Treatment of Depression Collaborative Research Program. J Consult Clin Psychol 64(3):532–539, 1996 8698947

Lake J, Turner MS: Urgent need for improved mental health care and a more collaborative model of care. Perm J 21:17–024, 2017 28898197

Laughon MM, Benjamin DK Jr, Capparelli EV, et al: Innovative clinical trial design for pediatric therapeutics. Expert Rev Clin Pharmacol 4(5):643–652, 2011 21980319

Lebowitz BD, Vitiello B, Norquist GS: Approaches to multisite clinical trials: the National Institute of Mental Health perspective. Schizophr Bull 29(1):7–13, 2003 12908657

Lim A, Cranswick N: Clinical trials, ethical issues and patient recruitment: an Australian perspective. Paediatr Perinat Drug Ther 5(4):183–187, 2003

March JS, Silva SG, Compton S, et al: The Child and Adolescent Psychiatry Trials Network (CAPTN). J Am Acad Child Adolesc Psychiatry 43(5):515–518, 2004 15100557

Mehler-Wex C, Kölch M, Kirchheiner J, et al: Drug monitoring in child and adolescent psychiatry for improved efficacy and safety of psychopharmacotherapy. Child Adolesc Psychiatry Ment Health 3(1):14, 2009 19358696

Mikkelsen EJ, Rapoport JL: Enuresis: psychopathology, sleep stage, and drug response. Urol Clin North Am 7(2):361–377, 1980 6996271

Miller FG, Brody H: A critique of clinical equipoise: therapeutic misconception in the ethics of clinical trials. Hastings Cent Rep 33(3):19–28, 2003 12854452

Morales-Olivas FJ, Morales-Carpi C: Clinical trials in children. Rev Recent Clin Trials 1(3):251–258, 2006 18473977

Murthy S, Mandl KD, Bourgeois F: Analysis of pediatric clinical drug trials for neuropsychiatric conditions. Pediatrics 131(6):1125–1131, 2013 23650305

National Commission for the Protection of Human Subjects of Biomedical and Behavioral Research: Belmont report: ethical principles and guidelines for the protection of human subjects of research. Rockville, MD, U.S. Department of Health and Human Services, 1978

Office for Human Research Protections: Federal Policy for the Protection of Human Subjects ("Common Rule"). n.d. Available at: www.hhs.gov/ohrp/regulations-and-policy/regulations/common-rule/index.html. Accessed March 21, 2020.

Pine DS, Helfinstein SM, Bar-Haim Y, et al: Challenges in developing novel treatments for childhood disorders: lessons from research on anxiety. Neuropsychopharmacology 34(1):213–228, 2009 18754004

Posner J: The role of precision medicine in child psychiatry: what can we expect and when? J Am Acad Child Adolesc Psychiatry 57(11):813–817, 2018 30392618

Pruett KD, Joshi SV, Martin A: Thinking about prescribing: the psychology of psychopharmacology, in Pediatric Psychopharmacology. Edited by Martin A, Scahill L, Kratochvil C. New York, Oxford University Press, 2010 pp 422–433

Puig-Antich J, Perel JM, Lupatkin W, et al: Imipramine in prepubertal major depressive disorders. Arch Gen Psychiatry 44(1):81–89, 1987 3541830

Rapoport JL: Pediatric psychopharmacology: too much or too little? World Psychiatry 12(2):118–123, 2013 23737413

Rapoport JL, Buchsbaum MS, Zahn TP, et al: Dextroamphetamine: cognitive and behavioral effects in normal prepubertal boys. Science 199(4328):560–563, 1978 341313

Rapoport JL, Buchsbaum MS, Weingartner H, et al: Dextroamphetamine: its cognitive and behavioral effects in normal and hyperactive boys and normal men. Arch Gen Psychiatry 37(8):933–943, 1980 7406657

Reeves G, Anthony B: Multimodal treatments versus pharmacotherapy alone in children with psychiatric disorders: implications of access, effectiveness, and contextual treatment. Paediatr Drugs 11(3):165–169, 2009 19445545

Reininghaus U, McCabe R, Slade M, et al: The validity of patient- and clinician-rated measures of needs and the therapeutic relationship in psychosis: a pooled analysis. Psychiatry Res 209(3):711–720, 2013 23452753

Rutherford BR, Sneed JR, Tandler JM, et al: Deconstructing pediatric depression trials: an analysis of the effects of expectancy and therapeutic contact. J Am Acad Child Adolesc Psychiatry 50(8):782–795, 2011 21784298

Shapiro M, Silva SG, Compton S, et al: The Child and Adolescent Psychiatry Trials Network (CAPTN): infrastructure development and lessons learned. Child Adolesc Psychiatry Ment Health 3(1):12, 2009 19320979

Shilling V, Young B: How do parents experience being asked to enter a child in a randomised controlled trial? BMC Med Ethics 10(1):1, 2009 19220889

Shirkey H: Therapeutic orphans. J Pediatr 72(1):119–120, 1968 5634934

Sinha I, Jones L, Smyth RL, Williamson PR: A systematic review of studies that aim to determine which outcomes to measure in clinical trials in children. PLoS Med 5(4):e96, 2008 18447577

Spencer T, Biederman J, Heiligenstein J, et al: An open-label, dose-ranging study of atomoxetine in children with attention deficit hyperactivity disorder. J Child Adolesc Psychopharmacol 11(3):251–265, 2001 11642475

Stringaris A: Trials and tribulations in child psychology and psychiatry: what is needed for evidence-based practice (editorial). J Child Psychol Psychiatry 55(11):1185–1186, 2014 25306851

Sultan RS, Correll CU, Zohar J, et al: What's in a name? Moving to neuroscience-based nomenclature in pediatric psychopharmacology. J Am Acad Child Adolesc Psychiatry 57(10):719–721, 2018 30274643

Swedo SE, Leonard HL, Rapoport JL: Childhood-onset obsessive compulsive disorder. Psychiatr Clin North Am 15(4):767–775, 1992 1461794

Turner MA, Attar S, de Wildt SN, et al: Roles of clinical research networks in pediatric drug development. Clin Ther 39(10):1939–1948, 2017 28943118

Viergever RF, Karam G, Reis A, Ghersi D: The quality of registration of clinical trials: still a problem. PLoS One 9(1):e84727, 2014 24427293

Washington HA: Medical Apartheid: The Dark History of Medical Experimentation on Black Americans From Colonial Times to the Present. New York, Harlem Moon, 2006

Wehry AM, Ramsey L, Dulemba SE, et al: Pharmacogenomic testing in child and adolescent psychiatry: an evidence-based review. Curr Probl Pediatr Adolesc Health Care 48(2):40–49, 2018 29325731

Weiss M, Gaston L, Propst A, et al: The role of the alliance in the pharmacologic treatment of depression. J Clin Psychiatry 58(5):196–204, 1997 9184613

Wells KC, Chi TC, Hinshaw SP, et al: Treatment-related changes in objectively measured parenting behaviors in the Multimodal Treatment Study of Children with Attention-Deficit/Hyperactivity Disorder. J Consult Clin Psychol 74(4):649–657, 2006 16881772

Witcher JW, Long A, Smith B, et al: Atomoxetine pharmacokinetics in children and adolescents with attention deficit hyperactivity disorder. J Child Adolesc Psychopharmacol 13(1):53–63, 2003 12804126

World Medical Association: WMA Declaration of Helsinki: Ethical Principles for Medical Research Involving Human Subjects. 64th WMA General Assembly, Fortaleza, Brazil, October 2013. Available at: www.wma.net/policies-post/wma-declaration-of-helsinki-ethical-principles-for-medical-research-involving-human-subjects. Accessed February 28, 2021.

Young ME, Bell ZE, Fristad MA: Validation of a brief structured interview: the Children's Interview for Psychiatric Syndromes (ChIPS). J Clin Psychol Med Settings 23(4):327–340, 2016 27761777

Zion SR, Crum AJ: Mindsets matter: a new framework for harnessing the placebo effect in modern medicine. Int Rev Neurobiol 138:137–160, 2018

Zito JM, Safer DJ, de Jong-van den Berg LT, et al: A three-country comparison of psychotropic medication prevalence in youth. Child Adolesc Psychiatry Ment Health 2(1):26, 2008 18817536

CHAPTER | 16

THE POWER OF PLACEBO

Jeffrey R. Strawn, M.D.
Jeffrey A. Mills, Ph.D.
Tara S. Paris, Ph.D.
John T. Walkup, M.D.

Placebo response (i.e., the improvement that patients perceive or experience in response to inert therapeutic agents) occurs commonly across clinical trials for both adult and child psychopathology (March et al. 2004; Pediatric OCD Treatment Study Team 2004; Walkup et al. 2008; Rutherford and Roose 2013). With rates ranging from 20% to 60%, high placebo response is one of the most significant barriers to detecting treatment effects in both pediatric and adult clinical trials (Rutherford and Roose 2013; Walkup 2017). At the same time, the value of placebo response to improvement in the clinic is undeniable. Placebo response in clinical trials and clinical practice has been attributed to nonspecific aspects of treatment (e.g., alliance, diagnostic formulation, and benefit of symptom tracking) as well as, in clinical trials, study design. However, this conceptualization fails to account for individual factors that exist within patients and their families that contribute to placebo response. Patients vary in how much they expect treatments to work and how much they believe that they can improve, and these are powerful drivers of clinical response. In this chapter, we review placebo response in children and adolescents with anxiety and depressive disorders and explore developmental, patient-specific, and family-specific factors that influence placebo response. We then discuss placebo response in terms of maximizing day-to-day outcomes in child and adolescent psychiatry and include vignettes.

Nonspecific Factors That May Affect Placebo Response in Clinical Trials

The placebo effect is conceptualized as a psychological response to receiving treatment rather than a response to an intervention itself. In clinical trials, it may be due to generic intervention elements (i.e., psychoeducation and instructions to monitor symptoms), which result in patients and families learning to 1) understand the clinical presentation of the illness, 2) recognize specific symptoms, and 3) attend to the fluctuation in these symptoms over time and in response to precipitating factors. Several factors contribute to this response, including the patient's experience of the therapeutic relationship, the patient-family therapist alliance, and the collaborative development of treatment goals. Interestingly, in clinical trials in adults with major depressive disorder (MDD), these factors, as they pertain to the treating psychiatrist, accounted for nearly 10% of the variance in treatment response (triple the variance associated with the medication) (McKay et al. 2006). Thus, nonspecific factors that drive placebo response are commonly discussed within the context of clinical trials but not often discussed as an important factor in routine clinical care.

Temporal Course of Placebo Response in Pediatric Anxiety Disorders, Obsessive-Compulsive Disorder, and Major Depressive Disorder

Placebo response in children and adolescents with MDD, obsessive-compulsive disorder (OCD), and generalized, separation, and social anxiety disorders emerges early and is logarithmic (Strawn et al. 2017; Varigonda et al. 2015) (Figure 16–1). For example, in the Child/Adolescent Anxiety Multimodal Study (CAMS), sertraline, sertraline plus cognitive-behavioral therapy (CBT), and CBT is associated with an increased probability of response over time; for placebo, the probability of response plateaued between 4 and 8 weeks of treatment and decreased thereafter (Strawn et al. 2017). In clinical trials in youth with MDD, placebo response emerges early but does not diminish over time in the same way that it does in those with anxiety disorders (Varigonda et al. 2016). However, the temporal course of placebo response has not been examined to the same extent in youth with MDD compared with those with anxiety disorders.

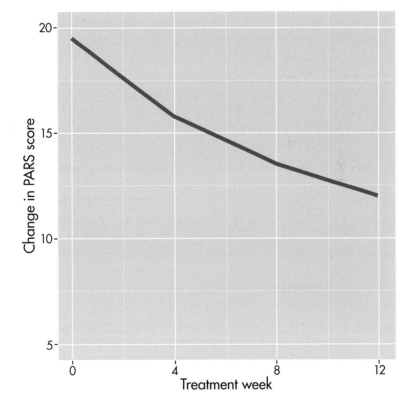

Figure 16–1. Trajectory of placebo response in pediatric anxiety disorders.

Note. Similar to medication-related improvement, placebo-related improvement occurs within the first several weeks. PARS=Pediatric Anxiety Rating Scale.
Source. Data from Walkup et al. 2008.

Clinical Trial Design and Placebo Response

Placebo response rates in clinical trials of antidepressants in youth are increasing and now reach 40%–50% in some pediatric trials (da Costa et al. 2013; Emslie et al. 2014; Wagner et al. 2004). In these clinical trials, placebo response remains poorly understood despite reports of clinical predictors of placebo response in children and adolescents with MDD and anxiety disorders (Cohen et al. 2010; Dobson and Strawn 2016; Locher et al. 2017; Nakonezny et al. 2015). The extant evidence suggests that the magnitude of placebo response relates to the disorder being studied (e.g., anxiety disorder vs. depressive disorder), the age of patients being studied (Cohen et al. 2010; Dobson and Strawn 2016), the funding source (Mossman et al. 2021; Walkup 2017), and the trial design (e.g., number of study sites, total number of subjects, randomization pattern, trial duration).

Several meta-analyses have examined clinical trial design and placebo response in youth with anxiety and depressive disorders (Bridge et al. 2009; Cohen et al. 2010; Mills et al. 2019; Mossman et al. 2021; Rutherford and Roose 2013; Strawn et al. 2017). In the first of these, Bridge et al. (2009) examined 12 studies ($N=2,862$) of youth with MDD and noted that placebo response increased as a function of the number of study sites and in younger patients and was inversely related to depressive symptom severity at baseline. A second meta-analysis found that depressed youth who had more contact with research staff had a greater placebo response. A third examination of studies of pediatric patients with depressive disorders, anxiety disorders, and OCD, including 10 studies of anxious youth ($N=634$), found that patients with anxiety disorders had higher response rates relative to youth with OCD but lower placebo response rates relative to those with MDD (Cohen et al. 2010). In this analysis, whereas placebo response was negatively associated with Caucasian status and the percentage of male participants, the presence of a washout decreased placebo response. In a more recent meta-analysis, which examined 14 trials (9 medications) in pediatric patients ($N=2,230$) with anxiety disorders, higher placebo response rates were associated with a greater number of study sites and fewer patients per site (Dobson and Strawn 2016). Finally, federally funded studies, studies conducted in the United States, and studies of patients with anxiety disorders (compared with those with depressive disorders) have lower placebo response rates (Mossman et al. 2021; Walkup 2017).

A number of methodological factors related to the measurement of symptoms also potentially affect observed placebo response in pediatric studies. Although these factors have been more extensively examined in adults (Papakostas et al. 2015), the findings are likely applicable in pediatric patients. Briefly, it has been suggested that some dimensional measures of symptoms may not reflect global severity (Bech et al. 1975) and that these measures are unidimensional (Bech et al. 1981, 2011). Papakostas et al. (2015) raise the possibility that "using the total score of the scale is problematic from a mathematical and statistical perspective." Creating a unidimensional measure of overall symptom severity as a linear combination (i.e., average or sum) of measurement across multiple symptom dimensions can be highly misleading. Improvement in some symptoms may be more important for overall improvement than improvement in others, and symptoms can interact in complex ways.

Problems With Unidimensionality and Measuring Improvement

Suppose the overall measure consists of two symptom category measures. The first captures generalized anxiety severity, and the second more reflects separation anxiety severity. Now consider two patients: Bobby is a 12-year-old boy with a generalized anxiety symptom severity of 5 and a separation anxiety score of 2 (Table 16–1). Emily is a 12-year-old girl with a generalized anxiety score of 2 and a separation anxiety score of 5. Both Emily and Bobby have total anxiety scores of 7 before starting treatment.

Table 16–1. Generalized anxiety symptom, separation anxiety, and total anxiety scores for two patients

	Generalized anxiety symptom score		Separation anxiety symptom score		Total anxiety severity score	
Pt.	**Baseline**	**Post-treat**	**Baseline**	**Post-treat**	**Baseline**	**Post-treat**
Bobby	5	4	2	1	7	5
Emily	2	1	5	1	7	2

After treatment with CBT, Bobby's symptoms are reduced to a total anxiety symptom score of 5 (Table 16–1), and Emily's symptom severity is reduced to a total anxiety symptom score of 2. However, Emily's improvement is due to the reduction in separation anxiety symptoms, and neither Emily nor Bobby had significant improvement in generalized anxiety disorder (GAD) symptoms. As more dimensions are added to the overall symptom score, these measurement problems can increase substantially and degrade our ability to identify treatment-related effects or may result in our interpreting improvement as related to placebo.

A related concern is that certain youth who have "depression" experience symptoms that are driven by exogenous factors—life struggles, adversity, and chronic variable stress—that boost scores on some measures. Thus, core symptoms do not drive these symptom rating scores; rather, they are driven by impairment. These factors, as well as the unidimensionality of these rating scales, increase placebo response rates in clinical trials that rely on these measures.

Placebo Response in Pediatric Anxiety Disorders

In clinical trials involving youth with anxiety disorders, placebo response is generally lower than in youth with OCD, PTSD, or MDD. Additionally, in this population, its trajectory and predictors differ from those seen in clinical trials involving youth with depression and other internalizing disorders. In CAMS (Walkup et al. 2008), placebo-related improvement in Pediatric Anxiety Rating Scale (PARS) score was predicted by a diagnosis of ADHD or separation anxiety disorder, parent and child expectations for treatment, and socioeconomic status ($P=0.0002$). In this sample, separation anxiety disorder was the strongest predictor of placebo response. Similarly, for the categorical definition of placebo response (Clinical Global Impression—Improvement [CGI-I] score), 18 patients (27%) were classified as responders, and 48 patients (72%) were classified as nonresponders. No statistically significant differences were observed between responders and nonresponders for age ($P=0.217$), sex ($P=0.979$), race ($P=0.743$), or socioeconomic status ($P=0.748$) or in the number of individuals who continued in open-label treatment after the acute treatment phase ($P=0.673$) (Strawn et al. 2017). Additionally, in this analysis (Strawn et al. 2017), cognitive factors were explored, including the amount of anxious self-talk (before treatment), as reflected by Negative Affect Self-Statement Questionnaire (NASSQ) score. However,

NASSQ scores did not differ between placebo responders and nonresponders ($P=0.500$). As with the continuous measure of response (PARS), the expectation of treatment efficacy was significantly higher in placebo responders compared with nonresponders ($P<0.001$; Figure 16–2), and expectation of treatment efficacy as reported by the patients' parents was also higher in placebo responders compared with nonresponders (Strawn et al. 2017).

Placebo Response in Pediatric Depressive Disorders

Relative to pediatric anxiety disorders, placebo response in patients with MDD has received considerably more attention. Taken together, the extant evidence suggests that placebo response differs by funding source and that a number of factors that differ between industry-funded studies and those funded by the federal government (e.g., number of sites, financial incentives, and design restrictions of the U.S. Food and Drug Administration Modernization Act) also affect placebo response. The severity of depressive symptoms at baseline is also an important predictor of placebo response because less ill patients have greater placebo-related improvement (Nakonezny et al. 2015). Additionally, in some studies of pediatric patients with MDD, the number of sites and the duration of the trial were also associated with enhanced placebo response (Cohen et al. 2010). Last, in most studies of children and adolescents, younger patients tend to have greater placebo response rates than adolescents, although not all studies have demonstrated this effect (Emslie et al. 2002).

Expectation and Placebo Response

The expectation of therapeutic benefit powerfully influences treatment outcome (Krell et al. 2004; Strawn et al. 2017). For anxious youth, this effect is mediated by treatment adherence, such that youth who expect CBT to work are more adherent with task demands, in turn improving outcomes (Wu et al. 2020). The expectation of treatment benefit directly influencing treatment adherence has been a focus of prior evaluations of placebo response and has been considered a key factor in placebo response (Benedetti et al. 2011). That said, this effect differs between youth with depressive disorders (Rutherford et al. 2011) and those with anxiety

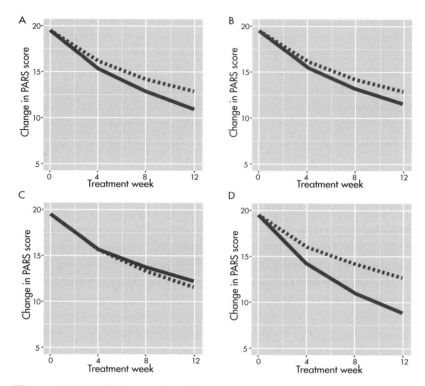

Figure 16-2. Trajectories of placebo response in the largest double-blind, placebo-controlled trial for pediatric anxiety disorders (*N*=76).

Note. Treatment expectations significantly influence the trajectory of placebo-related improvement. Patients who expected less improvement (*dotted line*) did not improve as much as those who expected greater improvement (*solid line*) (**A**). In panel **B**, age did not significantly influence the trajectory of improvement, with the *solid* and *dotted lines* representing patients 12 years or older and those youth younger than 12 years, respectively. Similarly, sex did not significantly influence the trajectory of response (**C**). Finally, having social anxiety disorder (*dotted line*) was associated with decreased placebo response (**D**). PARS=Pediatric Anxiety Rating Scale.
Source. Data from Walkup et al. 2008.

disorders (Strawn et al. 2017). Such expectations are associated with a number of cognitive factors that are germane to anxious pediatric patients, including "cognitive reassessment with positive expectation that may result in adaptation of behavior or symptom expression" (Benedetti et al. 2011). Additionally, the expectation of a positive effect of treatment in and of itself may decrease anxiety (Benedetti et al. 2011). Thus, patients' expectations for treatment success may represent a cognitive trait that reflects their ability to be impacted by the therapeutic structure of a clinical trial. From a clinical standpoint, additional studies are needed to understand the potential for augmenting treatment as part of routine care for anxious youth. It is also noteworthy that negative expectations, or threat bias, are often present in anxious youth (Britton et al. 2011; Roy et al. 2008) and may be associated with poorer response to treatment. In this regard, the neural response to this bias, as assessed with functional MRI, was observed in a randomized clinical trial in youth with generalized, social, or separation anxiety disorder to predict positive response to both CBT and sertraline (Kujawa et al. 2016). In pediatric patients with anxiety disorders, those with a greater expectation of benefit experienced more pronounced improvement over time (Figure 16–2).

In clinical trials, wherein the likelihood of receiving placebo (vs. active medication) varies as a function of the trial design, the randomization ratio influences placebo response (Rutherford and Roose 2013). Khan and colleagues (2004) observed that trials with more treatment arms are less likely to be "successful" or to demonstrate placebo-medication differences. The more likely a patient is to be randomized to receive medication, the greater the expectation on the part of the patient of responding. However, the influence of "expectancy" on placebo response in clinical trials is, with one exception (Strawn et al. 2017), mostly examined in trials of adults (Krell et al. 2004; Meyer et al. 2002; Rutherford et al. 2013). Consistent with the trial of anxious youth discussed earlier (Strawn et al. 2017), adult patients' expectations predict greater improvement during the course of the trial. One trial directly examined expectation by manipulating the randomization ratio (Mossman et al. 2021). In this study, patients could receive placebo-controlled treatment (i.e., there was a one in two chance of being randomly assigned to receive medication) or active treatment (i.e., they would receive active medication, with no chance of receiving placebo). Randomization to the active treatment comparison condition resulted in greater expectancy and patients had greater improvement in depressive symptoms—a finding that correlates with the degree of expectation effect (Rutherford et al. 2013).

Therapeutic Setting and Placebo Response

Rutherford and colleagues (2013) examined the degree of "therapeutic contact" in pediatric studies of youth with MDD and observed that more therapeutic contact was associated with larger placebo response (Rutherford and Roose 2013). This suggests that some degree of placebo response relates to depressed adolescents who experience "social isolation and de-

creased activity levels as part of their depressive illness enter[ing] a behaviorally activating and interpersonally rich new environment"
associated with the clinical trial. Furthermore, in an analysis of nine open
and four active comparators, as well as 18 placebo-controlled studies of
youth with depressive disorders, there was a significant interaction of age
and contact frequency, suggesting that this effect is nuanced and influenced not just by age or frequency of visits but also by a synergistic relationship between these two factors (Rutherford et al. 2011). Of note, in
many pediatric clinical trials in children and adolescents, patients may be
seen on a weekly basis or (during the initial phase of the trial) even more
frequently.

Natural Course of Anxiety and Depressive Disorders and Placebo Response

It is well established that the developmental trajectory of anxiety and depressive disorders differs in youth compared with adults (Wehry et al.
2015). In fact, these illnesses may remit or, depending on external factors,
may become less impairing or worsen. In children and adolescents, these
disorders may be associated with shifts in the development of comorbidity
(Beesdo-Baum and Knappe 2012; Bittner et al. 2004). In clinical trials involving children and adolescents, there has been less attention paid to
these shifts, although one study of adolescents with selective serotonin reuptake inhibitor (SSRI)–resistant depression who were randomized either
to venlafaxine or to an SSRI (with or without psychotherapy) (Brent et al.
2008) observed that when patients completed the study in the summer,
they had better outcomes (Shamseddeen et al. 2011). Furthermore, given
that symptoms fluctuate and that patients and their families may be more
likely to seek treatment during times characterized by more distress or impairment, it has been hypothesized that some of the placebo response in
adults with depressive disorders relates to the "natural waning of symptoms or alleviation in the precipitating stressors irrespective of the treatment they are provided" (Rutherford and Roose 2013).

Developmental Considerations and Placebo Response

The impact of age on placebo response has been examined in studies of
youth with depressive and anxiety disorders. In pediatric anxiety disor-

ders, some studies have suggested that age influences placebo response, although this appears to be more dependent on the measure used to define response. In CAMS (Walkup et al. 2008), age did not significantly affect categorical response based on CGI scores but did influence the trajectory of improvement based on PARS scores—younger patients had more improvement in anxiety symptoms at a threshold of $P=0.05$. In depressive disorders, younger patients have tended to have more placebo response.

Mechanisms of Placebo Response

The mechanisms of placebo response have received limited attention in children, adolescents, and adults. However, several interesting lines of research have examined placebo by proxy, which may be particularly important in youth (Czerniak et al. 2020; Grelotti and Kaptchuk 2011). Put simply, this placebo-related improvement occurs secondary to parents, family members, and perhaps even clinicians feeling better because the patient is receiving treatment. Thus, placebo by proxy results from an interaction "between a patient and an effect from proxies such as parents, caregivers, physicians or even the media" (Czerniak et al. 2020). As a fundamentally reciprocal phenomenon, placebo by proxy reflects improvement in the caregiver (through distress reduction and increased support from treatment) that may also allow the parent to change their behavior toward their child, which results in or accentuates clinical improvement. These factors—which are fundamentally contextual—drive changes in the proxy (e.g., parent) that facilitate the improvement rather than driving direct improvement in the child (Czerniak et al. 2020).

Finding neurofunctional predictors of placebo response represents an interesting line of investigation to improve our ability to detect medication-placebo differences in clinical trials. Distinct fingerprints of both static and dynamic functional connectivity variability robustly predict placebo response in adolescents with GAD (Lu et al. 2020). This fingerprint characterized by variable dynamic but "weak" static connectivity in the salience, default mode, frontoparietal, and ventral attention networks provides granular evidence of how circuit-based biotypes could mechanistically relate to placebo response in youth. Ultimately, finding biosignatures that predict placebo response represents an interesting line of investigation to potentially improve our ability to detect medication-placebo differences in clinical trials.

Implications for Treatment

The relationship between patients' expectations of clinical improvement and outcome, in particular, has direct clinical implications that have recently been systematically evaluated (Rutherford et al. 2017) and discussed (Linden 2017) in adults with depressive disorders. Assessing patients' expectations of treatment response may prove helpful in that psychoeducational or psychotherapeutic interventions that address threat bias, as well as those that increase a patient's positive expectation with regard to treatment, may bolster the "placebo response" that is part of "medication response." Strategies have been suggested to capture the placebo response with an active psychopharmacological treatment and to maximize the effect of a moderator of placebo response expectation (Linden 2017). Accordingly, clinicians might present treatments in a way that "enhances patient expectancy, which may involve educating patients about the effectiveness of the prescribed medication and utilizing a confident...interpersonal style" (Linden 2017, pp. 91–92). Moreover, given that multiple factors contribute to expectation (e.g., optimism, tolerance of uncertainty), clinicians could actively address these factors. For example, clinicians might 1) help patients to recognize positive changes, 2) work to induce and bolster hope and optimism (Linden 2017), and 3) actively explore the patient's expectation of therapeutic outcome as well as the expectations of the patient's family.

CASE EXAMPLE I

Sophie, a 11-year-old with one major depressive episode, experienced the onset of depressive symptoms approximately 18 months before presentation. Currently, her depressive symptoms are accompanied by intermittent anxiety, and she also has a history of separation anxiety disorder that began when she was 7½ years old. Her pediatrician discusses a trial of fluoxetine to help with her significant depressive symptoms, and the family is eager for her to begin the medication. Her mother and father both read a recent report in a national newspaper that fluoxetine was "the most effective antidepressant in kids." Her parents have a very good relationship, and Sophie has no externalizing pathology.

As her pediatrician listens to Sophie's history, he is aware that there are a number of aspects of Sophie's course that portend good improvement and placebo response. First, Sophie has separation anxiety disorder, which has been associated with a greater likelihood of placebo response. Second, she has a diagnosis of a major depressive episode and is prepubertal. Both of these are associated with placebo response. Finally, as is the case in anxiety disorders, the caregivers' expectation of improvement represents a strong predictor of placebo response.

CASE EXAMPLE 2

James, a 15-year-old with generalized and social anxiety disorders, has experienced significant anxiety since age 8 years. He began CBT approximately 5 months ago and completed 16 sessions that included behavioral exposures. He has noted improvement, and his mother notes that she feels a sense of relief in that James is "talking with his therapist every week" and that his therapist "listens to" her and consistently makes time for her concerns. However, James remains unable to engage in group projects at school, cannot eat at restaurants with his family, and finds himself continuing to worry about the future, college, and past events, as well as his parents and siblings, for several hours daily. His worries are present at least 6 days per week and frequently interfere with his schoolwork as well as social and family activities.

His psychotherapist refers James to a child and adolescent psychiatrist for consultation. During the discussion of escitalopram with James and his family, James comments: "I don't think it will actually work." The child and adolescent psychiatrist explores James's expectation and is surprised when his mother adds: "I think he's right…this isn't something that a medication can help."

Knowing that among the most important predictors of placebo response are patient and caregivers' expectation of improvement (see Figure 16–2), James' psychiatrist is concerned. She shifts to an exploratory approach to understand the family's beliefs regarding medication. James's psychiatrist learns that the family recently read on a blog that "antidepressants are no more effective than placebo in kids." After learning this, James's psychiatrist provides psychoeducation regarding the efficacy of SSRIs in pediatric anxiety disorders and discusses the relative efficacy of SSRIs in depressed youth relative to those with anxiety disorders, like James. She also helps the family to understand that the medication choice also influences its effectiveness and tolerability. In addition, James's psychiatrist, as she listens to James's mother, notes that she has felt a sense of relief as James began psychotherapy and is hopeful that, now in the context of their visit, some degree of placebo-by-proxy improvement may occur by her discussing treatment and providing a psychopharmacological consultation. Should this consultation result in James's mother feeling better about treatment through contextual factors as well as distress reduction and increased support, James's mother may change her behavior toward her child, which could accentuates clinical improvement.

Discussion

Placebo response represents a complex phenomenon (Figure 16–3) that has not received the careful exploration and characterization that it deserves, particularly given that high placebo response rates make it difficult to identify whether an active treatment can be demonstrated as "efficacious" in clinical trials (Mossman et al. 2021; Walkup 2017).

As clinicians, we are aware that across studies and across the life span, a number of factors are associated with enhanced placebo response, including 1) patient and family expectation, 2) the frequency of contact with treatment and the duration of treatment 3) age, and (4) comorbidity patterns (Figure 16–3). Among these, patient and family expectation and the frequency of contact appear to be the two factors most amenable to intervention. Sometimes clinicians believe the evidence for our interventions especially for depression is lukewarm, which diminishes patients' expectations as well as those of their families. Moreover, in considering the evidence for these interventions, we are often handicapped by the same placebo response that we are trying to accentuate in clinical practice. In talking with our patients and their families, it is important to remember that the effect sizes of interventions in the relatively large federally funded trials are less plagued by larger-than-life placebo response rates that are common in recent industry-funded studies.

Conclusion

In pediatric patients with anxiety and depressive disorders, the phenomenon of high placebo response represents a formidable challenge in clinical trials but a largely untapped resource in clinical practice. In working to increase the positive expectation of treatment success, clinicians must address optimism as well as intolerance of uncertainty. Psychologically, both of these may be affected in pediatric depressive and anxiety disorders in general, as well as OCD specifically. We must facilitate our patients' identifying positive changes and improvement and actively explore their expectation for the success of a given treatment.

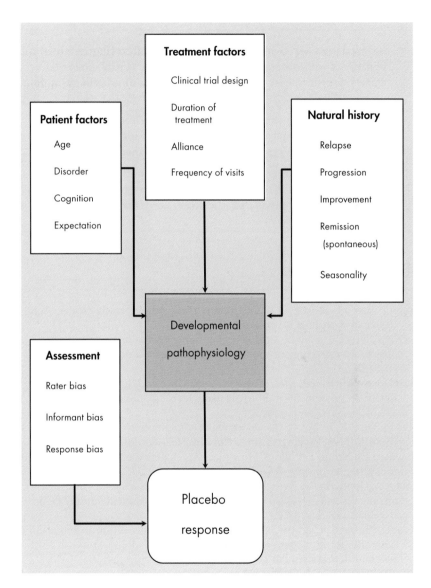

Figure 16–3. Factors that potentially affect placebo response in pediatric patients with depressive and anxiety disorders.

Source. Adapted from Rutherford and Roose 2013.

TAKE-AWAY POINTS

- In clinical trials with children and adolescents, placebo response is lowest in patients with obsessive-compulsive disorder (OCD), followed by anxiety disorders more broadly, and is greatest in those with major depressive disorder.

- Placebo response in children and adolescents with anxiety and depressive disorders as well as in those with OCD is logarithmic. In other words, most of the response occurs early and then plateaus.

- Placebo response in anxious youth relates to both parents' and patients' expectation of treatment success. The role of parent and child treatment expectations in pediatric depression is unclear as of the time of this writing.

References

Bech P, Gram LF, Dein E, et al: Quantitative rating of depressive states. Acta Psychiatr Scand 51(3):161–170, 1975 1136841

Bech P, Allerup P, Gram LF, et al: The Hamilton Depression Scale: evaluation of objectivity using logistic models. Acta Psychiatr Scand 63(3):290–299, 1981 7015793

Bech P, Fava M, Trivedi MH, et al: Factor structure and dimensionality of the two depression scales in STAR*D using level 1 datasets. J Affect Disord 132(3):396–400, 2011 21440308

Beesdo-Baum K, Knappe S: Developmental epidemiology of anxiety disorders. Child Adolesc Psychiatr Clin N Am 21(3):457–478, 2012 22800989

Benedetti F, Carlino E, Pollo A: How placebos change the patient's brain. Neuropsychopharmacology 36(1):339–354, 2011 20592717

Bittner A, Goodwin RD, Wittchen HU, et al: What characteristics of primary anxiety disorders predict subsequent major depressive disorder? J Clin Psychiatry 65(5):618–626, 2004 15163247

Brent D, Emslie G, Clarke G, et al: Switching to another SSRI or to venlafaxine with or without cognitive behavioral therapy for adolescents with SSRI-resistant depression: the TORDIA randomized controlled trial. JAMA 299(8):901–913, 2008 18314433

Bridge JA, Birmaher B, Iyengar S, et al: Placebo response in randomized controlled trials of antidepressants for pediatric major depressive disorder. Am J Psychiatry 166(1):42–49, 2009 19047322

Britton JC, Lissek S, Grillon C, et al: Development of anxiety: the role of threat appraisal and fear learning. Depress Anxiety 28(1):5–17, 2011 20734364

Cohen D, Consoli A, Bodeau N, et al: Predictors of placebo response in randomized controlled trials of psychotropic drugs for children and adolescents with internalizing disorders. J Child Adolesc Psychopharmacol 20(1):39–47, 2010 20166795

Czerniak E, Oberlander TF, Weimer K, et al: "Placebo by proxy" and "nocebo by proxy" in children: a review of parents' role in treatment outcomes. Front Psychiatry 11:169, 2020 32218746

da Costa CZG, de Morais RMCB, Zanetta DMT, et al: Comparison among clomipramine, fluoxetine, and placebo for the treatment of anxiety disorders in children and adolescents. J Child Adolesc Psychopharmacol 23(10):687–692, 2013 24350814

Dobson ET, Strawn JR: Placebo response in pediatric anxiety disorders: implications for clinical trial design and interpretation. J Child Adolesc Psychopharmacol 26(8):686–693, 2016 27027330

Emslie GJ, Heiligenstein JH, Wagner KD, et al: Fluoxetine for acute treatment of depression in children and adolescents: a placebo-controlled, randomized clinical trial. J Am Acad Child Adolesc Psychiatry 41(10):1205–1215, 2002 12364842

Emslie GJ, Prakash A, Zhang Q, et al: A double-blind efficacy and safety study of duloxetine fixed doses in children and adolescents with major depressive disorder. J Child Adolesc Psychopharmacol 24(4):170–179, 2014 24815533

Grelotti DJ, Kaptchuk TJ: Placebo by proxy: clinicians' and family members' feelings and perceptions about a treatment may influence their judgements about its effectiveness (editorial). BMJ 343:d4345, 2011 21835868

Khan A, Kolts RL, Thase ME, et al: Research design features and patient characteristics associated with the outcome of antidepressant clinical trials. Am J Psychiatry 161(11):2045–2049, 2004 15514405

Krell HV, Leuchter AF, Morgan M, et al: Subject expectations of treatment effectiveness and outcome of treatment with an experimental antidepressant. J Clin Psychiatry 65(9):1174–1179, 2004 15367043

Kujawa A, Swain JE, Hanna GL, et al: Prefrontal reactivity to social signals of threat as a predictor of treatment response in anxious youth. Neuropsychopharmacology 41(8):1983–1990, 2016 26708107

Linden M: Placebo: unsolved problems for science, and simple conclusions for clinical practice. Am J Psychiatry 174(2):91–92, 2017 28142273

Locher C, Koechlin H, Zion SR, et al: Efficacy and safety of selective serotonin reuptake inhibitors, serotonin-norepinephrine reuptake inhibitors, and placebo for common psychiatric disorders among children and adolescents: a systematic review and meta-analysis. JAMA Psychiatry 74(10):1011–1020, 2017 28854296

Lu L, Li H, Mills JA, et al: Greater dynamic and lower static functional brain connectivity prospectively predict placebo response in pediatric generalized anxiety disorder. J Child Adolesc Psychopharmacol 30(10):606–616, 2020 32721213

March JS, Silva SG, Compton S, et al: The Child and Adolescent Psychiatry Trials Network (CAPTN). J Am Acad Child Adolesc Psychiatry 43(5):515–518, 2004 15100557

McKay KM, Imel ZE, Wampold BE: Psychiatrist effects in the psychopharmacological treatment of depression. J Affect Disord 92(2–3):287–290, 2006 16503356

Meyer B, Pilkonis PA, Krupnick JL, et al: Treatment expectancies, patient alliance, and outcome: further analyses from the National Institute of Mental Health Treatment of Depression Collaborative Research Program. J Consult Clin Psychol 70(4):1051–1055, 2002 12182269

Mills JA, Mossman S, Strawn JR: The impact of funding source on antidepressant trial outcomes in pediatric depressive and anxiety disorders. J Am Acad Child Adolesc Psychiatry 58(10):S253, 2019

Mossman SA, Mills JA, Walkup JT, Strawn JR: The impact of failed antidepressant trials on outcomes in children and adolescents with anxiety and depression: a systematics review and meta-analysis. J Child Adolesc Psychopharmacol 31(4):259–267, 2021 33887154

Nakonezny PA, Mayes TL, Byerly MJ, Emslie GJ: Predicting placebo response in adolescents with major depressive disorder: the Adolescent Placebo Impact Composite Score (APICS). J Psychiatr Res 68:346–353, 2015 26028546

Papakostas GI, Østergaard SD, Iovieno N: The nature of placebo response in clinical studies of major depressive disorder. J Clin Psychiatry 76(4):456–466, 2015 25700292

Pediatric OCD Treatment Study Team: Cognitive-behavior therapy, sertraline, and their combination for children and adolescents with obsessive-compulsive disorder: the Pediatric OCD Treatment Study (POTS) randomized controlled trial. JAMA 292(16):1969–1976, 2004 15507582

Roy AK, Vasa RA, Bruck M, et al: Attention bias toward threat in pediatric anxiety disorders. J Am Acad Child Adolesc Psychiatry 47(10):1189–1196, 2008 18698266

Rutherford BR, Roose SP: A model of placebo response in antidepressant clinical trials. Am J Psychiatry 170(7):723–733, 2013

Rutherford BR, Sneed JR, Tandler JM, et al: Deconstructing pediatric depression trials: an analysis of the effects of expectancy and therapeutic contact. J Am Acad Child Adolesc Psychiatry 50(8):782–795, 2011 21784298

Rutherford BR, Marcus SM, Wang P, et al: A randomized, prospective pilot study of patient expectancy and antidepressant outcome. Psychol Med 43(5):975–982, 2013 22971472

Rutherford BR, Wall MM, Brown PJ, et al: Patient expectancy as a mediator of placebo effects in antidepressant clinical trials. Am J Psychiatry 174(2):135–142, 2017 27609242

Shamseddeen W, Clarke G, Wagner KD, et al: Treatment-resistant depressed youth show a higher response rate if treatment ends during summer school break. J Am Acad Child Adolesc Psychiatry 50(11):1140–1148, 2011 22024002

Strawn JR, Dobson ET, Mills JA, et al: Placebo response in pediatric anxiety disorders: results from the Child/Adolescent Anxiety Multimodal Study. J Child Adolesc Psychopharmacol 27(6):501–508, 2017 28384010

Varigonda AL, Jakubovski E, Taylor MJ, et al: Systematic review and meta-analysis: early treatment responses of selective serotonin reuptake inhibitors in pediatric major depressive disorder. J Am Acad Child Adolesc Psychiatry 54(7):557–564, 2015 26088660

Varigonda AL, Jakubovski E, Bloch MH: Systematic review and meta-analysis: early treatment responses of selective serotonin reuptake inhibitors and clomipramine in pediatric obsessive-compulsive disorder. J Am Acad Child Adolesc Psychiatry 55(10):851–859, 2016 27663940

Wagner KD, Berard R, Stein MB, et al: A multicenter, randomized, double-blind, placebo-controlled trial of paroxetine in children and adolescents with social anxiety disorder. Arch Gen Psychiatry 61(11):1153–1162, 2004 15520363

Walkup JT: Antidepressant efficacy for depression in children and adolescents: industry- and NIMH-funded studies. Am J Psychiatry 174(5):430–437, 2017 28253735

Walkup JT, Albano AM, Piacentini J, et al: Cognitive behavioral therapy, sertraline, or a combination in childhood anxiety. N Engl J Med 359(26):2753–2766, 2008 18974308

Wehry AM, Beesdo-Baum K, Hennelly MM, et al: Assessment and treatment of anxiety disorders in children and adolescents. Curr Psychiatry Rep 17(7):52, 2015 25980507

Wu Q, Li J, Parrott S, et al: Cost-effectiveness of different formats for delivery of cognitive behavioral therapy for depression: a systematic review based economic model. Value Health 23(12):1662–1670, 2020 33248522

PART VI

BECOMING

CHAPTER | 17

THE "GOOD ENOUGH" PEDIATRIC PSYCHO-PHARMACOTHERAPIST

Practical Pointers in Six Parables

Ian Tofler, M.B.B.S.

From Nothing to Something or When Less Is Much More... Except When It Is Not: The "Nail Soup" Treatment Model

"Nail Soup" is a Scandinavian fairy story that neatly encapsulates the role a child pharmacotherapist must adopt to be successful (Great Books Foundation 2015). To that end, we must cast ourselves in the role of the tramp at the center of this wonderful story. Through creativity and by being both proactive and a little crafty, the tramp is able to triumph in a "win-win" situation by "adding a little this and a little that" to miraculously transform the thin, watery soup of an old woman in payment for free food and lodging. We, as members of the relatively new subspecialty of pediatric psychopharmacology, can likewise creatively but modestly contribute to the treatment, and hopefully to the future functional lives, of our patients and their families. By synthesizing our knowledge of the environment, the phenotypic and genotypic presentation of the child or teen, and our diagnostic formulation, we are well placed to help manage these challenges.

We must make the most of our sometimes very fragile and tenuous connection to the child, teen, or family. Our relationship often begins mired in the irritation, suspicion, stigma, and downright hostility shown by the old woman in "Nail Soup." This is not always the most fertile ground for positive change. Our humble but noble role and goal is not to shy away from this hostility but to produce something hopefully helpful but not always "miraculous" with our "bent nail" pharmacotherapy and family engagement skills. Of course, we would like the end result to be beneficial. But this is only possible through ongoing, consistent hard work for the patient, reflected through an alliance with the family and community systems, in addition to ongoing adherence with the administered medications.

And we should not forget our hard-earned physician skills either. Sometimes a medical intervention, dysmorphic feature assessment, careful historical re-review, or timely referral to a pediatric subspecialist can make a big difference in a patient's life experience and in building a solid alliance (American Academy of Child and Adolescent Psychiatry 2019; Hoyme et al. 2016; Shapira et al. 2019). All of these components may create a positive perturbation in the youth's social system. This will, we hope, spread reciprocally to all the systems the youth touches, amplifying positive feelings and responses in the family, school, and community milieu. Our own therapeutic programs may also consist of layers of nursing, case management and administration follow-up; individual, family, and group therapies; parental educational interventions; or "wraparound" intensive community interventions. This constructive positivity can spread in a virtuous cycle because our teams help develop child and family self-efficacy and resilience skills, facilitated, we hope, by our toolkit of interventions. In the final analysis, if we are successful in the long term, we will be comfortable with returning to a consultative role because our patients can developmentally "age out" of requiring our active treatment.

The words and concepts of pediatrician and pioneering child psychiatrist Donald Winnicott ring true in pediatric pharmacotherapy. We aim to improve the positive self-regulation of the child or adolescent, just like the "good enough" mothering (parenting) he describes in his early work (Winnicott 1971). In parallel, the treatment we provide not only facilitates the individuation of the child but also affirms and assists in the individuation of the always learning and curious "good enough" pediatric pharmacotherapist.

The Developmental Trajectory of the Pediatric Pharmacotherapist

First as medical students, then as doctors and psychiatrists, and finally as child and adolescent psychiatrists, we go through a very long apprenticeship. After such a long gestation period, it is not surprising that the initial "product" is so sophisticated, slightly unbalanced, and yet ready to function at a high level. This sophistication does come with inherent risks and rewards, as this unusual developmental trajectory shows.

1. *Newly minted.* The newly minted child and adolescent psychiatrist displays genius—confident, omnipotent, omniscient—with powerful theoretical knowledge of neurotransmitters and neuropsychiatry, often far greater than their seniors'. They are willing to take "risks" with a patient and push the envelope in treatment. They have not witnessed many "failures" of their treatment, and those that they have experienced could be attributed to teachers and supervisors.

2. *The magician or "Doctor Strange" phase.* Early successes breed further confidence that burgeons. Overconfidence can produce the risks for major, even catastrophic, side effects, which can sometimes go unnoticed until too late, if at all. For example, heroic (excessively high) lithium levels, severe weight gain with olanzapine (producing good psychiatric response despite severe metabolic side effects), or subjective changes in personality or decreased libido can be rationalized away in the setting of a "good clinical response." The use or misuse of alcohol and cannabis in a comorbidly ill teenager may be "winked at" by a cool psychiatrist as being a simple part of growing up. An overemphasis on the alliance with the patient over that with the family may prove to be a difficult balancing act for all psychiatrists. The patient's family will often "fire" the "magician" psychiatrist and move to another.

3. *Master tradesman or tradeswoman.* Results are generally good, but the tradesperson understands their limitations much more, does not "oversell" a product, and thoughtfully looks at their role within a larger system, in which communication and therapy exceed the significant but still limited role played by medication interventions.

The tradesperson may have been sued, knows firsthand the importance of good legal back-up, may have had complaints lodged by patients, and may have even withstood some poor reviews; they do not always go for "outside the box" treatments if possible but still have great new ideas to implement when the need arises.

4. *The "emeritus" senior pharmacotherapist.* The senior pharmacotherapist still enjoys clinical work, values learning new skills, and uses subtle medication "tweaks" and combinations; their contribution is valued, but they are prepared to leave the innovations and pioneering ways to others. They make up for some lost skills by reading and keeping up with journals and continue to attend conferences and have peer support. The senior pharmacotherapist tends to "undersell" their interventions, emphasizing instead the need for adherence by the family, and the child in particular. They are comfortable with redundant interventions, options, and opportunities to optimize treatment response. They still have much to contribute, value the relationship with the patient and family, and endeavor to develop it significantly more than the medication "tools of the trade." The senior pharmacotherapist applies new medication options, is aware that major change in psychiatry is generally slow, and values the expression *plus ça change, plus c'est la même chose* ("The more things change, the more they stay the same"). They take advantage of the opportunity provided by urgent or emergent situations to make a difference, hopefully with long-term positive consequences.

Preconceptions, Misconceptions, and Some Perhaps Accurate Perceptions About Medications and Pharmacotherapy

The psychiatrist-patient relationship, in all of its transferential and countertransferential glory, is equally rich in the pediatric psychopharmacological context. There is no tabula rasa here. It can be more like entering the fire swamp in the film *The Princess Bride*, beset with quicksand and nasty surprises. A pediatric pharmacotherapist must be ready to address and cope with all these relationship twists and turns. If possible, we should be able to use our psychological skills and, judo-like, turn such challenges to our advantage. The partial and incomplete listing in Table 17–1 summarizes some of the more common misconceptions that we may be called on to deal with.

Table 17–1. Common preconceptions and misconceptions (and perhaps some accurate perceptions)

1. Medications are bad, especially for children; in fact, they should never be used in children.

2. Medications are great. Nothing else has worked. I don't like it but will try anything you say. We need to see some improvement in her behavior; it's totally out of control. I trust you to do whatever you think is right, Doc.

3. Doctors are not to be trusted; let's face it, they are liars, or in Big Pharma's pocket.

4. I only go to doctors in an emergency (or when forced by social services or by school "edicts").

5. This *is* an emergency, so medications may be an imperative, at least temporarily (or until systemic supervision decreases).

6. This is not going to be a long-term thing. There is no intention of following up or continuing treatment after the emergency has been dealt with.

7. Where is the research to back this up? You are just experimenting on my little one.

8. They forced him to go into the hospital, and they gave him who knows what medications that just put him to sleep. You call that good treatment? And I couldn't visit, either; the hospital was too far away.

9. Do you really know what you're doing? Would you give these meds to your own family?

10. I read about this medication on the internet. I know it's no good. I wouldn't want anyone I know on this medication.

11. All psychiatrists are a little unsteady. It's like the blind leading the blind here.

12. You never tell us all the side effects. What about antidepressants making kids more suicidal? You never talk about that. How do we deal with that?

13. Your medicine is good, but I don't like giving my child medications every day, so I only give it twice a week. It helps that way, sometimes. Maybe.

14. Don't you think medications are the easy way out when you can't connect with a kid?

15. And what about the long-term side effects? Don't tell me you really know all about them. What's going to happen to my child when he grows up after taking all these medications?

16. I heard you use the term *discontinuation syndrome* and then say these medicines are not addictive or cause withdrawal. Which one is it, or are you using "scientific" terms to make yourself feel better?

Medications Are Sometimes the Only Solution, and Sometimes They Are Just Plain Wrong

Suffice it to say, our medication interventions, like it or not, are often useful and important, but so are our general assessment and deep knowledge of nonmedication recommendations. We are all familiar with the psychopharmacology consultation. What appears to be an urgent crisis can rapidly become bogged down in a polemic about the merits and ethics of prescribing medications to children—or not. As scientifically disciplined and trained prescribers, we often find ourselves justifying medication initiation in ways that would be quite unusual in other medical disciplines. We can still be taken aback when the parental decision makers are "shocked, shocked" that they are even discussing medications with a psychiatrist. "I really thought you were going to do something medical, like a brain scan or blood tests. Maybe we should just come back when things get really bad. I'm sure she will do well just with therapy for the time being. I've just heard so many really bad things about these medications."

It is wise to don our systemic therapy glasses and see our roles and repertoires through the bigger clinical picture or narrative for the child. The "Lone Ranger" pediatric psychiatrist may find it easier to simply address the narrowly defined diagnosis, rather than stepping back and thoughtfully formulating a case fully. Looking at the patient in their milieu may help us realize that medications are rarely the only solution, not always the panacea, and often not what is most necessary for the child. After all, our patients may have experienced trauma, early attachment problems, or prenatal substance exposure; they may be presenting at times of extreme crisis. It is true that the right medication intervention could still help lead toward a brighter developmental future. Medications can, for example, enable or enhance impulse control and thereby improve communication ability, and facilitate trust with caregivers and teachers.

By the very nature of medicalizing a clinical interaction, pharmacotherapy provides an overarching, at times calming, and more objective biological nexus for the patient's multidisciplinary treatment plan. In a well-functioning multidisciplinary mental health system, the psychiatrist is involved, often in a fit of exasperation or desperation. The "big-gun" psychopharmacologist may be consulted early on but is generally consulted only after months or more of individual and family therapy by well-qualified social work, counseling, or psychology staff. The very act of consultation can indeed jump-start or reify a significantly positive strategic treatment intervention. We may at times function less through chemicals than as usefully authoritative "transitional objects" covered by insurance.

Saying "No" to Psychopharmacological Intervention

Saying no to or delaying a decision on a psychopharmacological intervention can be as important a task as starting a medication. And it may be a more advanced developmental task for the clinician, who, after all, has been trained to prescribe rather than to *not* prescribe. There can be a crescendo of systemic pressure built up when a child first comes in for a psychopharmacology evaluation. There is usually an acute agenda, but just because of this drive, do we, the professionals, need to respond in an equally acute or reflexive manner? We do not always have a full history with sufficient collateral input available. The diagnosis may be uncertain, and we sometimes may need to gather further information, which may require additional time or ancillary testing. A prescribed medication can be the right (or at least the quickest) solution to the wrong question. Some of the instances in which we should "just say no to drugs" or at the very least delay the decision to start psychiatric medications are summarized in Table 17–2.

Pro Re Nata (PRN): Blunt Instrumentation, As Needed

Pediatric psychiatrists should always be very cognizant of the competing interests and systemic "secondary gain" of the young person being medicated and how to respond in these situations. Patients who present to us often embody a "crisis." We can use this crisis to help our patients and to institute a consistent, even long-term, treatment in the form of a psychopharmacological intervention. Like it or not, the PRN may be the only game in town versus a comprehensive, well-thought-out (but sometimes static) intervention that comes with adherence problems (Saito et al. 2019). This "crisis" is often precipitated by issues in the school setting, as when a child or teen with severe suicidal ideation represents a major

Table 17–2. When should we say "no" (or at least feel comfortable delaying medication administration)?

1. When the diagnosis is uncertain and requires more history, evaluation, or testing

2. When behavioral interventions may be indicated instead

3. When there are clear, stark differences of approach between custodial parents and the patient is ambivalent about taking medication

4. When the child himself or herself is strongly against medication and will fight its administration

5. When there is no clear way of monitoring the child's response to medication

6. When school demands medication before allowing the child to return to school

7. When judicious use of over-the-counter options can be just as helpful, for sleep in particular

crisis. Taking this opportunity to begin medication with the cooperation and permission of the parents may be, to some degree, coerced by the school system. Most parents do want their children back in the school system. Some, of course, take this opportunity to place their child in a home-schooling arrangement, staving off the need for imminent medication intervention.

PRN medication options may be for some patients a good opportunity as well for the psychiatrist to establish an alliance with them (Saito et al. 2019). A child with increased self-efficacy could play an instrumental role in daily administration, choosing the time or need for medications. PRNs, in particular, are administered with their awareness and active input for a school or home context. It is often a good place to start a minimalist intervention to cultivate a pharmacotherapeutic alliance. It is true that in many circumstances, behavioral interventions, cognitive-behavioral therapy, calming strategies, time-outs, and mindful meditation skills may be just as successful and can be presented as demonstrating more self-efficacy skills for the young person negotiating within a particular school or justice system. However, when a child or teen presents in true emergency to the clinician or to the emergency department, often these interventions have already been exhausted.

PRN intervention may be a blunt instrument. But it does demonstrate eloquently to the child, adolescent, and young adult—and often to the delighted surprise of supervisory adults—that control akin to a computer reboot is still attainable even in the most dire of public situations. The young person does not always require inpatient or partial hospital psychiatry admission or placement outside the house in a residential program setting. In some cases, this intervention can create a major "win-win" situation. Another counterintuitive positive factor involved in the PRN as first medication intervention is that by producing confidence within the parent-child dyad, the supporting alliance among school-doctor-parent and child may set the stage for a suitable daily routine medication regimen (Feinstein et al. 2009).

Conclusion

Being a pediatric pharmacotherapist is a privilege. On a daily basis, we have the opportunity to proactively impact and reorient the developmental trajectories of vulnerable children, teens, and young adults. We can also help reverse problematic behavioral pathways and impulsive constellations in these patients as well.

In the limited time windows we see a patient—every few weeks or months for the most part—we can slowly and organically establish rapport and alliances with an individual child or teen and their family members. Through this clinical engine, we can enable positive change and relief in a system with built-up allostatic load (McEwen 2003). This can occur through improved adaptation or social problem solving, improved impulse control, enhanced attentional focus and goal attainment, improved intrusive thought management, or diminished substance use and misuse.

Not surprisingly, many, if not most, of these behaviors can be finessed through multimodal systemic interventions that do not always require medications. Our psychopharmacology, that rusty nail in the nail soup, can certainly make a dramatic impact—that is, when we use it wisely and judiciously, intermittently or routinely, within a trusting, "good enough" professional relationship. As we progress through all the stages of our career, it is incumbent upon us to use (but not overuse) our hard-won skills with care and with the strongest integrity.

References

American Academy of Child and Adolescent Psychiatry: 2019 Pediatric Psychopharmacology Update Institute Notebook. Washington, DC, American Academy of Child and Adolescent Psychiatry, 2019. Available at: www.aacap.org/ItemDetail?iProductCode=PH-19andCategory=JAN-NOTEandWebsiteKey=a2785385–0ccf-4047-b76a-64b4094ae07f. Accessed December 3, 2020.

Feinstein NR, Fielding K, Udvari-Solner A, Joshi SV: The supporting alliance in child and adolescent treatment: enhancing collaboration among therapists, parents, and teachers. Am J Psychother 63(4):319–344, 2009 20131741

Great Books Foundation: Nail Soup. Chicago, IL, Great Books Foundation, 2015. Available at: www.greatbooks.org/wp-content/uploads/2015/08/Nail-Soup_OER_FINAL.pdf. Accessed December 3, 2020.

Hoyme HE, Kalberg WO, Elliott AJ, et al: Updated clinical guidelines for diagnosing fetal alcohol spectrum disorders. Pediatrics 138(2):e20154256, 2016 27464676

McEwen BS: Mood disorders and allostatic load. Biol Psychiatry 54(3):200–207, 2003 12893096

Saito E, Eng S, Grosso C, et al: Pro re nata Medication use in acute care adolescent psychiatric unit. J Child Adolesc Psychopharmacol 30(4):250–260, 2019

Shapira SK, Tian LH, Aylsworth AS, et al: A novel approach to dysmorphology to enhance the phenotypic classification of autism spectrum disorder in the study to explore early development. J Autism Dev Disord 49(5):2184–2202, 2019 30783897

Winnicott DW: Playing and Reality. London, Routledge, 1971

CHAPTER | 18

TEACHING AND MENTORING THE NEXT GENERATION OF PEDIATRIC PSYCHO-PHARMACOTHERAPISTS

Dorothy Stubbe, M.D.
Isheeta Zalpuri, M.D.
Mandeep Kaur Kapur, M.D.
Donald M. Hilty, M.D., M.B.A.

> Education is not the filling of a pail,
> but the lighting of a fire.
>
> *Attributed to William Butler Yeats*

Child and adolescent psychiatry fellowship training programs have made substantial changes to their learning objectives over the past several decades. These changes are in large part due to the advances made in neurobiology and pharmacology, leading to a shift in curriculum emphasis from psychotherapy to psychopharmacology (Bluestone et al. 1999; Rubin and Zorumski 2003). Despite this shift by training programs, the Accreditation Council for Graduate Medical Education (ACGME) has maintained resident and fellow Milestone competency requirements in brief and long-term individual therapies, including supportive, psychodynamic, and cognitive-behavioral psychotherapy, family therapy, and group therapy, in addition to pharmacotherapy (Accreditation Council for Graduate Medical Education 2015). In contrast to past surveys, in which program directors requested less ACGME-mandated psychotherapy training (Marriage and Halasz 1991), more recent data suggest that child and adolescent program directors support psychotherapy training as integral to the fellowship, although this competency has been hard to verify (Kitts et al. 2019).

In all fields of medicine, the doctor-patient relationship has been and remains the keystone of good medical care. It is the medium through which symptom data are gathered, diagnoses made, and issues of adherence addressed (Ha and Longnecker 2010). In psychiatry, a meaningful doctor-patient relationship starts with the psychological assessment of the patient and family to advance an accurate and meaningful diagnostic formulation (Perry et al. 1987). The biopsychosocial model (Engel 1980) is still a useful approach for clinical practices. Adaptations (i.e., culturally informed biopsychosocial-developmental-spiritual) emphasize the influence of contextual and psychosocial factors, illness, and trauma on personality development and current behavior—all important for child and adolescent psychiatry—along with weighing risk and protective factors for stabilizing the patient's symptoms and well-being and for preventing future disability (Hilty 2015).

With burgeoning scientific data, there is increasingly more for trainees to learn during their two-year child and adolescent psychiatry fellowship. Today's trainee must integrate an understanding of developmental psychopathology, genetics, environment, culture, psychosocial context, neuroimaging, epidemiology, and medicolegal and ethics issues while also learning to navigate various systems of care (Stubbe 2002) and demonstrating psychotherapeutic and pharmacotherapeutic competence. This daunting task requires a comprehensive curriculum that uses multiple teaching techniques, accommodates disparate learning styles, and optimizes opportunities for formulation of complex concepts.

Trainees may graduate without a full appreciation of the psychological meaning of medications and the power of the therapeutic prescribing clinician–patient relationship. The inadvertent separation of psychopharmacology and psychotherapy training may contribute to a "split treatment" model in which the fellow is the psychopharmacologist and another clinician is the psychotherapist. Supervision of psychotherapy and psychopharmacology is typically provided by different supervisors at separate supervisory meetings. One way that fellows may integrate psychotherapy and psychopharmacology roles is through group intakes and ongoing treatment case conferences. Addressing issues of split treatment in interprofessional team meetings requires sufficient time and the availability of adept supervisors—difficult to accomplish in many programs. See Chapter 7 ("Pharmacotherapy or Psychopharmacotherapy: When Therapist and Pharmacologist Are Different People—or the Same Person") for a full discussion of these topics.

Child and adolescent psychiatry fellows and the faculty who do a significant amount of teaching, supervision, and role modeling are juggling many professional activities: clinical care, academic scholarship, teaching, mentorship, and administration (Teshima et al. 2019). Events occurring outside of the career, including family, financial, and other factors, are also salient. This chapter focuses on four themes relevant to the teaching and mentorship of psychopharmacology training within a biopsychosocial-developmental-cultural framework: 1) curricular methods that incorporate principles of adult learning and evidence-based practice to prepare graduates for independent practice; 2) the therapeutic relationship and psychological meaning of medication for the patient, family, and treaters; 3) systems of care skills, including working in the context of a split treatment model and teaching multidisciplinary collaboration skills; and 4) the characteristics of effective teachers and mentors.

Psychopharmacology Training Curriculum

The goal of a training curriculum is "to help educators produce competent psychopharmacology clinicians schooled in the latest evidence, capable of keeping up with new knowledge as it becomes available, and practicing both the art and science of expert clinical care" (Zisook et al. 2008, p. 96). There have been a limited number of studies, with no consensus, on an effective curriculum to teach psychiatry trainees the nuances

Table 18–1.   Core adult learning principles

1. Involved learners	Adult learners desire engagement in planning course and methods of learning.
2. Adult learners' experience	New learning activates and builds on prior experience.
3. Relevance to and impact on learners' lives	Learning needs to be useful and relevant to current needs, with greater autonomy as skills are mastered.
4. Problem centered	Learning is optimized when it is experiential, active, and involves problem solving.

Source.   Adapted from Knowles et al. 2012.

of pharmacotherapy. Although there have been models proposed in the past, such as Balint groups (Balint 1957), Beitman's curriculum (Beitman 2003), and Mintz's curriculum for teaching psychodynamic psychopharmacology (Mintz 2005), none has had widespread implementation. More commonly, trainees participate in lecture-based didactics followed by supervised clinical experience to learn prescribing skills.

Acknowledging the limitations of lecture-based teaching of psychopharmacology, Kavanagh and colleagues (2017) conducted a study of an interactive workshop format to teach psychiatry residents how to talk to patients about medications. Using principles of adult learning, they constructed a curriculum that is practical, active and interactive, and relevant; builds on prior experiences; and solves real-life problems (Knowles et al. 2012) (Table 18–1). The residents participated in facilitated group discussions with role-playing exercises to mock-prescribe, explain mechanisms of therapeutic action, and provide informed consent for various medication classes. The course also addressed communication skills, ethics, therapeutic process, and professional identity. After implementation of this protocol at one site, it was disseminated to another, with 144 residents participating over 6 years. The pre- and postsurveys showed significant improvement in comfort with various aspects of prescribing and a strong preference for the protocol over lecture-based didactics (Kavanagh et al. 2017).

Surveys of trainees and early-career psychiatrists have provided the field with preliminary data on how prepared they feel to manage child and adolescent pharmacotherapy. Hutchison and colleagues (2020) surveyed ACGME-accredited child and adolescent psychiatry trainees to assess comfort and confidence with prescribing skills and concepts. Preliminary data from 63 respondents (7.2%) suggested that child and adolescent psychiatry trainees leave their programs with confidence in basic psychopharmacology skills (i.e., initiating, titrating, and discontinuing psychotropic medications) but lack confidence in more complex skills (managing polypharmacy, off-label prescribing, and de-prescribing). The amount of psychopharmacology supervision received was associated with significantly higher training satisfaction and enhanced comfort with medication titration, discussing side effects, and de-prescribing.

In a 2002 survey, early-career child and adolescent psychiatrists ($N=$ 392) reported high-quality training overall. Clinical experiences, supervisors and mentors, and a well-rounded program were all crucial components of their training (Stubbe 2002). The experiences ranked from highest to lowest in quality were the inpatient experience, outpatient supervision, psychopharmacology teaching, electives, outpatient individual psychotherapy experience, didactics, and inpatient supervision. Although psychopharmacology was ranked third in quality, early-career psychiatrists ranked it as the most relevant training experience related to their current work, with outpatient supervision and outpatient individual psychotherapy experience ranking second and fourth in relevance, respectively. These studies highlight psychopharmacology experience and psychotherapy supervision and experience as among the most valuable aspects of training in preparing psychiatric residents and trainees for independent practice.

Evidence-Based Practice

Medical education is charged with training a workforce to keep pace with the burgeoning scientific literature that informs the practice of medicine. Skills in evidence-based medicine (EBM) help physicians identify the best available clinical evidence to inform treatment decisions. EBM skills include developing appropriate clinical questions, searching the literature, and critically appraising studies (Straus et al. 2019). Pediatric psychopharmacotherapists apply EBM to inform decisions regarding individual patient care when using medications, conducting psychotherapy, or recommending specific psychosocial treatments (Chrisman et al. 2007). When the evidence is incomplete (which is often the case in pediatric psychopharmacology), setting realistic expectations for patients and families based on the best available scientific evidence helps establish a strong therapeutic alliance and improves adherence to treatment.

The evidence for effective treatments in psychiatry expands beyond that of biological interventions. A growing body of evidence suggests that psychological meaning effects of medication, such as the placebo response, may be at least as potent as, if not more potent than, the "active" chemical agents in medications (Kirsch et al. 2002). Patient variables such as attachment style, locus of control, treatment preferences, and readiness to change impact prognosis. Patients who are ready to change have particularly positive prognoses even if they receive a placebo in a randomized controlled trial (Lewis et al. 2009). Mallo and Mintz (2013) advocate for considering all of the variables affecting prescribing, including psychological and interpersonal aspects of medication response. "Residents attuned to pill, patient, provider, and partnership variables that affect treatment outcome are better equipped to prescribe in a way that fosters the patient's overall adaptive capacity," (p. 31) and this promotes health. For a full discussion of the placebo effect in pediatric pharmacotherapy, see Chapter 16 ("The Power of Placebo").

The Therapeutic Relationship and Meaning of Medication

THE THERAPEUTIC ALLIANCE

The patient-experienced quality of the therapeutic alliance has repeatedly been demonstrated to be the most robust predictor of therapy outcome, surpassing the impact of specific therapeutic techniques (Gabbard and Westen 2003). The pediatric pharmacotherapist forms a bond with patients and families that has often been underappreciated. In completing a thorough psychiatric evaluation, cultural, spiritual, and biopsychosocial factors are revealed in the context of a therapeutic alliance (Chubinsky and Hojman 2013). Psychodynamic concepts, such as therapeutic alliance, unconscious fantasy and symbolic meaning, transference, and countertransference, also impact psychopharmacological treatment. The therapeutic relationship facilitates shared decision making, which reflects equalization of the informational and power symmetry between doctors and patients (Schauer et al. 2007). A positive placebo effect relates to the strength of the therapeutic alliance. *This may also be true of the nocebo response,* in which a patient demonstrates a poorer-than-expected response to treatment because of negative expectations from medication treatment, or of the psychodynamic factors that may elicit resistance to improvement—often related to anticipated harm from authority figures (Mintz 2005).

Trainees use skillful supervision to identify strengths and potential impediments to forming an authentic rapport with patients and families. Awareness of the patient's psychological factors that may enhance or interfere with successful treatment must be evaluated. In addition, the supervisor should inquire about the resident's potential counter-transference issues that may interfere with effectively treating the patient (Mintz 2005). Unconscious bias about culture, lifestyle, ethnicity, gender identity, and other factors may be difficult to elicit but are grist for the mill in terms of supervisory attention. Helping trainees identify these unconscious processes in themselves promotes personal and professional growth.

The importance of the therapeutic alliance is accentuated during times of transition. Graduation or a switch in rotation of the psychopharmacology fellows may elicit in the patient a sense of loss and abandonment, which can be as strong as when losing their psychotherapist. It can also be a recurring event for families who obtain treatment in a teaching clinic and needs to be addressed with both patient and parents. In 2000, a survey of 38 psychiatric residents found that nearly one-third of their patients were negatively affected by treatment transfer or termination (Mischoulon et al. 2000). Transference from patients or families can lead to a worsening of symptoms, reports of new symptoms, and anger toward or detachment from the terminating child and adolescent psychiatry fellow, often also eliciting feelings of guilt or frustration on the part of the fellow. The transition period is also a time when the supervisor and new fellow are adapting to each other's practice styles and forming their own working relationship (Young and Wachter 2009). Informing families at the beginning of their treatment relationship about the fellow's training and its length can facilitate the inevitable transition. The psychological impact of termination on patients, their parents, and the fellow should be addressed in the curriculum and supervision.

DEVELOPMENTAL CONSIDERATIONS

All psychiatrists need an understanding of normal development and risk and resilience factors that may alter this trajectory. Osofsky and colleagues (2017) have advocated for incorporating principles and practices from the field of infant mental health into all child and adolescent psychiatry training programs. The role of development is essential in considerations of treatment recommendations, parent interventions, and psychopharmacology. The biopsychosocial-developmental-cultural perspective remains relevant throughout the life cycle.

A developmental perspective is crucial in diagnostics. Young children more commonly present with autism, developmental disorders, sleep disorders, and feeding disorders. Collaborative models of care and parent-child treatments are relevant in training across the developmental perspective as well. Diagnosis and treatment constitute a complex phenomenon with changing meanings for children, their families, and their community (Chubinsky and Hojman 2013; McCabe 1996). Medications may reduce symptoms and enhance functioning or impact self-image and self-esteem in negative ways. At any age, taking medication is laced with meaning. For example, a young child who is prescribed a stimulant medication for ADHD may perceive that he takes medication because he is "bad." An adolescent may be reluctant to take medication because it is perceived as acquiescing to adult authority. Another child may want to take a medication to avoid taking responsibility for their hurtful actions.

Parents also imbue medications with meaning. Psychiatry educators help trainees maintain curiosity and openness to understanding patients (and their caregivers') preferences, collaborating around the important decisions regarding their care. Psychopharmacology supervisors have the important role of promoting a comprehensive understanding of treatment mechanisms—that medication treatment involves more than the physiological response. A patient-centered approach that allows time for discussion about hopes, concerns, and readiness for medication with children, adolescents, and their caregivers will build trust, foster adherence, and improve outcomes (Mallo and Mintz 2013).

SPLIT TREATMENT

With a shortage of child and adolescent psychiatrists, there is an impetus to allocate the psychiatrist to the prescriber role. The most common model in clinics and group practices is of a "split model" of treatment whereby medication is prescribed by a psychopharmacologist while psychotherapies of various types are provided by a clinician, typically a psychologist or social worker (Chubinsky and Hojman 2013). Trainees must acquire excellent collaborative and communication skills to ensure that both treaters are on the same page, with a similar conceptualization of the focus of treatment—both in domains of treating disability as well as fostering resilience (Riba and Balon 2005).

Under the ACGME competencies of patient care and systems-based practice, supervisors can assist trainees in considering the complexities of collaboration in the patient's treatment. For example, a therapist who is frustrated with a lack of progress may trigger the psychiatrist to prescribe medication. A child and adolescent psychiatrist may overidealize therapy when the medication is not working well. There is an ever-potential risk of "splitting" in split treatment patient care—meaning that one treater may be perceived as "all good and helpful," while the other is devalued. An astute supervisor will highlight these dynamics to help treaters work together as a supportive "holding environment" for the patient and patient's caregivers (Chubinsky and Hojman 2013; Iannitelli et al. 2019). With busy clinics and limited time, inattention to treater communication and collaboration in a split treatment model may sabotage treatment (Pellegrini 2010). However, most training programs in the United States still strive to help train and nurture the next generation of psychopharmacotherapists, in which newly minted child and adolescent psychiatrists can "prescribe" psychotherapy (which they can conduct) as readily as writing an e-Rx for a selective serotonin reuptake inhibitor. For a more detailed discussion on the issues involving split and combined treatments, please see Chapter 7, by Kurahashi and colleagues, in this book.

Patient-parent-trainee-supervisor dynamics are also important. For example, parents may look past the trainee to the supervisor, who is more senior and experienced, for guidance when making medication decisions. This dynamic, if not addressed appropriately, can disrupt the trainee's therapeutic relationship with the family and lead to feelings of resentment or inadequacy. Supervisors must be attentive to when they need to be actively present to provide guidance and support, as well as when to draw back to promote the fellow's confidence and skill.

Systems of Care

Child and adolescent psychiatrists are systems-based providers. "Our patients exist in a world of expanding systems, from internal processes to a wide array of external interactions, which include not only areas under the direct purview of mental health systems but also families, school, social service, community groups, legal systems, health care systems, and beyond" (Chrisman et al. 2007, p. 170). Interprofessional education is key to training health care professionals (World Health Organization 2010). Interprofessional education promotes active skill building in health care competencies during and after formal professional education. It also helps fellows develop crucially important and relevant skills with care coordination and collaborative health care.

In the pediatric setting, effective communication—empathic listening; building rapport; providing clear, culturally sensitive and developmentally appropriate explanations and recommendations—involves a parent, teacher, social worker, and others as well as the child or adolescent. As Stubbe (2016) notes, "This requires having specialized expertise for engagement, a high level of sensitivity to the parent-child dynamic, and attention to the needs and preferences of the parents while appropriately advocating for and protecting the confidences of the youth. This can be a fine line to tread, especially for the older child and adolescent" (p. 60). Mintz (2005) describes the "triadic alliance" as the dynamics between the patient, psychiatrist, and caregivers involved in reaching treatment goals. For trainees and skilled supervisors, understanding and addressing the parent's and child's understanding, concerns, and desires for treatment—and helping to come to a shared goal—may be the most challenging, and essential, aspects of psychopharmacotherapy.

A particularly taxing time for patients and caregivers is the transition from the pediatric health and mental health systems to those of adults. Child and adolescent psychiatrists must gain ease in accessing these resources to anticipate and mobilize a system of care for adolescents as they transition to adulthood (Institute of Medicine 2006).

Teachers and Mentors

Effective teachers model patient engagement skills, provide timely and specific feedback, and offer a safe venue in which to discuss the vicissitudes of the art and science of treatment. Valuable mentors focus on the professional development of an individual mentee "in a deliberate and future-oriented way, electing to harness the potential of another over one's personal goals" (Martin 2005, p. 1227).

TEACHERS

Residency and fellowship training assume a primacy of faculty teaching and trainee learning. However, learning is not a one-way process from teacher to student. Rather, adult learners need to be optimally engaged in their learning plan to retain knowledge, gain skills, and hone professional attitudes (Stahl and Davis 2009). Research and writing in the field of medical education have increasingly emphasized that teaching and learning occur within the context of a relationship—the educational or teaching alliance (Telio et al. 2015; Ursano et al. 2007). A good supervisor-supervisee relationship depends on setting clear expectations, active and engaged participation from both parties, mutual respect, and mutual responsibility. The teaching supervisor establishes a safe learning environment and identifies an "educational diagnosis"—the focus for skill improvement. One frequently diagnosed skill deficit is ambiguity tolerance. This important skill can be facilitated by a reflective practice journal that not only addresses emotional responses and cultural effectiveness but also can enhance leadership (Hilty et al. 2013).

Ursano et al. (2007) compare the teaching alliance and the therapeutic alliance, noting that in both, insight into one's own and others' limitations is paired with empathy and understanding to facilitate goal attainment. A strong educational alliance enhances the likelihood that feedback will be incorporated productively into future practice.

MENTORS

Mentorship is widely acknowledged to play a significant role in career development across disciplines. Despite the powerful nature of the mentor-mentee relationship, it is difficult to find a succinct definition. Mentorship may be formal, with a more senior individual paired with a more junior, for academic and career guidance. However, informal mentoring relationships (based on mutual identification) often lead to greater benefits for protégés than do formal arrangements. Desired characteristics of mentors include being honest, trustworthy, accessible, dedicated, a "good match," well respected in one's field, knowledgeable, and experienced. Protégés look to mentors to create a safe environment for open expression, support, and guidance in the processes of career planning, vision building, and goal setting (Martin 2005; Williams et al. 2004).

Peer mentorship may be used in lieu of or in conjunction with dyadic academic mentorship to produce greater productivity, career satisfaction, and collaboration (Teshima et al. 2019). Another essential component of early-career development is networking with mentors in other institutions. This may be facilitated by faculty or professional organizations. Technology facilitates easy communication and collaboration across institutions. Table 18–2 compares the roles and attributes of a good teacher/supervisor and a good mentor.

Discussion

Residency and fellowship training in psychiatry require a coherent curriculum that is designed within the context of ACGME requirements to ensure graduate competency in the Milestones of Patient Care, Medical Knowledge, Practice-Based Learning and Improvement, Systems-Based Practice, Interpersonal and Communication Skills, and Professionalism. These Milestones provide the foundation on which knowledge, skills, and professional attitudes are built. Time, efficiency, and financial forces, however, are increasingly compartmentalizing psychiatrists' role as that of psychopharmacological evaluation and treatment monitoring, while other mental health providers deliver psychosocial treat-

Table 18–2. Comparison of roles and attributes of a good teacher/supervisor and a good mentor

Teacher/supervisor	Mentor
Is preassigned teaching role on the basis of an educational enterprise; student "takes a course" or "is assigned a supervisor"	May be informally developed from mutual identification (often more effective than assigned formal mentor)
Forms a teaching alliance bounded by the goals and procedures of the joint undertaking	Establishes relationship based on professional and personal interests and commitment to mutually agreed-on objectives
Uses adult learning principles to optimize learning	Respects mentee and does not expect servitude or personal gain
Devotes necessary time and energy to agreed-on goals	Devotes necessary time and energy to agreed-on goals
Co-constructs goals of teaching	Assists mentee in defining and reaching goals
Keeps learning relevant	Helps mentee identify skills needed to succeed
Is able to take the learner's perspective	Demonstrates a deep interest in and identifies strengths and positive potential in mentee
Provides timely and objective feedback	Fosters autonomy
Makes an educational diagnosis—identifies impediments to learning	Works with mentee to identify path best (or worst) suited to career
Actively engages the learner	Is actively engaged by the mentee
Teaches the student	Learns from mentee about as much as mentee learns from mentor
Carries out role in usually time-limited framework based on educational goals of coursework or rotation	May establish long-term relationship for career development

ments. Integrated care models are also proliferating. These models have advantages for patients and payers, but there is the risk of losing the therapeutic alliance between patients and doctors. Teaching the art of medicine, with attention to psychological, social, developmental, cultural, and biological mechanisms, is a critical challenge for psychiatric educators on the path to train the next generation of pediatric psychopharmacotherapists.

The pediatric pharmacotherapy curriculum must specify goals and objectives to direct the choice of curricular content. Ensuring a broad-based curriculum guides didactics and clinical work. Graduates with an integrated biopsychosocial, developmental, cultural, spiritual, and health care disparities and equity curriculum will be well trained to address the complexity of mental health issues facing the population we serve. Table 18–3 identifies model Milestone Goals and Objectives for a comprehensive pediatric pharmacotherapy curriculum, addressing the six core competency areas.

Medical education is moving toward practice-based learning methods to address the needs of adult learners. Identifying and fostering the personal characteristics and teaching styles that optimize learning are ongoing areas for investigation. Further research is required to fully understand the crucial components of effective postgraduate education. With the pressures of large-volume patient care, our field needs to investigate models of cost-effective care that ensure the time and expertise to teach psychiatry trainees not to be just "med managers"—banish the thought (and banish the term "med check"; see Chapter 6, by Rosen and Glowinski, in this book)—but physicians well trained to treat the whole person.

Conclusion

Medical educators wear many hats. They are clinicians, teachers, mentors, academics, advocates, and trainee-performance monitors. Training the next generation of psychiatrists to embrace their role as psychopharmacotherapists and use evidence-based principles of care to optimize treatment outcomes requires attention to the evidence supporting a strong therapeutic alliance and consideration of the meaning of medication for patients and their caregivers in addition to physiological medication efficacy.

A comprehensive psychopharmacology curriculum incorporates all core aspects of training (Table 18–4). The didactic curriculum uses adult learning principles to teach practical skills. Pharmacogenetics and genomics may eventually assist in considering risk for adverse effects, as well as provide hope for personalized medicine. The impact of culture on mental health treatment, mental health care access disparities, and trends in prescribing related to race and gender need to be considered. Incorporating multiple aspects of an individual (e.g., sociocultural context, biology, environment, experience, psychodynamics) may be facilitated by multidisciplinary case conferences that highlight integrated formu-

Table 18–3. Milestone goals and objectives for comprehensive pediatric pharmacotherapy

Learning objective	Teaching method	Assessment
Patient care		
Form a therapeutic working relationship with patients and guardians.	Interactive psychopharmacology class with role-play exercises (Kavanagh et al. 2017)	Clinical Skills Exam
Provide a thorough and culturally sensitive, developmentally appropriate psychiatric evaluation.	Psychology of pharmacology: case-based didactic sessions on eliciting meaning of medication for patients, families, and prescribers	Clinical Skills Exam
Formulate a biopsychosocial-developmental-cultural formulation, incorporating strengths as well as pathology.	Supervised clinical experience with observed evaluations, formulations, and treatment planning	Annual clinical examination
Elicit patient and family goals and motivation for medication treatment.	Observed informed consent process with timely feedback from supervisors	Feedback from peers and faculty about strengths and areas for improvement in role-played medication discussion
Consider psychological mechanisms that may enhance or detract from therapeutic engagement.	Teaching alliance: a teaching and learning "contract"	Clinic supervisor on-site feedback and collaborator ratings
Recognize and manage treatment impasses and medication nonadherence.	Active supervisory discussions about transference, countertransference, and optimizing treatment engagement	Patient ratings and self-evaluation
Describe and appropriately manage countertransference that may impact treatment.	Reflective practice journaling and supervisory discussion	Journaling and reflective practice exercise

Table 18–3. Milestone goals and objectives for comprehensive pediatric pharmacotherapy (*continued*)

Learning objective	Teaching method	Assessment
Patient care (*continued*)		
Devise individualized, developmentally sensitive, and biologically informed treatment plans.	Schwartz Rounds case discussion on the emotional impact of patient care on care-team members	Supervision with feedback
Engage in a fully informed consent or assent process with families and patients.	Interdisciplinary complex case discussion from various theoretical viewpoints	Supervisor-observed consent process with feedback
Appropriately titrate dosages and prevent and manage adverse effects.		Psychiatry Resident-in-Training Examination (PRITE) scores
Ensure thorough risk assessment, including risks of medication overdose, and interventions to mitigate risk.		Supervisor-observed interview and chart review
Medical knowledge		
Discuss strengths and limitations of the evidence supporting the use of medication in treatment of children and adolescents, including off-label indications and developmental considerations.	Interactive psychopharmacology class with role-playing exercises	PRITE scores
Demonstrate knowledge of risk and resilience factors and components of a thorough diagnostic evaluation.	Case-based didactic sessions to foster understanding and elicit the meaning of medication for patients, families, and prescribers	Annual clinical examination

Table 18–3. Milestone goals and objectives for comprehensive pediatric pharmacotherapy (*continued*)

Learning objective	Teaching method	Assessment
Medical knowledge (*continued*)		
Describe mechanism of action, indications, dosing, expected benefits, potential side effects, and necessary workup and follow-up for medications of multiple classes.	Evidence-based medicine didactics Journal club Case conference or treatment review, morbidity and mortality conference	Psychopharmacology clinic supervisor on-site feedback and formal evaluation ratings Self-evaluations
Systems-based practice		
Engage with multidisciplinary team in treatment planning.	Team patient-safety root-cause analysis	Collaborator feedback
Discuss the pros and cons of split treatment and integrated care models.	Multidisciplinary team case discussions about appropriate level of care	Annual clinical examination
Collaborate effectively with community systems, including physicians, mental health providers, educators, and other community-based service providers.	Didactics–psychopharmacology treatment as component of systems of care	On-site feedback Milestone ratings from supervisors Ratings and feedback from collaborators
Practice-based learning and improvement		
Review the evidence-based literature to inform treatment planning decisions for patients.	Journal club presentations	PRITE scores
Demonstrate a process to keep up with relevant changes in medical management and standards of care.	Team projects and coursework on reviewing the quality of the evidence base in literature Teaching with feedback	On-site feedback Milestone ratings Self-evaluation Teaching ratings

Table 18–3. Milestone goals and objectives for comprehensive pediatric pharmacotherapy *(continued)*

Learning objective	Teaching method	Assessment
Professionalism		
Incorporate ethical issues into case discussions and clinical care.	Psychopharmacology interactive didactics to include ethical and work environment issues on care	Direct feedback from supervisor in clinic
Manage conflicting opinions in the treatment to develop a mutually agreeable plan of care that addresses patient and family treatment goals.	Supervised clinical experience with observed patient interactions and conflict management skills, with feedback	Patient ratings
Optimize clinical care and the work environment by appropriately prioritizing and balancing interests of patients, coworkers, family, self, and others.	Reflective practice Schwartz Rounds	Collaborator ratings Peer ratings Self-evaluation Journaling
Interpersonal and communication skills		
Manage therapeutic relationships via proactive communication about interruptions or transitions of care.	Cultural competency interactive didactics	Clinic supervisor feedback
Collaborate effectively in multidisciplinary team and with therapist in split treatment.	Multidisciplinary team participation	Collaborator ratings
Ensure appropriate cultural and linguistic communication with patients and caregivers.	Feedback on documentation clarity	Patient ratings
Document medication management and rationale behind decisions.	Planning for transitions in care with supervision	Peer ratings Self-evaluations Journaling; reflective practice

Table 18–4.   Model components of a psychopharmacology
                   curriculum

Didactics

Psychopharmacology prescribing workshops	Reading: Kavanagh et al. 2017 Facilitated group discussion combined with role-play exercises of talking to patients about medications and informed consent
Psychology of psychopharmacology	Readings: Mallo and Mintz 2013; Pruett et al. 2011 Case-based interactive discussions about meaning of medication; impact of the therapeutic relationship
Evidence-based medicine seminar and journal clubs	Readings: Chrisman et al. 2007; Straus et al. 2005 Discussion of evidence-based medicine and critical reading of the scientific literature
Ethnopsychopharmacology and pharmacogenomics	Reading: Silva 2013 Groups at risk for adverse reactions; limitations of pharmacogenomics
Ethics and psychopharmacology	Readings: Geppert 2007; Stein 2012 Pharmaceutical influence Medication for enhancement
Mental health care disparities and pediatric psychopharmacology	Readings: Institute of Medicine 2006; Leslie et al. 2003 How implicit bias and sociodemographics impact access and treatment
Culture and prescribing	Reading: Parens and Johnston 2008 Cultural humility in the psychiatric encounter
Interdisciplinary case conferences	Complex case presentation by clinician and fellow; discussion from multiple theoretical viewpoints: biological, psychodynamic, developmental, cultural, and social determinants of health and health equity
Schwartz Rounds	Case or theme related to the emotional impact of patient care on care-team members

Table 18–4. Model components of a psychopharmacology curriculum *(continued)*

Clinical supervision

CAFÉ (Collaborative Attending Fellow Educational) model, a well-supervised psychopharmacology clinic at Stanford University as part of child and adolescent psychiatry fellowship. It includes protected time for psychopharmacology supervisors to teach two fellows. Fellows begin the year with more time per new evaluation and more intensive supervision, while demonstrating competence and taking on more independence in later training.	CAFÉ model: 1) supervisor initially models new psychiatric evaluations, 2) peer learning from the other fellow at the clinic in small group supervision, and 3) graduated responsibility and autonomy. Advantages: 1) fellows observe their supervisors' clinical expertise in real time, 2) there is timely individual feedback, 3) there are opportunities to discuss the case from the attendings' and fellows' perspective
Individual supervision	On-site supervision of fellows in psychopharmacology clinic
Group supervision and clinic rounds	Small group supervision and rounds with psychotherapist and child and adolescent psychiatry fellow to enhance communication and integrate formulations and treatment plans

lations. Clinical supervision is optimized when a strong teaching alliance encourages ongoing feedback to boost skills.

Educators and mentors of psychiatry residents and fellows have the daunting but enlivening task of preparing the next generation of leaders to have a broad understanding of the powerful biopsychosocial-developmental-cultural-health equity and access forces impacting the prognosis of our patients and guiding them in how to integrate this understanding to advance the field.

References

Accreditation Council for Graduate Medical Education: The Child & Adolescent Psychiatry Milestone Project. July 2015. Available at: www.acgme.org/Portals/0/PDFs/Milestones/ChildandAdolescentPsychiatryMilestones.pdf?ver=2015-11-06-120533-753. Accessed March 25, 2021.

Balint M: The Doctor, His Patient and the Illness. London, Pitman Medical Publishing, 1957

Beitman BD (ed): Integrating Psychotherapy and Pharmacotherapy: Dissolving the Mind-Brain Barrier. New York, WW Norton, 2003

Bluestone H, Clemens NA, Meyerson AT: Should clinical training in long-term psychodynamic psychotherapy be mandatory in residency training? A debate. J Psychother Pract Res 8(2):162–165, 1999 10079463

Chrisman AK, Enderlin HT, Landry KL, et al: Teaching evidence-based medicine pediatric psychopharmacology: integrating psychopharmacologic treatment into the broad spectrum of care. Child Adolesc Psychiatr Clin N Am 16:165–181, 2007 17141123

Chubinsky P, Hojman H: Psychodynamic perspectives on psychotropic medications for children and adolescents. Child Adolesc Psychiatr Clin N Am 22(2):351–366, 2013 23538017

Engel GL: The clinical application of the biopsychosocial model. Am J Psychiatry 137(5):535–544, 1980 7369396

Gabbard GO, Westen D: Rethinking therapeutic action. Int J Psychoanal 84 (Pt 4):823–841, 2003 13678491

Geppert CMA: Medical education and the pharmaceutical industry: a review of ethical guidelines and their implications for psychiatric training. Acad Psychiatry 31(1):32–39, 2007 17242050

Ha JF, Longnecker N: Doctor-patient communication: a review. Ochsner J 10(1):38–43, 2010 21603354

Hilty DM: Advancing science, clinical care and education: shall we update Engel's biopsychosocial model to a bio-psycho-socio-cultural model? Psychol Cogn Sci 1(1):1–6, 2015

Hilty DM, Srinivasan M, Xiong GL, et al: Lessons from psychiatry and psychiatric education for medical learners and teachers. Int Rev Psychiatry 25(3):329–337, 2013 23859096

Hutchison L, Clark M, Gnerre C, et al: Child and adolescent psychiatry trainees' attitudes toward prescribing and managing psychotropic medications. Acad Psychiatry 44(3):277–282, 2020 31907786

Iannitelli A, Parnanzone S, Pizziconi G, et al: Psychodynamically oriented psychopharmacotherapy: towards a necessary synthesis. Front Hum Neurosci 13:15, 2019 30766484

Institute of Medicine: Adaptation to Mental Health and Addictive Disorders: Improving the Quality of Health Care for Mental and Substance-Use Conditions. Washington, DC, National Academies Press, 2006

Kavanagh EP, Cahill J, Arbuckle MR, et al: Psychopharmacology prescribing workshops: a novel method for teaching psychiatry residents how to talk to patients about medications. Acad Psychiatry 41(4):491–496, 2017 28194682

Kirsch I, Moore TJ, Scorboria A, Nicholls SS: The emperor's new drugs: an analysis of antidepressant medication data submitted to the US Food and Drug Administration. Prevention & Treatment 5(1):23, 2002

Kitts RL, Isberg RS, Lee PC, et al: Child psychotherapy training in the United States: a national survey of child and adolescent psychiatry fellowship program directors. Acad Psychiatry 43(1):23–27, 2019 30411233

Knowles MS, Holton EF, Swanson RA: The Adult Learner. New York, Routledge, 2012

Leslie LK, Weckerly J, Landsverk J, et al: Racial/ethnic differences in the use of psychotropic medication in high-risk children and adolescents. J Am Acad Child Adolesc Psychiatry 42(12):1433–1442, 2003 14627878

Lewis CC, Simons AD, Silva SG, et al: The role of readiness to change in response to treatment of adolescent depression. J Consult Clin Psychol 77(3):422–428, 2009 19485584

Mallo CJ, Mintz DL: Teaching all the evidence bases: reintegrating psychodynamic aspects of prescribing into psychopharmacology training. Psychodyn Psychiatry 41(1):13–37, 2013 23480158

Marriage K, Halasz G: A 13 year follow-up of child psychiatry training. Aust N Z J Psychiatry 25(2):270–276, 1991 1877964

Martin A: Ignition sequence: on mentorship. J Am Acad Child Adolesc Psychiatry 44(12):1225–1229, 2005 16292113

McCabe MA: Involving children and adolescents in medical decision making: developmental and clinical considerations. J Pediatr Psychol 21(4):505–516, 1996 8863460

Mintz DL: Teaching the prescriber's role: the psychology of psychopharmacology. Acad Psychiatry 29(2):187–194, 2005 15937266

Mischoulon D, Rosenbaum JF, Messner E: Transfer to a new psychopharmacologist. Acad Psychiatry 24:156–163, 2000

Osofsky JD, Drell MJ, Osofsky HJ, et al: Infant mental health training for child and adolescent psychiatry: a comprehensive model. Acad Psychiatry 41(5):592–595, 2017 27561276

Parens E, Johnston J: Understanding the agreements and controversies surrounding childhood psychopharmacology. Child Adolesc Psychiatry Ment Health 2(1):5–39, 2008 18261228

Pellegrini DW: Splitting and projection: drawing on psychodynamics in educational psychology practice. Educ Psychol Pract 26(3):251–260, 2010

Perry S, Cooper AM, Michels R: The psychodynamic formulation: its purpose, structure, and clinical application. Am J Psychiatry 144(5):543–550, 1987 3578562

Pruett KD, Joshi SV, Martin A: Thinking about prescribing: the psychology of psychopharmacology, in Pediatric Psychopharmacology: Principles and Practice. Edited by Martin A, Scahill L, Kratochvil CJ. New York, Oxford University Press, 2011, pp 432–434

Riba M, Balon R: Competency in Combining Pharmacotherapy and Psychotherapy: Integrated and Split Treatment. Washington, DC, American Psychiatric Publishing, 2005

Rubin EH, Zorumski CF: Psychiatric education in an era of rapidly occurring scientific advances. Acad Med 78(4):351–354, 2003 12691960

Schauer C, Everett A, del Vecchio P, Anderson L: Promoting the value and practice of shared decision-making in mental health care. Psychiatr Rehabil J 31(1):54–61, 2007 17694716

Silva H: Ethnopsychopharmacology and pharmacogenomics. Adv Psychosom Med 33:88–96, 2013 23816866

Stahl SM, Davis RL: Applying the principles of adult learning to the teaching of psychopharmacology: overview and finding the focus. CNS Spectr 14(4):179–182, 2009 19407729

Stein DJ: Psychopharmacological enhancement: a conceptual framework. Philos Ethics Humanit Med 7:5, 2012 22244084

Straus SE, Ball C, Balcombe N, et al: Teaching evidence-based medicine skills can change practice in a community hospital. J Gen Intern Med 20(4):340–343, 2005 15857491

Straus SE, Glasziou P, Richardson WS, Haynes RB: Evidence-Based Medicine: How to Practice and Teach EBM, 5th Edition. New York, Elsevier, 2019

Stubbe DE: Preparation for practice: child and adolescent psychiatry graduates' assessment of training experiences. J Am Acad Child Adolesc Psychiatry 41(2):131–139, 2002 11837402

Stubbe DE: The doublespeak dilemma: effectively communicating with children and adolescents and their caregivers. Focus (Am Psychiatr Publ) 14(1):60–63, 2016 31975796

Telio S, Ajjawi R, Regehr G: The "educational alliance" as a framework for reconceptualizing feedback in medical education. Acad Med 90(5):609–614, 2015 25406607

Teshima J, McKean AJS, Myint MT, et al: Developmental approaches to faculty development. Psychiatr Clin North Am 42(3):375–387, 2019 31358118

Ursano AM, Kartheiser PH, Ursano RJ: The teaching alliance: a perspective on the good teacher and effective learning. Psychiatry 70(3):187–194, 2007 17937516

Williams LL, Levine JB, Malhotra S, Holtzheimer P: The good-enough mentoring relationship. Acad Psychiatry 28(2):111–115, 2004 15298862

World Health Organization: Framework for Action on Interprofessional Education & Collaborative Practice. Geneva, World Health Organization, 2010. Available at: https://apps.who.int/iris/bitstream/handle/10665/70185/WHO_HRH_HPN_10.3_eng.pdf?sequence=1. Accessed December 23, 2020.

Young JQ, Wachter RM: Academic year-end transfers of outpatients from outgoing to incoming residents: an unaddressed patient safety issue. JAMA 302(12):1327–1329, 2009 19773568

Zisook S, Glick ID, Jefferson JW, et al: Teaching psychopharmacology: what works and what doesn't. J Clin Psychopharmacol 28(1):96–100, 2008 18204350

GRATITUDE

This project has been under construction (in my mind) for years.

Thank you to the dedicated authors who contributed their diverse clinical experiences and research to this book, which was launched from an invitation and early enthusiasm from Laura Roberts, my prolific Chair of Psychiatry at Stanford University, and Andrés Martin, my gifted and creative coeditor at Yale University. I especially appreciate our patient and wise managing editor (Greg Kuny) for his guidance through the entire writing and production process, and the editorial and marketing staff at American Psychiatric Association Publishing (Erika Parker and Christie Couture). A special thanks goes to Simone Hasselmo, whose unique artistic talent captured just what the doctor(s) ordered for the cover and introduction.

There were many influences and experiences along the way for which I have enormous gratitude, and I am listing a few of the most indelible. This is by no means an exhaustive list.

As a medical student at Baylor College of Medicine in Houston, I witnessed the profound effects that emotional support and psychiatric treatment could have on human suffering during my very first clinical rotation at the Ben Taub Hospital, working with Drs. Octavio Pinell and James Lomax. When I was a resident and fellow in pediatrics and psychiatry at Albert Einstein College of Medicine in the Bronx in the 1990s, many others influenced my thinking regarding medication for children and teens, its meaning, and the social and cultural context of psychiatry. I am forever grateful to my early supervisors and colleagues in pharmacotherapy at the Bronx Children's Psychiatric Center (Ginny Gerbino-Rosen, Joe Youngerman, Harvey Kranzler, Harlan Spitz, Linda Chokroverty, Laurence Katz, Juhi Chawla, Naomi Najman, Victor Sierra, Pedro Castaíng, Gary Pawl, Liz Charney), Jacobi Hospital (Ed Sperling,

John Constantino, Tami Benton, Jill Joseph, Alex Okun, Peter Belamarich), and Montefiore Hospital (Audrey Walker, Louise Ruberman), and the many other supervisors, nurses (especially Linda Gilbert), social workers (especially Maria Portalatín and Venecia Marchena), psychologists (especially Will Ansorge and William Meyers), case managers, and milieu therapists (especially Devory Gibson from House 8). Most of all, I am deeply grateful to the patients and families from the Bronx who trusted me to care for them, learn from their experiences, and invite me into their everyday lives.

Crucial in my path to child and adolescent psychiatry was identification as a pediatrician through the Einstein Triple Board Program: Michael Cohen, Steven Shelov, Henry Adam, Ruth Stein, Nathan Litman, Marguerite Mayers, Maris Rosenberg, Robert Marion, Philip Ozuah, and so many others from the Social Pediatrics program with whom we co-trained.

Thanks for the expert curation of Lawrence Nii Nartey from *The African Show* (WKCR) during my weekends on call, DJ Mush 1 and the many other rudies of the *Tunnel One Ska and Rocksteady Show* (WNYU) [Tuesday nights], and the inimitable Phil Schaap at WKCR for starting my weekday morning commutes with a dose of Charlie Parker over many years.

My move to Stanford University in 1999 facilitated new academic collaborations in the practice and teaching of relational psychopharmacology. Leston Havens encouraged me to stay true to my career goals as a *doctor of the psyche*, and to remember that each interaction with patients carries potential therapeutic meaning. Many others deserve credit for first influencing me about the relational aspects of psychopharmacology, including John Schowalter ("Psychodynamics and Medication," *JAACAP* [1989]); Allan Tasman, Michelle Riba, Kenneth Silk, and their contributing authors (*The Doctor-Patient Relationship in Pharmacotherapy* [2000]); Alex Sabo, Leston Havens, and their contributing authors (*The Real World Guide to Psychotherapy Practice* [2000]); Glen Elliott (*Medicating Young Minds* [2006]); and, most recently, David Mintz (*Psychodynamic Psychopharmacology: Caring for the Treatment-Resistant Patient* [2021]) and Warren Kinghorn and Abraham Nussbaum (*Prescribing Together: A Relational Guide to Psychopharmacology* [2021]). As we emerge from the darkest days of COVID-19, the latter duo invites pharmacotherapists to consider both the inside-out and outside-in conceptualization of mental disorders:

> The inside-out view correlates with the question, "To what extent is my patient's problem something that starts in their body and brain, and

then shows up in the world of relationship, community, and culture?" The outside-in view correlates with the question, "To what extent does my patient's problem start in their relationships, community, and culture, and then show up in their body and brain?" Rarely is either perspective entirely sufficient; both are generally required. But the perspective that we take makes a big difference for the kind of therapies that we are likely to recommend. An inside-out perspective most often correlates with the dispenser model, leading to a search for a medication that will correct the underlying (inside) problem. But using both perspectives facilitates use of the collaborator model, in which the clinician is a collaborator and guide, using medication not as a fix but rather as a tool that may be useful in helping the patient to realize their purposes and goals. (p. 22)

I thank the many elder generatives who gave my ideas an audience: Saul Levine from UCSD (who invited me to give my first grand rounds on the topic of the therapeutic alliance in pediatric psychopharmacology); David DeMaso from Children's Hospital Boston ("Someday you'll write a book about this"); Alan Schatzberg and Allan Reiss (who recruited me to Stanford in the late 1990s and let me follow my own path); the early collaborators on this topic who believed strongly in the moment-to-moment relational transactions between doctor, patient, and parents/caregivers: Carl Feinstein, Leon Wanerman, Donald Mordecai, Steven Shirk, Jeffrey Bostic, Margaret Weiss, Noah Feinstein; and the many teacher scholars from the Harvard Macy Institute, who helped me weave together my interests in clinical teaching, culture, school mental health, and psychotherapy. Special thanks to the departmental and community leaders who have been crucial partners in my faculty development at Stanford over the past 22 years:

Steven Adelsheim, Antonio Hardan, Victor Carrión, Richard Shaw, Alan Louie, Cheryl Gore-Felton, Cheryl Koopman, Christine Blasey Ford, Hans Steiner, James Lock, Mary Sanders, Linda Lotspeich, Sharon Williams, Frances Wren, Jennifer Derenne, Grace Gengoux, Victoria Cosgrove, Daryn Reicherter (and all students of the Stoke), Steve Sust, Dan Becker, Ryan Matlow, Kiki Chang, and Robyn O'Byrne (Coach of coaches)

From Lucile Packard Children's Hospital: Sherri Sager, Lynne Huffman, James McGough, Chris Dawes, Harvey Cohen, Fernando Mendoza, Elizabeth Stuart, Lee Sanders, Rebecca Blankenberg, Carrie Rassbach, Heidi Feldman, and Mary Leonard

From the Schools at the University: Dean Deborah Stipek, Dean Dan Schwartz, Teresa LaFromboise (Graduate School of Education),

Dean Phil Pizzo, Dean Charles Prober, and Dean Lloyd Minor (School of Medicine), Jennifer Brody (Center for Comparative Studies in Race & Ethnicity), Harry Elam, Sarah Church, Sharon Palmer, and Warren Chiang (Office of the Vice Provost of Undergraduate Education)

From the graduate medical education world: Ola Golovinsky, Maryam Mossadeghian, Claire Remy, Lawanda Mills, Isheeta Zalpuri, David Hong, Glen Elliott, Michelle Goldsmith, Mario Mercurio, Chris Hayward, Belinda Bandstra, Sallie De Golia, Ann Dohn, Nancy Piro, and Larry Katznelson

From the SF Bay Area community: Carol Zepecki, Rob DeGeus, Mary and Vic Ojakian, Amy Heneghan, Meg Durbin, Linda Lenoir, Wes Cedros, Erica Weitz, Jasmine Lopez, Nadia Jassim, Ivan Rodriguez, Mego Lien, Joyce Chu, Sita Patel, Brian Gerrard, Jorge Wong, Becky Beacom, Mary Gloner, Bill Johnson, Elena Kadvany, Monica Nepomuceno, Amika Guillaume, and Lorna Chiu

Others who have been highly impactful in my thinking about doctoring, teaching, and writing include Kelley Skeff and Georgette Stratos from the Stanford Faculty Development Center, Liz Armstrong and Bob Kegan at the Harvard Macy Institute, Donald Hilty (UC Davis), Andrés Pumariega (U Florida), David Kaye (U Buffalo), Tony Rostain (U Penn), Chris Varley (U Washington), Jeff Hunt (Brown U), Gene Beresin (MGH Clay Center), Geri Fox (U Illinois Chicago), Dorothy Stubbe (Yale), John Krumboltz (Stanford, Happenstance Learning Theory), and the inimitable Tom Anders (Mentor of mentors)

A Very Special Thanks goes to:

My immediate family (Sanjan, Amrit, Aanand, Mala, and Luna) for their patience in tolerating my work schedule and my penchant for writing on nights and weekends, and even while on vacation ("that #%&*@ book is, like, part of the family at this point!")

My parents (Vishnu and Neelu Joshi), sister (Sheelu Joshi Flegal), and parents-in-law (Veluppillai and Indira Sivapalasingam) for their unwavering enthusiasm for my academic work, wherever it has led me

The numerous students, residents, fellows, and colleagues who have allowed me to be part of their career journey

Linda Shapiro, Marianne Ault-Riché, and Andrea Throndson for the model holding environments

Jane Flegal and Eric Dougherty for the writing studio in Redwood City

Big Ups to the bands and artists whose music kept me going late into the night, through numerous writing deadlines for this book: The janitor and audiophile (I wish I knew his name) who recorded Thelonious Monk at Palo Alto High School in 1968, and to Danny Scher for bringing it to us in 2020; Cal Tjader, Bobby Hutcherson, Lambert, Hendricks, Ross and Bavan, the Tritonics, Franconero, Slackers, Aggrolites, Hepcat, Lions, Frightnrs, Clash, Mikey Dread, Scratch the Upsetter, Specials, Selecter, English Beat, Bandulus, Boss 501, Victor Rice, King Chango Family, Dr. Wood's Soundsystem, Mexican Institute of Sound, Blur, St. Etienne, Joe Jackson Band, Elvis Costello and (all the iterations), Pizzicato 5, Questlove, Guru, Thievery Corporation, United Future Organization, DJs Fat Boy Slim, Quantic, Ticklah, Binki, Nightmares on Wax, Flamingosis & Nickodemus, the entire genre of Krishnacore, and so many others. (All my playlists from this book writing period are public: Search 1355 ECR on Spotify.)

Finally, to **you**, for reading our book and remembering that each interaction with patients and families is at its core relational, transcultural, and potentially transformational.

With deep appreciation,

Shashank V. Joshi
Palo Alto, California 2021

INDEX

Page numbers printed in **boldface** *type refer to tables or figures.*